Cognitive-Behavioral Therapy for Refractory Cases

Cognitive-Behavioral Therapy for Refractory Cases

Turning Failure Into Success

Edited by
Dean McKay,
Jonathan S. Abramowitz,
and Steven Taylor

American Psychological Association • Washington, DC

Published by
American Psychological Association
750 First Street, NE
Washington, DC 20002
www.apa.org

To order
APA Order Department
P.O. Box 92984
Washington, DC 20090-2984
Tel: (800) 374-2721; Direct: (202) 336-5510
Fax: (202) 336-5502; TDD/TTY: (202) 336-6123
Online: www.apa.org/books/
E-mail: order@apa.org

In the U.K., Europe, Africa, and the Middle East, copies may be ordered from
American Psychological Association
3 Henrietta Street
Covent Garden, London
WC2E 8LU England

Typeset in Goudy by Stephen McDougal, Mechanicsville, MD

Printer: Maple-Vail Book Manufacturing Group, York, PA
Cover Designer: Mercury Publishing Services, Rockville, MD
Technical/Production Editor: Devon Bourexis

The opinions and statements published are the responsibility of the authors, and such opinions and statements do not necessarily represent the policies of the American Psychological Association.

Library of Congress Cataloging-in-Publication Data

Cognitive-behavioral therapy for refractory cases : turning failure into success / edited by Dean McKay, Jonathan S. Abramowitz, and Steven Taylor. — 1st ed.
    p. cm.
  Includes bibliographical references and index.
  ISBN-13: 978-1-4338-0472-4
  ISBN-10: 1-4338-0472-7
  1. Cognitive therapy—Case studies. I. McKay, Dean, 1966– II. Abramowitz, Jonathan S. III. Taylor, Steven, 1960–

  RC489.C63C6416 2010
  616.89'1425—dc22
                                             2009008177

British Library Cataloguing-in-Publication Data
A CIP record is available from the British Library.

Printed in the United States of America
First Edition

To Dawn and Rebecca
—*Dean McKay*

To Stacy, Emily, and Miriam
—*Jonathan S. Abramowitz*

To Anna, Alex, and Amy
—*Steven Taylor*

CONTENTS

CONTRIBUTORS

Jonathan S. Abramowitz, PhD, ABPP, Department of Psychology, University of North Carolina at Chapel Hill

Martin M. Antony, PhD, ABPP, Department of Psychology, Ryerson University, Toronto, Ontario, Canada; Anxiety Treatment and Research Centre, Hamilton, Ontario, Canada

Bruce A. Arnow, PhD, Department of Psychiatry and Behavioral Sciences, Stanford University School of Medicine, Stanford, CA

Michelle A. Blackmore, MA, Department of Psychology, Adult Anxiety Clinic, Temple University, Philadelphia, PA

Alexander L. Chapman, PhD, Department of Psychology, Simon Fraser University, Burnaby, British Columbia, Canada

Michelle G. Craske, PhD, Department of Psychology, University of California, Los Angeles

Peter J. de Jong, PhD, Department of Clinical and Developmental Psychology, University of Groningen, Groningen, the Netherlands

Hermien J. Elgersma, MSc, Department of Psychiatry, University Medical Centre Groningen, Groningen, the Netherlands

Joanna Fava, MA, Department of Psychology, Fordham University, Bronx, NY

Anita Federici, PhD, Centre for Addiction and Mental Health, Toronto, Ontario, Canada

J. Paul Fedoroff, MD, Institute of Mental Health Research, University of Ottawa, Ottawa, Ontario, Canada

Virginia Fineran, MA, Department of Psychology, John Jay College of Criminal Justice, New York, NY

Michele Galietta, PhD, Department of Psychology, John Jay College of Criminal Justice, New York, NY

Ata Ghaderi, PhD, Department of Psychology, Uppsala University, Uppsala, Sweden

Jon E. Grant, MD, JD, MPH, Department of Psychiatry, University of Minnesota Medical School, Minneapolis

Allison G. Harvey, PhD, Department of Psychology, Sleep and Psychological Disorders Laboratory, University of California, Berkeley

Richard G. Heimberg, PhD, Department of Psychology, Adult Anxiety Clinic, Temple University, Philadelphia, PA

Steven D. Hollon, PhD, Department of Psychology, Vanderbilt University, Nashville, TN

Howard Kassinove, PhD, ABPP, Department of Psychology, Hofstra University, Hempstead, NY

Jacques van Lankveld, PhD, Department of Clinical Psychological Science, University of Maastricht, Maastricht, the Netherlands

Deborah Roth Ledley, PhD, Department of Psychology, Adult Anxiety Clinic, Temple University, Philadelphia, PA

Melissa M. Magaro, PhD, Department of Psychology, University of California, Los Angeles

W. L. Marshall, PhD, Institute of Mental Health Research, University of Ottawa, Ottawa, Ontario, Canada

Dean McKay, PhD, ABPP, Department of Psychology, Fordham University, Bronx, NY

Roisin M. O'Connor, PhD, Departments of Psychiatry and Psychology, Dalhousie University, Halifax, Nova Scotia, Canada

Brian L. Odlaug, BA, Department of Psychiatry, University of Minnesota Medical School, Minneapolis

Lisa I. Post, PhD, Department of Psychiatry and Behavioral Sciences, Stanford University School of Medicine, Stanford, CA

Michael R. Ritter, PhD, Department of Psychology, Adult Anxiety Clinic, Temple University, Philadelphia, PA

Anna Rosenberg, MA, Department of Psychology, Adult Anxiety Clinic, Temple University, Philadelphia, PA

Barry Rosenfeld, PhD, ABPP, Department of Psychology, Fordham University, Bronx, NY

Karen Rowa, PhD, Anxiety Treatment and Research Centre, St. Joseph's Healthcare; Department of Psychiatry and Behavioural Neurosciences, McMaster University, Hamilton, Ontario, Canada

Sherry H. Stewart, PhD, Departments of Psychiatry and Psychology, Dalhousie University, Halifax, Nova Scotia, Canada

Raymond Chip Tafrate, PhD, Department of Criminology and Criminal Justice, Central Connecticut State University, New Britain

Steven Taylor, PhD, ABPP, Department of Psychiatry, University of British Columbia, Vancouver, British Columbia, Canada

FOREWORD

STEVEN D. HOLLON

Clients do not fail therapies; therapies (or therapists) fail clients. Nonresponse or noncompliance may be (in part) a consequence of the difficulties with which clients present or their reluctance or inability to do the things that the therapy requires, but any good and useful treatment will find ways to work around (or through) these impediments. The chapters that follow provide a lively and stimulating discussion of some of the many factors (some client- or therapist related) that contribute to instances when treatment fails. The authors describe efforts to identify, understand, and deal with a variety of problems that can arise in dealing with instances in which treatment does not provide as much benefit as might be desired. It is a rich and provocative discussion.

But I want to get back to the original point. *Merriam-Webster's Online Dictionary* (n.d.)[1] defines *refractory* as "resistant to treatment or cure," which would be fine if the reference were to the disorder, but it also defines *refractory* as "resisting control or authority," which can be taken to imply a motivational problem on the part of the person who has the disorder. That is where the problem lies. When a client does not respond to a given intervention, the problem lies with the intervention (or how it was applied) and not with the client. It may be that no suitable intervention has yet been developed to deal with the problem at hand or that the wrong intervention has been selected to be applied or that the right intervention has been applied in the wrong fashion, but it is never the case that the client is to blame. Some

---

[1]Refractory. (n.d.). In *Merriam-Webster's online dictionary*. Retrieved March 13, 2009, from http://www.merriam-webster.com/dictionary/refractory

problems are more difficult to treat than others (e.g., schizophrenia vs. depression), and some clients are tougher to treat than others with the same disorder (meaning that they walk into therapy with beliefs and behaviors that serve them poorly in that context), but no client is ever to blame if things do not go well. Recognizing the source of an impediment is not the same as ascribing moral culpability; clients may behave in ways that make it tough for treatment to succeed, but when they do, there always are reasons that make sense in terms of their past experience and basic principles of learning. As the authors in this text so richly describe, these processes can often be uncovered and worked through if the therapist only takes the time to inquire.

Most of us come to the helping professions filled with good intentions. We want to help, and we want to make a difference in people's lives. There is nothing wrong with that; it is one of the things that I like most about the people with whom I share the profession. However, we are only human, and it is all too easy to blame the other person in the room when things do not go the way that we desire. Nonetheless, blaming the client is rarely therapeutic and even more rarely accurate. Therapy is not a natural state of existence (Woody Allen notwithstanding), and most people come into treatment because they are not happy with the way things are going in their lives (or because someone in their lives is not happy with them). If people who entered therapy had the capacity to relieve their own distress (or to change their own beliefs or to modify their own behavior) to make things go better in their lives, they would. That is not to say that they do not have any of those capacities, just that they do not know they do when they first enter therapy, and it is the therapist's job to bring that out. People with complicated problems or persistent pervasive pathological ways of dealing with other people (what the current nomenclature would term *personality disorders*) tend to elicit distress in their therapists (because therapists want to help), and it can be all too easy to blame the client for coming to therapy with problems that frustrate the therapist's natural desire to help. As the contributors of this volume repeatedly describe across a number of different problem areas and from a variety of different perspectives, this is rarely helpful, never accurate, and largely unnecessary.

Several principles have helped me deal with instances in which my own efforts at therapy did not appear to work. They are as follows.

1. *Ask your client what is going on if things are not going well.* Clients who participate fully in the treatment are more likely to get better than clients who do not. The only thing that is surprising about that statement is that it comes as a revelation to the field. There usually are good reasons when a client does not comply with treatment (at least from the client's perspective), and it is often useful to lay them out. I had a client in Philadelphia who was underemployed and clearly capable of finding a better job but yet was curiously unwilling to carry through the strategies that we laid out. When I

asked him to sit back and tell me what would happen if he did get a better job, the first thing that popped into his head was an image of being ridiculed by coworkers when his presumed inadequacies were exposed on the job. Some clients engage in a passive noncompliance because they cannot imagine things working out (the sine qua non of depression), and others engage in an active resistance because they think that taking steps to change will make things worse (the sine qua non of anxiety). Passive noncompliance is easier to deal with because all it requires is effort on the part of the client, whereas active resistance is harder to overcome because it requires taking on added risk, but both are easier to deal with if they are out on the table. It would be foolish to waste time doing things that will not work, but it would be tragic to miss opportunities for reward merely because you underestimate your chances for success. Similarly, no one would willingly put himself or herself in a situation in which the dangers are high and exceed his or her ability to cope. Nonetheless, people often overestimate the dangers and underestimate their resources. As a consequence, they live a life filled with anxious dread of things that never happen. I have been struck with just how rational my clients tend to be; if they are not doing something that I have asked them to do, it is usually because they have a good reason that I do not yet understand.

2. *If problems persist, inquire about the nature of the relationship.* We are social animals, and everything we do occurs in an interpersonal context. That does not mean that the therapeutic relationship needs to be the primary mechanism of change, but if things are not going well it is often useful to inquire about how you are coming across to your client. In cognitive therapy we talk about going to the "third leg of the stool" (the first leg being a central focus on current life difficulties and the second being a limited reconstruction of those earlier life events that gave rise to current beliefs and behavior patterns). The authors of the chapter on depression provide a nice example of a client who was largely noncompliant with treatment because he feared that if he tried to do what was suggested, his inadequacies would be exposed and his therapist would reject him. You do not have to have a psychodynamic orientation to recognize that people have habitual ways of relating to other people and that these patterns often center on clusters of thoughts and feelings that can get in the way of treatment. I do not bother to inquire about the working relationship if things are going well, other than to check at the end of each session to see whether anything I said or did raised concerns for my client and to make a point of inviting clients to tell me something that they think I do not want to hear early in the course of treatment just to be sure that the client would be comfortable doing so later on if the need arises. However, if things are not going well in treatment, I do make a point of checking in to see whether there is something of an interpersonal nature going on. I make a special point of doing so if my client has chronic difficulties getting along with others. A client in a recent trial with a lot of borderline features had a history of engaging in provocative behaviors in relation-

ships and then acting out impulsively when she thought she was being criticized. I had agreed to see her on an evening when I did not typically come in to work, and she showed up late for the session with a steaming cup of coffee that she had obviously just purchased along the way. I expressed my displeasure that she had kept me waiting when I had gone out of my way to accommodate her schedule, and she first became upset, then got angry with me, and then wanted very much to leave. We had talked about this kind of pattern in her intimate relationships outside of therapy, and it was good to get an example of the process that we could work on in the session. We started by exploring my behavior and what she thought it meant (that I was angry with her and would abandon her to her distress) and then moved on to her behavior (putting her preferences ahead of mine when I was doing her a favor and then getting angry when I pointed that out). I would not do it often, but the opportunity was just too good to pass up as it afforded us an opportunity to explore the kinds of thoughts and feelings that often led her to act out and to practice dealing assertively with problems in a relationship.

3. *If problems still persist, ask a colleague to consult.* When I took my first job at the University of Minnesota I was asked by a colleague to help out with a client with whom therapy had gotten stuck. The client was a pleasant but avoidant lady who had been raised by an extremely labile father with bipolar disorder and a mother who tried to placate him in every way she could. The client grew up being hesitant to speak up for herself (or to even express normal good spirits), but she adjusted well enough to a quiet life as a secretary at the university until she married a prominent academic. When they proved unable to have children, she entered therapy to discover the cause and ended up deteriorating in the care of an overbearing male psychiatrist. By the time she reached my colleague, she was prone to breaking down and becoming mute in the midst of sessions and then calling throughout the night seeking relief from her profound distress. I was called in to provide advice regarding the problems in their working relationship. The client found me much less intimidating to work with than my colleague and against my better judgment, switched to work with me instead of him. Within a couple of months, we were locked in the same pattern, and I was calling on my colleague to come in and consult regarding what was going wrong in our therapeutic relationship. What we found over time was that she was so avoidant of interpersonal conflict that if either of us said something to which she took offense, she could not deal directly with the offending party (that was when she would become mute in individual sessions) but could turn to the other therapist in the room to lay out her concerns. Whereas before we had only one therapist in the room at a time (who would invariably cause offense that would take days of phone conversations to resolve), when both therapists were present at every session we were able to move to a process in which the therapist who did not cause offense could mediate between the client and the one who did. It was an unusual way to do therapy, but it worked

better than what we had tried to do before. Over time the client was able to recognize the role that her own misperceptions played in the process and became more comfortable dealing with the therapist who had caused offense in a direct and assertive manner. In essence, what we had done was to replicate the family dynamics from her childhood in which we each took turns playing her mother's role of mediating between the client and her irascible father, but doing so in a way that helped her examine the accuracy of her own beliefs and develop skills in standing up for herself in an appropriately assertive fashion. I remember how pleased and proud I was the first time that she got angry at me in a session for something that she thought that I implied instead of becoming mute and going home in a suicidal crisis. The therapy stretched over the course of several years, but the client made great strides and eventually took to the road each winter in a recreational vehicle to travel across the southwest, making new friends at campgrounds along the way.

4. *If problems still persist but you are on the right track, keep trying.* Some problems are tougher to treat than others, and some clients just take longer to treat. Some of that variance may be related to problems in treatment selection or implementation, but some are driven by individual differences in the clients that we treat. The client with borderline features previously described entered our randomized controlled trial with a history of chronic depression that stretched back to a traumatic sexual assault in her early adolescence. In recent years she had married a man who was overbearing and controlling and then left him impulsively for someone that she met on the Internet. At the time she entered treatment, she was despondent about throwing her marriage away and was convinced that no decent man would have anything to do with her because she was "sullied" by the prior abuse. Protocol gave us only 16 weeks to help her get better, and she finished treatment in the study no less depressed than when she entered. At the same time, there were signs that we were making progress; she entered treatment convinced that she was a "bad person" who always hurt the people she got close to (as a consequence of the earlier sexual trauma) but had become intrigued by the prospect that someone else might see her differently. It took 3 months to get to the point at which we were both comfortable enough to relive her adolescent trauma. When we did, we were both surprised to find that part of the reason that she clung so tenaciously to the belief that she was "bad" was that it was even more frightening for her to think that something so awful could happen to someone who had done nothing to deserve such a fate. Although she was somewhat reassured that I did not run screaming out of the room, it was several months before she could bring herself to describe to a close female friend what had happened and several months more before she was able to do the same with a young man she was dating. Their reaction was much the same as mine; neither held her responsible in any way for the event, and neither saw her as damaged or defiled as a consequence. What she once had viewed as a shameful secret that had come to dominate her life, she slowly

began to view as an unfortunate event that she was lucky to survive and that held no further power over her or what others thought about her. It took time to work all this through (about 16 months rather than 16 weeks), and from the perspective of the research she was one of the least responsive patients in the trial, but the long-term clinical outcome was gratifying both to her and to me. Some patients just take longer to treat than others, and although I would not have wanted to keep her from something that might have worked better for her, what we were doing had coherence and seemed to be on target both to me and to the colleagues I consulted. I always try to do intensive treatment targeted at producing change as rapidly as I can, but rapid change can take a long time to achieve when clients have complicated problems.

5. *If problems still persist and you do not know why, try something else.* I had another client in Philadelphia whom I never did succeed in treating successfully. She had been a patient in one of our early trials who had not gotten better on medications alone. After her time in the trial was done, she was referred to one of my colleagues for a course of cognitive therapy, to which she also did not respond. About 6 months into treatment my colleague moved out of town, and she started seeing me, all the while continuing on medication. We worked together for another several months before she suddenly started to improve. The passive and quiet young woman I had been working with for half a year came in one day looking alert and energetic and much more self-possessed. I could not attribute the change to anything that we had done in therapy; she did her homework faithfully (both for me and for her earlier therapist), but nothing seemed to produce much change. What turned out to be the case was that her prescribing clinician had changed her medications and put her on a monoamine oxidase inhibitor, having run through the tricyclics in widespread use at that time. The change in the client was dramatic. It is possible that I was not doing adequate cognitive therapy, and it is possible that the same was true for the therapist who first worked with her. My sense was that, for this client, what we had to offer was just not enough and that the same was true for the first class of medications she had tried.

The contributors of this volume describe a number of tough cases that they approached with compassion and in an innovative fashion. They are remarkably nondefensive in describing the problems that they encountered, and they do a marvelous job of not blaming their clients for the lack of progress that was made. It takes great courage to describe the clients who do not at first get better, and the contributors are to be commended for their willingness to do so and the progress that they made. I learned a lot from reading the chapters, and I suspect that the reader will as well.

This volume should have a real impact on the field. Working with refractory patients is difficult and makes special demands on the therapists. Such patients elicit frustration in their therapists that only makes the treatment process that much more difficult. The contributors have done a marvelous job of providing a framework for describing what to do when patients do not get better. The chapters that follow provide a rich context for working with refractory patients in both clinical and research contexts.

PREFACE

Cognitive–behavioral therapy (CBT) has achieved unparalleled dominance in the arena of empirically supported psychotherapies (Barlow, Hayes, & Nelson-Gray, 1999; Nathan & Gorman, 2007).[1] The development of CBT protocols began as far back as (at least) the 1940s and 1950s (e.g., Ellis, 1958; Salter, 1949; Wolpe, 1958).[2] Treatment studies began to appear in the 1960s, with the number of studies increasing dramatically over the ensuing decades. The push for empirically supported treatments met with much initial resistance. Some practitioners argued that empirical research on treatment efficacy would demean the human nature of psychological treatment (see Salter, 1952, for a discussion).[3] Others argued—and some continue to argue today—that clinical experience is far more important in the choice of treatments than the findings from randomized controlled treatment studies (Garb & Boyle, 2003).[4] To be sure, clinical experience is important, but to rely entirely on one's unsystematic clinical observations, which are inevitably biased by one's theoretical perspective and preconceptions, is clinically irresponsible, especially when there is a large corpus of published research to guide treatment decisions.

Despite the empirical support for CBT, even highly skilled practitioners have their fair share of treatment failures. This can occur for cases in

---

[1]Barlow, D. H., Hayes, S. C., & Nelson-Gray, R. O. (1999). *The scientist–practitioner: Research and accountability in the age of managed care.* Boston: Allyn & Bacon.
Nathan, P. E., & Gorman, J. M. (2007). *A guide to treatments that work* (3rd ed.). New York: Oxford University Press.
[2]Ellis, A. (1958). Rational psychotherapy. *Journal of General Psychology, 59,* 35–49.
Salter, A. (1949). *Conditioned reflect therapy.* New York: Creative Age Press.
Wolpe, J. (1958). *Psychotherapy by reciprocal inhibition.* Stanford, CA: Stanford University Press.
[3]Salter, A. (1952). *The case against psychoanalysis.* New York: Citadel Press.
[4]Garb, H. N., & Boyle, P. A. (2003). Understanding why some clinicians use pseudoscientific methods: Findings from research on clinical judgment. In S. O. Lilienfeld, S. J. Lynn, & J. M. Lohr (Eds.), *Science and pseudoscience in clinical psychology* (pp. 17–38). New York: Guilford Press.

which there are empirically supported protocols and for cases (e.g., unusual clinical conditions) for which sound protocols have not yet been developed. For the latter cases, the odds of treatment failure are high, especially if the therapist fails to develop a good working understanding of the nature of the client's problems (i.e., a good case formulation).

The further development of protocols or strategies for dealing with seemingly refractory cases is an important step in expanding the scope of empirically supported treatments. There has been a growing interest in developing ways of addressing this problem. To illustrate, a search of the PsycINFO database on March, 25 2009, using the key words *treatment failure* or *treatment failures*, yielded 590 citations, the vast majority of which were journal articles. The number of articles containing these key words has steadily risen over the past 6 decades. This is illustrated by the mean number of articles per year containing these key words for the following decades: 1950s mean < 1 article/year; 1960s mean = 1; 1970s mean = 6; 1980s mean = 12; 1990s mean = 15; and 2000 through 2009 mean = 41.

Although there has been growing interest in systematically determining factors that contribute to limited response in treatment, there are few texts on the topic to guide clinicians. The classic text on this issue in the cognitive–behavioral field was Foa and Emmelkamp's 1983 edited volume, *Failures in Behavior Therapy*.[5] This book was regarded as a "splendid text" when reviewed the year after its publication in the APA journal *Contemporary Psychology: A Journal of Reviews* (Barbrack & Franks, 1984, p. 381).[6] Nevertheless, the book is over 2 decades old. Many important treatment advances have occurred since its publication, and the nature of treatment challenges has similarly changed.

The goal of the present volume is to review the current state of knowledge on complicating factors for a wide variety of psychological conditions that cognitive–behavioral therapists may encounter in clinical practice. The contributors are all well-known researchers in treatment development and implementation of CBT. Their expertise covers a wide range of psychiatric problems.

Given that CBT is a theory-driven approach, with identifiable mechanisms of action as well as interventions that emerge from the theory, Part I of the book describes factors that would be predicted from the theory to lead to nonresponse. Included in Part I is a chapter on major approaches to modifying interventions to meet the needs of clients who do not neatly fit the "textbook" client. Part II covers the challenges sometimes encountered in treating those major psychological disorders that are generally associated with

---

[5]Foa, E. B., & Emmelkamp, P. M. G. (1983). *Failures in behavior therapy*. New York: Wiley.
[6]Barbrack, C. R., & Franks, C. M. (1984). The virtue of failure in behavior therapy. *Contemporary Psychology: APA Review of Books*, 29, 381–382.

positive treatment outcome. The chapters in Part II consider the implications of poor prognostic signs for disorders that otherwise are effectively treated with CBT. Part III covers psychological treatment for conditions that clinicians typically view as difficult to treat or refractory regardless of intervention (e.g., antisocial personality disorder). To illustrate how treatment response may be improved, the chapters in Parts II and III include case examples (with client identities masked to maintain anonymity) in which treatment methods are adapted to deal with challenging clinical presentations.

Our aim in assembling this text was to bring additional nuance to the existing empirically supported treatment protocols in order to address the complex problems clinicians face in everyday practice. In that way, this book is oriented primarily to practitioners and researchers who are developing protocols that will build on existing methods. Graduate students and therapists in training will benefit from this text, as it highlights both the primary empirically supported methods for treating major psychiatric problems and also common problems that interfere with the implementation of treatment.

It is our hope that by bringing together experts on a wide array of major psychological disorders to describe limitations in treatment and methods for overcoming poor prognostic indicators, additional research will accrue and lead to more effective interventions.

I

THE NATURE OF REFRACTORY CLIENTS AND THEIR IMPACT ON THE PRACTICE OF COGNITIVE–BEHAVIORAL THERAPY

1

COGNITIVE–BEHAVIORAL THERAPY AND REFRACTORY CASES: WHAT FACTORS LEAD TO LIMITED TREATMENT RESPONSE?

DEAN McKAY, STEVEN TAYLOR, AND JONATHAN S. ABRAMOWITZ

In the 1990s, a growing movement was underway in psychotherapy to define and identify treatment protocols that had empirical support. Candidate therapies had to demonstrate efficacy according to a set of carefully specified criteria (Chambless & Hollon, 1998; Chambless & Ollendick, 2001). These standards remain in effect as of this writing. They apply not only to established treatments but also to interventions in various stages of development. Specifically, treatments that appear promising but have not yet been shown efficacious in randomized controlled trials or a large body of single cases experiments are called *probably efficacious*. Other plausible but untested treatments are referred to as *experimental*.

Most empirically supported treatments have established this standing by controlled trials with carefully selected clients. Many forms of cognitive–behavioral therapy (CBT) now have a rightful claim to being empirically supported (Nathan & Gorman, 2007). But what happens in everyday clinical practice? When clinicians in the field modify protocols to meet the spe-

3

cial needs of their clients but still have a rightful claim to refer to their interventions as *cognitive–behavioral*, can they still also claim to practice an empirically supported approach to therapy? It is in this regard that many treatments, in everyday practice, revert back to "experimental" on the basis of the criteria for empirically supported treatments. That is, the treatment approach deviates far enough from the empirically supported protocol that it is no longer considered similar to the original. These modifications are put in place by practitioners when clients present with problems that are not necessarily in line with the diagnoses for which the original empirically supported treatment arose. Despite this fact, many CBT practitioners consider their approaches to be empirically informed. In our opinion, these clinicians are correct in their assumption. However, the need for modifications to existing empirically supported interventions also highlights some inherent challenges in the description of practice. At the most basic level, those who practice CBT and refer to their work as *empirically informed* are unified by a reliance on scientific standards rather than a retreat to pseudoscientific practices with limited theoretical basis (cf. Garb & Boyle, 2003; Garske & Anderson, 2003). In this way, clinicians often identify theoretically relevant factors that could lead to poor outcome if the original empirically supported protocols are strictly followed. Several major generalities associated with poorer outcome are described here.

CLIENT VARIABLES THEORETICALLY RELATED TO POORER TREATMENT RESPONSE

An important focus of research attention has been on factors that might plausibly interfere with treatment delivery and response. A substantial literature has accumulated on this topic, much of it devoted to specific diagnoses listed in the *Diagnostic and Statistical Manual of Mental Disorders* (4th ed., text rev.; American Psychiatric Association, 2000). However, some generalities emerge from the basic theoretical underpinnings of CBT.

Low Cognitive or Intellectual Functioning

One theoretical claim for CBT (and for many other psychotherapies) is the requirement that the client have at least average intellectual functioning. This is based on the twofold assumption that with higher intellectual functioning comes an ability to understand the verbal information imparted in therapy and that the client can profitably use that information to alter emotion and behavior. Recent data have partially supported this, where higher fluid intelligence was associated with greater improvement for depression and anxiety in a sample of older adults seeking psychotherapy with CBT (Doubleday, King, & Papageorgiou, 2002). This study did not include participants with particularly low levels of intellectual functioning (i.e., in the borderline or mentally retarded range). However, people with below-average cognitive abilities can benefit from CBT. Here, the types of interventions are tailored to the particular client. For example, for a depressed person who also has mild mental retardation, behavioral interventions would be used instead of more sophisticated interventions such as cognitive restructuring (e.g., Klein-Tasman & Albano, 2007). There is also promising preliminary evidence that CBT can improve functioning in people with dementia (e.g., Walker, 2004). Nevertheless, it can be challenging to effectively administer CBT for, say, mood or anxiety disorders, to cognitively impaired people, aside from the most rudimentary interventions such as ward-based contingency management programs.

Problems With Insight

For many years, it was assumed that for the CBT practitioner to effectively deliver CBT, the client had to possess insight. This simply meant that the client had the ability to draw connections between his or her thought processes and resultant behavior. Although this assumption is still prevalent, the data have not supported it. For example, it has been shown that CBT may be used for psychosis (Haddock & Slade, 1996), for bipolar disorder (Miklowitz, 2008), and for many childhood disorders (Van Hasselt & Hersen, 1998), all conditions or populations in which insight is often impaired or inadequately developed. However, at this point, the interfering aspects of poor insight depend in part on the condition being treated. For example, it is still the case that poor insight can interfere with the effective CBT for many disorders, such as obsessive–compulsive disorder and hypochondriasis (e.g., Abramowitz, 2008; McKay & Gruner, 2008; Taylor & Asmundson, 2004).

Comorbid Axis I and Axis II Diagnoses

In many randomized controlled trials, clients are selected who have minimal additional diagnoses, or if present, a diagnosis can be reasonably assumed to exist as secondary to the primary diagnosis. The data have been inconsistent in showing a relation between comorbid Axis I diagnoses and treatment outcome. On the one hand, comorbid mood disorder has been equivocal in predicting treatment outcome for panic disorder (Mennin & Heimberg, 2000) and posttraumatic stress disorder (Taylor, 2006). On the other hand, major depression and severity of depression have been more consistently associated with negative treatment outcome for obsessive–compulsive disorder (Keeley, Storch, Merlo, & Geffken, 2008). In treatment for borderline personality disorder, the presence of substance use disorder adversely affects treatment outcome and is a significant factor in treatment dropout, but severity of mood disturbance does not have these negative effects on therapy (Bornovalova & Daughters, 2007).

Randomized controlled trials are typically conducted with exclusion criteria for Axis II disorders (personality disorders) or at the least exclude those clients for whom the presence of a personality disorder interferes with the treatment for the target Axis I diagnosis. If the presence of a personality disorder does not rule out participation, then the exclusion may be based on whether the severity of the personality disorder is high enough to interfere with treatment for the Axis I diagnosis. It is assumed that these personality problems will frequently appear at the most inopportune times, right when the therapist is making progress with the Axis I problem, assuming the therapist makes it that far with the personality disordered client.

Although the clinical lore suggests comorbid personality disorders interfere with treatment outcome, the data on this point have been less consistent than expected. For example, van den Hout, Brouwers, and Ooman (2006) found, in a large outpatient sample ($N = 421$), a substantial subsample had one or more personality disorders ($n = 289$). The authors found that the presence of additional personality disturbance did not significantly interfere with treatment outcome for Axis I diagnoses. However, Axis I diagnoses were more severe in those with personality disorders when treatment began. This study suggests that clinical lore is based on the perceived difficulty of treating severe cases, in which personality disturbance may be present, rather than the problem posed by the presence of personality disorders per se. In the case of specific Axis I diagnoses, personality disorders have been widely hypothesized as negatively impacting treatment, with inconsistent results. For example, in obsessive–compulsive (Keeley et al., 2008), hypochondriasis (Taylor & Asmundson, 2004), and posttraumatic stress disorder (Taylor, 2006), the literature has been inconsistent in showing a relation between personality disorders and treatment outcome. On the other hand, research on panic disorder has shown a more consistent association, with personality disorders a poor prognostic indicator for treatment outcome (Mennin & Heimberg, 2000).

THERAPIST FACTORS THAT INTERFERE WITH TREATMENT

The approach and attitude of the therapist has been an important subject of study in psychotherapy research. It has been suggested that, in general, negative outcomes in treatment often are due to a therapist effect (Hadley & Strupp, 1976). Foa, Steketee, Grayson, and Doppelt (1983) noted that in their service for obsessive–compulsive disorder using behavior therapy, dropouts and treatment refusal for many clients, at that time, were due to a single therapist whom clients rated low on warmth. Controlled investigations also show substantial therapist effects on determining outcome. For example,

Hedley, Thornes, Larsen, and Friis (2006) found that therapist insecurity was associated with poorer outcome in treatment for panic with agoraphobia. Interestingly, this has not been the subject of systematic investigation in CBT, whereas it has been the subject of investigation in general psychotherapy.

Therapist factors may exert their effects by shaping the nature of the therapeutic alliance. A poor alliance has been found to adversely affect CBT outcome for several disorders, including obsessive–compulsive disorder (Keeley et al., 2008), social anxiety disorder (Hayes, Hope, VanDyke, & Heimberg, 2007), and bulimia nervosa (Loeb et al., 2005). There have been mixed findings about the effects of therapeutic alliance on CBT outcome for mood disorders (e.g., Russell, Shirk, & Jungbluth, 2007; Saatsi, Hardy, & Cahill, 2007).

EMPIRICALLY SUPPORTED TREATMENT VERSUS EMPIRICALLY SUPPORTED PRACTICE

The movement to validate specific treatment protocols has been an important development in psychotherapy. It has offered clear guidelines for developing interventions in the treatment of often severe disorders. The movement to empirically validate treatment has allowed a larger percentage of clients to receive efficacious treatment. At the same time, because so many clients deviate substantially from those described in the treatment trials, practitioners have restricted their reliance on empirically supported treatments.

Practitioners of CBT, who primarily view their approach to therapy as empirically grounded and protocol driven, are returning to the roots of the theory. In this way, it becomes possible to consider specific types of interventions, derived from the theory underlying CBT, as empirically supported. This movement is empirically supported practice, and although it is relatively new in psychology, it has been in existence for many other professions. For example, engineers designing roads in different environments rely on principles associated with the environment to determine curvature of the road, material chosen, and manner of design for water runoff. It is not the case that these engineers have a single protocol for highway design and a separate specific protocol for a single rural lane through farmland.

The movement to empirically supported practice brings CBT full circle. The early behavior therapists tested specific hypotheses derived from theory with clients with a wide variety of different psychopathology. The hegemony of the psychiatric diagnostic system required that CBT practitioners show empirical support for specific diagnoses, leading to the movement for empirically supported treatments. The aforementioned limitations in applying these protocols to conditions has led in turn to reliance on theory to inform selection of specific interventions for clients with various diagnoses but presentations that deviate from the protocol (McKay & Tryon, 2002). This approach has been debated recently. Ruscio and Holohan (2006) argued that the problem has less to do with clients matching up poorly with the protocol and more to do with dissemination of the empirically supported intervention and the simultaneous development of rules for modifying the treatment package. Alternatively, Abramowitz (2006) noted that practitioners should instead return to functional analyses and make clear case conceptualization in developing treatment plans. These functional analyses may be informed by the empirically supported treatment, but rigid adherence and heuristics for modifying treatment packages may be unproductive and unnecessarily complicated. The coming years will likely witness additional developments in the effective application of empirically supported practice.

Research into the practice of CBT has grown significantly over the past several decades. Notably, the sophistication in developing treatment plans for complex cases has matured substantially, largely on the basis of the emphasis on empirical support for our interventions. However, it is clear that we have a long way yet to go in consistently providing symptom relief to a full range of clients. As the chapters in this volume amply demonstrate, significant numbers of clients either fail to benefit or respond in a limited degree to CBT, even when therapy is tailored extensively to meet the specific needs of the case. Foa et al. (1983) noted early in their book on treatment failures in behavior therapy that "failures are hard" (p. 3). The reason failures are hard is partly due to the powerlessness and demoralization that providers and clients may feel when it seems that "all the right things were done." For this reason, we must carefully study the treatment failures to learn how to better develop efficacious interventions and refine our empirically supported practices.

REFERENCES

Abramowitz, J. S. (2006). Toward a functional analytic approach to psychologically complex patients: A comment on Ruscio & Holohan (2006). *Clinical Psychology: Science and Practice, 13*, 163–166.

Abramowitz, J. S. (2008). Scrupulosity. In J. S. Abramowitz, D. McKay, & S. Taylor (Eds.), *Clinical handbook of obsessive–compulsive disorder and related problems* (pp. 156–172). Baltimore: Johns Hopkins University Press.

American Psychiatric Association. (2000). *Diagnostic and statistical manual of mental disorders* (4th ed., text rev.). Washington, DC: Author.

Bornovalova, M. A., & Daughters, S. B. (2007). How does dialectical behavior therapy facilitate treatment retention among individuals with comorbid borderline personality disorder and substance use disorders? *Clinical Psychology Review, 27*, 923–943.

Chambless, D. L., & Hollon, S. D. (1998). Defining empirically supported treatments. *Journal of Consulting and Clinical Psychology, 66*, 7–18.

Chambless, D. L., & Ollendick, T. H. (2001). Empirically supported psychological interventions: Controversies and evidence. *Annual Review of Psychology, 52,* 685–716.

Doubleday, E. K., King, P., & Papageorgiou, C. (2002). Relationship between fluid intelligence and ability to benefit from cognitive–behavioural therapy in older adults: A preliminary investigation. *British Journal of Clinical Psychology, 41,* 423–428.

Foa, E. B., Steketee, G., Grayson, J. B., & Doppelt, H. G. (1983). Treatment of obsessive–compulsives: When do we fail? In E. B Foa & P. M. G. Emmelkamp (Eds.), *Failures in behavior therapy* (pp. 10–34). New York: Wiley.

Garb, H. N., & Boyle, P. A. (2003). Understanding why some clinicians use pseudoscientific methods: Findings from research on clinical judgment. In S. O. Lilienfeld, S. J. Lynn, & J. M. Lohr (Eds.), *Science and pseudoscience in clinical psychology* (pp. 17–38). New York: Guilford Press.

Garske, J. P., & Anderson, T. (2003). Toward a science of psychotherapy research. In S. O. Lilienfeld, S. J. Lynn, & J. M. Lohr (Eds.), *Science and pseudoscience in clinical psychology* (pp. 145–175). New York: Guilford Press.

Haddock, G., & Slade, P. D. (1996). *Cognitive–behavioural interventions with psychotic disorders.* Hove, England: Routledge.

Hadley, S. W., & Strupp, H. H. (1976). Contemporary views of negative effects in psychotherapy: An integrated account. *Archives of General Psychiatry, 33,* 1291–1302.

Hayes, S. A., Hope, D. A., VanDyke, M. M., & Heimberg, R. G. (2007). Working alliance for clients with social anxiety disorder: Relationship with session helpfulness and within-session habituation. *Cognitive Behaviour Therapy, 36,* 34–42.

Hedley, L. M., Thornes, K., Larsen, S. M., & Friis, S. (2006). Therapists' emotional reactions to patients as a mediator in cognitive behavioural treatment of panic disorder with agoraphobia. *Cognitive Therapy and Research, 35,* 174–182.

Keeley, M. L., Storch, E. A., Merlo, L. J., & Geffken, G. R. (2008). Clinical predictors of response to cognitive–behavioral therapy for obsessive–compulsive disorder. *Clinical Psychology Review, 28,* 118–130.

Klein-Tasman, B. P., & Albano, A. M. (2007). Intensive, short-term cognitive–behavioral treatment of OCD-like behavior with a young adult with Williams syndrome. *Clinical Case Studies, 6,* 483–492.

Loeb, K. L., Wilson, G. T., Labouvie, E., Pratt, E. M., Hayaki, J., Walsh, B. T., et al. (2005). Therapeutic alliance and treatment adherence in two interventions for bulimia nervosa: A study of process and outcome. *Journal of Consulting and Clinical Psychology, 73,* 1097–1107.

McKay, D., & Gruner, P. (2008). Obsessive–compulsive disorder and schizotypy. In J. S. Abramowitz, D. McKay, & S. Taylor (Eds.), *Clinical handbook of obsessive–compulsive disorder and related problems* (pp. 126–138). Baltimore: Johns Hopkins University Press.

McKay, D., & Tryon, W. (2002). Behavior therapy: Theoretical bases. In W. Sledge & M. Hersen (Eds.), *Encyclopedia of psychotherapy* (Vol. 1, pp. 277–291). San Diego, CA: Academic Press.

Mennin, D. S., & Heimberg, R. G. (2000). The impact of comorbid mood and personality disorders in the cognitive–behavioral treatment of panic disorder. *Clinical Psychology Review, 20*, 339–357.

Miklowitz, D. J. (2008). Bipolar disorder. In D. H. Barlow (Ed.), *Clinical handbook of psychological disorders: A step-by-step treatment manual* (4th ed., pp. 421–462). New York: Guilford Press.

Nathan, P. E., & Gorman, J. M. (2007). *A guide to treatments that work* (3rd ed.). New York: Oxford University Press.

Ruscio, A. M., & Holohan, D. R. (2006). Applying empirically supported treatments to complex cases: Ethical, empirical, and practical considerations. *Clinical Psychology: Science and Practice, 13*, 146–162.

Russell, R., Shirk, S., & Jungbluth, N. (2007). First-session pathways to the working alliance in cognitive–behavioral therapy for adolescent depression. *Psychotherapy Research, 17*, 185–195.

Saatsi, S., Hardy, G. E., & Cahill, J. (2007). Predictors of outcome and completion in cognitive therapy for depression. *Psychotherapy Research, 17*, 185–195.

Taylor, S. (2006). *Clinician's guide to PTSD: A cognitive–behavioral approach.* New York: Guilford Press.

Taylor, S., & Asmundson, G. J. G. (2004). *Treating health anxiety: A cognitive–behavioral approach.* New York: Guilford Press.

van den Hout, M., Brouwers, C., & Ooman, J. (2006). Clinically diagnosed Axis II co-morbidity and the short term outcome of CBT for Axis I disorders. *Clinical Psychology and Psychotherapy, 13*, 56–63.

Van Hasselt, V. B., & Hersen, M. (1998). *Handbook of psychological treatment protocols for children and adolescents.* Mahwah, NJ: Erlbaum.

Walker, D. A. (2004). Cognitive behavioural therapy for depression in a person with Alzheimer's dementia. *Behavioural and Cognitive Psychotherapy, 32*, 495–500.

2

ADJUSTING TREATMENT FOR PARTIAL- OR NONRESPONSE TO CONTEMPORARY COGNITIVE–BEHAVIORAL THERAPY

ANITA FEDERICI, KAREN ROWA, AND MARTIN M. ANTONY

Although an extensive body of empirical data supports the use of cognitive–behavioral therapy (CBT) for numerous psychological disorders, a significant number of clients fail to respond adequately to mainstream CBT approaches. Partial or nonresponse to treatment is a significant issue that affects outcome across diagnostic groups. Clinicians working within a CBT framework often encounter ambivalence, poor homework compliance, and premature treatment dropout. Furthermore, a significant number of clients refuse treatment altogether, and many who do complete a course of CBT continue to struggle with residual symptoms posttreatment, which increases the risk of relapse (Westra & Dozois, 2006). In response to these issues, researchers have sought ways of improving outcome in CBT for greater numbers of individuals (Antony, Ledley, & Heimberg, 2005). In addition to modifying existing CBT protocols, the development of a so-called third wave of CBT interventions has evolved (Hayes, Follette, & Linehan, 2004), marking what proponents consider to be an exciting paradigmatic shift. As a field, and particularly for more complex clinical populations, psychology has begun to place greater emphasis on the flexible integration of change-oriented interventions with acceptance-based approaches. For example, the development of motivational interviewing (MI; Miller & Rollnick, 2002), acceptance and commitment therapy (ACT; Hayes, Luoma, Bond, Masuda, & Lillis, 2006), dialectical behavior therapy (DBT; Linehan, 1993a), and mindfulness-based cognitive therapy (MBCT; Segal, Williams, & Teasdale, 2002) offers clinicians promising new ways of conceptualizing and approaching psychological and behavioral change across diverse clinical populations.

Our goals for this chapter are twofold: First, we describe a variety of modifications to contemporary CBT protocols that may help to address poor treatment response. We discuss such topics as client suitability, treatment sequencing, enhancing homework compliance, and identifying and modifying therapist-related variables (e.g., the therapeutic alliance) that may be related to treatment outcome. Second, we describe innovative treatment strategies that are currently being added to CBT protocols to enhance treatment retention, engagement, and outcome. In many cases, data regarding these strategies are preliminary, and more research is needed to more definitively determine their effects.

FACTORS CONTRIBUTING TO POOR RESPONSE

In the sections that follow, we highlight some of the factors that have a negative impact on treatment outcome. The following discussion is not an exhaustive review of these factors given that subsequent chapters review these and other variables as they relate to specific disorders.

Client-Related Factors

Possibly one of the most important pieces of information for a therapist to continually keep in mind is that each client brings more than just his or her primary diagnosis to the treatment session. Unique familial histories, socioeconomic status, histories of trauma, past treatment experiences, beliefs about change, degree of insight, and level of motivation may significantly color the relative success of therapy (Freeman & McCloskey, 2003). For instance, studies have consistently shown that across diagnostic categories, motivation for change is significantly related to treatment outcome (Miller & Rollnick, 2002; Westen & Morrison, 2001). Ambivalence encountered in the therapeutic setting may emerge in the form of overt (e.g., arguing with the therapist, missing therapy sessions) or subtle (e.g., failure to complete homework, dissociating during therapy, refusing to answer questions) behaviors. Several key variables are considered to play a role in the development and maintenance of ambivalence. Clients who hold positive beliefs about their symptoms tend to be less motivated to change (e.g., "ruminating about my problems helps me find solutions"). Change-based interventions, like CBT, can be a frightening and overwhelming prospect for clients whose symptoms have become a reliable and integral part of their functioning.

Likewise, the specific beliefs and expectations that clients bring to therapy appear to play an important role in overall clinical outcome. Westra, Dozois, and Marcus (2007) found that positive expectations for change were predictive of greater homework compliance and initial therapeutic change in a CBT intervention. In essence, clients who do not expect to improve in treatment, disagree with the therapy rationale, or do not believe in their own capacity for change are significantly less likely to succeed in treatment. Researchers have also found that degree of insight regarding symptoms is predictive of outcome. This appears to be especially relevant for clients with obsessive–compulsive disorder (OCD; Foa, Abramowitz, Franklin, & Kozak, 1999) and psychotic disorders (Byerly, Fisher, Carmody, & Rush, 2005).

Therapist-Related Factors

Research has repeatedly shown that the therapist–client relationship is a robust predictor of outcome across diverse samples and therapeutic approaches (e.g., Castonguay, Goldfried, Wiser, Raue, & Hayes, 1996). Given that CBT is an action-oriented intervention that requires clients to be highly motivated and willing to confront anxiety-provoking and emotionally laden stimuli, the degree to which clients trust and feel comfortable with their therapists may greatly affect the course of treatment. Other clinician-related variables may also impede therapeutic progress, including lack of therapist skill or confidence in treatment delivery, inaccurate case conceptualization, unstated therapeutic goals, poor orientation and rationale of the therapy model, poorly timed interventions, unrealistic expectations for client improvement, the communication of pejorative beliefs about mental illness, ending sessions prematurely, and lack of a collaborative and empathic therapeutic stance (Freeman & McCloskey, 2003; Linehan, 1993a).

Diagnosis-Related Factors

Across numerous psychological disorders, studies have demonstrated a reliable relationship between symptom severity and treatment outcome. For example, greater pretreatment levels of depression, anger, and emotional numbing were predictive of partial or poor response to CBT for posttraumatic stress disorder (PTSD; Taylor et al., 2001). Similarly, clients with more severe levels of perfectionism (Blatt, Quinlan, Pilkonis, & Shea, 1995) or depression (Hamilton & Dobson, 2002) at baseline are less likely to respond favorably to treatment. In addition, certain diagnostic subtypes are associated with a more protracted course of treatment. Data suggest that clients with the generalized subtype of social phobia have a poorer response to treatment than do those with more circumscribed symptoms of social phobia (E. J. Brown, Heimberg, & Juster, 1995). Likewise, there is some indication that individuals with primary hoarding obsessions are less likely to improve or remain in treatment as compared with people with other OCD symptoms (Abramowitz, Franklin, Schwartz, & Furr, 2003).

Another major determinant of treatment outcome is the presence of comorbid diagnoses. Research has demonstrated that comorbid mood disorders, substance use, intellectual limitations, autism spectrum disorders, and anxiety disorders can interfere with treatment delivery and the client's ability to sufficiently engage in therapy sessions (Anderson & Morris, 2006; Chambless, Tran, & Glass, 1997). Comorbid Axis II disorders also significantly complicate treatment, and rates of comorbid personality disorders are significant among many clients with Axis I pathology (e.g., Hirschfeld, 1999). Furthermore, higher levels of neuroticism (O'Leary & Costello, 2001) and impulsivity (Wonderlich & Mitchel, 2001) have been associated with poor treatment response across several therapeutic interventions. Related to personality functioning is the issue of pervasive skill deficits. Individuals with Axis II disorders may lack the requisite skills required to successfully integrate and apply CBT concepts and directives. For instance, severe interpersonal and social skill deficits are observed among individuals with avoidant personality disorder (Stanley, Bundy, & Beberman, 2001). Similarly, clients with borderline personality disorder struggle to adaptively and skillfully regulate their emotions (Linehan, 1993a). These unique and enduring traits challenge the existing boundaries of contemporary CBT protocols.

Regardless of the presence of an Axis II diagnosis, significant emotion regulation difficulties can complicate treatment for numerous psychological disorders (Kashdan, Barrios, Forsyth, & Steger, 2006; Mennin, Heimberg, Turk, & Fresco, 2005). Difficulties managing, identifying, coping with, and processing emotions pose significant challenges in CBT interventions. For example, exposure-based treatments for anxiety disorders require an individual to endure increasing levels of anxiety when encountering feared stimuli and situations. Cognitive interventions for depression and eating disorders require an individual to be able to notice, label, and think about strong negative emotions. Thus, difficulties with emotion identification and regulation may significantly interfere with the outcome of treatment and may contribute to nonresponse or early dropout in CBT.

MODIFYING COGNITIVE–BEHAVIORAL THERAPY INTERVENTIONS FOR TREATMENT-RESISTANT CLIENTS

When confronted with poor or nonresponse to standard CBT interventions, one option is to modify these interventions to best help a particular client or a particular population. In the sections that follow, we review some examples of how CBT can be modified to maximize gains and outcome for those who show minimal or no response to treatment.

Assessing Suitability for Cognitive–Behavioral Therapy

Even before therapy begins, it may be helpful to assess a client's suitability for an active, structured intervention such as CBT. If there is little fit between client and intervention strategy, perhaps alternative interventions should be considered, or CBT strategies should be modified. Suitability interviewing may have the added benefit of enhancing a client's readiness for a brief, focused treatment like CBT. For example, clients may begin to consider explanations for their symptoms that they had not considered before, simply by having to answer questions about the main components of a CBT intervention. Phrasing of questions may encourage clients to take responsibility for symptoms over which they had previously felt little control.

Although the idea of screening clients' suitability for CBT is appealing, there are few interviews or tools available for this purpose. Safran and Segal (1990) provided a suitability interview for CBT that rates suitability across 10 dimensions, including the client's ability to notice automatic thoughts, the client's awareness of emotions and ability to discriminate between various emotional states, and the degree to which clients accept responsibility for change. Scores on this instrument have shown moderate correlations with both client and therapist ratings of success in treatment (Safran & Segal, 1990).

Modifying Content of Cognitive–Behavioral Therapy Sessions

If clients are not responding to treatment, therapists can modify the content of CBT sessions in a number of ways. An initial strategy might be to find out how well a client understands the model and rationale for CBT, and to modify or expand this information if the client does not have a ready grasp of why he or she is being asked to complete particular assignments or tasks. Indeed, research has suggested that the more a client accepts the treatment rationale, the better the outcome in CBT for depression (Addis & Jacobson, 2000). Therefore, if nonacceptance of the rationale is a barrier to treatment success, it would be useful to review the rationale, provide concrete examples to aid clients in their understanding, provide a variety of self-help or psychoeducational materials for the client to read, use visual as well as verbal teaching methods, and use metaphors or analogies to explain concepts.

Many of these strategies may also be useful if poor outcome in CBT is due to cognitive or language limitations. Research has found that CBT can be an effective therapy for people with mild cognitive deficits, with some practical modifications (Haaga, DeRubeis, Stewart, & Beck, 1991). Expectations regarding material to be covered in sessions and for homework may need to be tempered. Similarly, concepts can be simplified and then reinforced with regular repetition. If the client has some difficulty using the first language of the therapist, CBT techniques could be modified to be more visual and simplified, and the therapist could take advantage of self-help materials available in the client's first language.

Similarly, the content of CBT sessions should be modified to address a client's cultural beliefs and practices. For example, Hinton, Safren, Pollack, and Tran (2006) described a culturally sensitive form of CBT for PTSD and panic attacks in Vietnamese refugees. Their treatment focuses on the relationship between somatic sensations (e.g., headaches) and trauma memories, on culturally specific cognitive distortions, and on the semantic differences between English and Vietnamese. This type of work should be broadly applied.

CBT therapists can also adapt manual or treatment protocols to account for a client's beliefs and comprehension level. For example, it may be fruitless to continually focus on cognitive interventions for a client who firmly believes his or her symptoms are the result of biology, genetics, or a "chemical imbalance." Instead, a therapist could focus on using a biopsychosocial model to conceptualize the person's symptoms, in which biological and environmental factors affect each other in various ways. Further, the therapist could provide examples of research studies in which psychological interventions cause changes in brain functioning (e.g., Goldapple et al., 2004). He or she could shift the focus of treatment toward more behavioral interventions, which might be more easily tolerated by someone who strongly believes in the biology of their symptoms. In this sense, CBT techniques are presented as ways to "retrain" the ways in which the mind and body respond.

Modification may also be necessary if clients have experienced a number of feared outcomes or stressful life events that relate to their symptoms. For example, some clients with OCD have experienced their feared consequences at some point and may have developed their symptoms as a result (Rhéaume, Freeston, Léger, & Ladouceur, 1998). In these cases, it might be fruitless or potentially damaging to try to "convince" the person that feared events will not occur. Instead, CBT techniques can be used to estimate realistic future risk, provide support, solve problems that the client is facing, and enhance his or her coping resources. It is important to remember that CBT can be effective for "realistic" problems (e.g., depression based on objectively difficult circumstances), as long as the content of sessions is modified to reflect these circumstances (Moorey, 1996).

Emphasizing Expectations and Homework Completion

CBT protocols can be modified to place even greater emphasis on the importance of completing between-session work. Homework completion appears to have a relationship with therapy outcome (e.g., Neimeyer & Feixas, 1990; Persons, Burns, & Perloff, 1988). Research has also suggested that homework completion is affected by the client's expectancies about treatment outcome (Westra et al., 2007), implying that enhancing expectations for change may be important for individuals who are not responding to CBT. The importance of patient expectations on treatment outcome has been highlighted across multiple therapies (R. P. Greenberg, Constantino, & Bruce, 2006). Thus, CBT could be modified both to enhance individuals' expectations for change and to emphasize the importance of homework completion. Modifications may include strategies such as having clients who are just beginning the process of therapy talk with clients who have succeeded with CBT, providing research evidence that CBT is effective for a particular problem, providing a clear rationale for homework assignments, soliciting client involvement in planning and monitoring homework efforts, and making it a priority to ensure homework is being done to the best of a client's ability.

Modifying Service Delivery Factors

It may be useful to not only change the content of therapy sessions to best suit a client but also to modify other factors in the delivery of CBT. For example, some studies have suggested that the number of sessions can have an impact on outcome. Length of treatment has generally shown a positive relationship with therapy outcome (Howard, Kopta, Krause, & Orlinsky, 1986), although this relationship does not appear to be linear—doubling the number of sessions does not appear to double the treatment effect (Barkham et al., 1996). Number of sessions of CBT for panic disorder in primary care (ranging from 0 to 6) showed a positive relationship with some outcome measures (Craske et al., 2006), as did number of group sessions for panic disorder in an outpatient population (Bowen, South, Fischer, & Looman, 1994). Indeed, most clinicians can likely think of a particular client who benefited from a few extra sessions or another full course of CBT. A large-scale review of treatment outcome found that between 13 and 18 sessions was associated with a 50% response rate for clinically significant change across a broad range of presenting problems (Hansen & Lambert, 2003). Thus, there is evidence that more may be better when it comes to number of treatment sessions.

On the other hand, studies of different disorders have found that when adding more sessions, the dose–response relationship often plateaus, and the relationship between number of sessions and outcome can be complex. For example, Kraft, Puschner, and Kordy (2006) found that neither number of sessions nor number of treatment interruptions had an impact on outcome in CBT in a general outpatient clinic. Himle et al. (2001) found similar outcomes for 7 versus 12 sessions of group CBT for OCD. Karatzias et al. (2007) found that a higher number of sessions actually predicted worse outcome in the treatment of PTSD, though this result was confounded by disorder severity. Reardon, Cukrowicz, Reeves, and Joiner (2002) found that the relationship between number of sessions and treatment outcome was complicated: For patients attending fewer sessions in a community outpatient program (i.e., 11 or fewer), a longer duration of treatment (i.e., when sessions were more spaced out across time) was associated with worse outcome, suggesting that the regularity of therapy attendance is an important variable to consider. Although the interventions used in this study were not described, the difficulties treated (e.g., the majority were anxiety and mood disorders) and the range of sessions offered suggested that cognitive–behavioral interventions were likely one modality used and that the results were likely applicable to a time-limited treatment such as CBT. Thus, there may be benefit in adding sessions for some clients; however, simply adding more sessions without addressing other barriers in treatment may exacerbate frustration in both client and therapist. At the current time, the ideal number of sessions for treatment-resistant or partially responding clients is unknown. However, existing research would suggest that sessions should be spaced closer together (i.e., at least weekly) and that nonresponders should be offered a longer course of therapy, with the understanding that there should be a limit to adding further sessions if there is no change.

It may also be helpful to consider the format of CBT. For example, studies have examined the relative efficacy of CBT in group versus individual formats. Group CBT is often used because it is assumed to be more cost-effective and provides a support network for participants. Meta-analyses and studies directly comparing group and individual CBT have generally found few differences in the effectiveness of these modalities for a variety of problems, though some studies have tended to favor one modality or the other (for a review, see Bieling, McCabe, & Antony, 2006).

Studies have also compared intensive CBT interventions versus more conventional weekly or twice-weekly sessions. Much of this work focuses on the treatment of OCD, a problem for which intensive treatments are frequently used. Studies of both adult and child populations have found that intensive and nonintensive (i.e., weekly or twice weekly) outpatient treatments are similarly effective, with some slight advantages for intensive treatment programs (Abramowitz, Foa, & Franklin, 2003; Storch et al., 2007). An intensive treatment for social phobia has been found to be effective, yielding medium to large effect sizes on outcome measures, though this study did not use a control or comparison group (Mörtberg, Berglund, & Sundin, 2005). Although the above-cited research suggested that the advantages of intensive treatments over less intensive treatments are small overall, it may be useful to try a more intensive form of CBT for nonresponders if traditional spacing of sessions has not produced results.

Similarly, a randomized controlled trial of home-based versus office-based therapy for OCD at our center found similar positive outcomes for both modalities of therapy (Rowa et al., 2007), suggesting that offering therapy in a person's natural environment (i.e., where symptoms occur) does not reliably lead to a significant advantage over traditional therapy offered in an office setting. However, a case series of individuals who did not respond to a trial of more typical office-based treatment showed that home or natural environment-based therapy for OCD was helpful for these clients (Rosqvist et al., 2001). Again, if clients do not respond to traditional office-based treatments for OCD or related problems, it may be useful to consider a trial of home-based CBT, at least in the case of OCD.

Sequencing Treatments for Comorbid Problems

Patients often present with multiple problems that require treatment, leaving clinicians to decide whether to treat all disorders or just the most predominant one, as well as whether to treat multiple conditions concurrently or to treat one problem at a time. In some cases, the answer is obvious. If one problem makes it virtually impossible to work on another, the initial problem needs to be dealt with first. For example, if a client is using excessive amounts of alcohol or other substances, it is almost impossible to diagnose an anxiety or mood disorder, let alone treat it. Similarly, it is impossible to diagnose or treat depression in someone with anorexia whose weight is compromised, as depressive symptoms appear to be a side effect of starvation and remit upon weight restoration (e.g., Meehan, Loeb, Roberto, & Attia, 2006).

There is minimal research examining the effectiveness of sequential versus concurrent CBT for multiple problems, though at least one study suggested that sequential treatment of comorbid panic and depression yields similar outcomes to the singular treatment of panic (McLean, Woody, Taylor, & Koch, 1998). Furthermore, treatment of a primary diagnosis often leads to improvements in comorbid problems, even those that were not the focus of treatment (e.g., T. A. Brown, Antony, & Barlow, 1995; Tsao, Mystkowski, Zucker, & Craske, 2005), though some research has found that CBT has little effect on anxiety with comorbid depressed symptoms (Joormann, Kosfelder, & Schulte, 2005). Craske et al. (2007) found that CBT focused specifically on the primary diagnosis of panic disorder with agoraphobia was generally more effective than CBT focused on the next most impairing comorbid problem, suggesting the importance of carefully considering which problem to treat first.

RECENT APPROACHES FOR ENHANCING COGNITIVE–BEHAVIORAL THERAPY

In addition to modifying traditional CBT protocols, a number of newer approaches to treatment have recently been the focus of attention. The sections that follow discuss some of the treatment approaches that are currently having the biggest impact on research and practice.

Motivational Enhancement Strategies

CBT interventions assume that clients are willing and motivated to change problematic thoughts and behaviors. Thus, the therapist, armed with an arsenal of empirically supported strategies, seeks to move the client toward more optimal and adaptive functioning. Although such a strategy may be ideal for clients who are ready to modify maladaptive behaviors, it may be detrimental for those who are less prepared to change. Indeed, many clients are not only fearful of change but may also believe that their symptoms are beneficial. For example, research in the area of generalized anxiety disorder (GAD) has shown that a significant proportion of clients view their worry as adaptive (e.g., for protecting oneself from danger; Borkovec & Roemer, 1995). Similarly, clients with anorexia nervosa often view their symptoms as highly egosyntonic and as crucial aspects of their identity (Vitousek & Watson, 1998). Thus, motivational issues are important to address in standard CBT interventions.

Enhancing motivation for change has received a great deal of clinical attention over the past 2 decades. One of the most influential contributions in this respect has been the development of the stages of change model (Prochaska & DiClemente, 1992). Although originally proposed as a way of conceptualizing the process of change in the addictions field, the stages of change model has been used to understand the complexity of change across numerous psychological disorders. The five stages of change, as outlined by Prochaska and DiClemente (1992), are as follows: (a) *precontemplation* (client is unaware of problem behavior and/or has no intention to change), (b) *contemplation* (client is aware that a problem exists, and is considering options for change, but no commitment to modify behavior has been made), (c) *preparation* (client has made a commitment and intends to change), (d) *action* (client actively makes necessary and adaptive changes to problem behavior), and (e) *maintenance* (client works on maintaining gains and preventing relapse). This model has important implications for CBT, which as an action-oriented therapy may initially appear ill-suited for clients who experience a great deal of uncertainty and ambivalence about their specific therapeutic goals.

MI (i.e., motivational interviewing) was designed to help therapists work more effectively with treatment resistance by providing a distinct way of conceptualizing and approaching ambivalence (Miller & Rollnick, 2002). In MI, reluctance and ambivalence toward treatment are regarded as natural and expected processes of change. MI emphasizes four key strategies to facilitate resolution of ambivalence: (a) expressing empathy, (b) developing discrepancy, (c) rolling with resistance, and (d) supporting self-efficacy (Miller

& Rollnick, 2002). Each strategy is used to increase the likelihood that clients will self-generate *pro*change talk. For example, agreeing with arguments for nonchange (rolling with resistance) tends to have the paradoxical effect of facilitating prochange arguments from the client. Miller and Rollnick (2002) emphasized, however, that MI is less about technique and more about the attitude or stance that a clinician brings to the therapy session. A motivational approach includes evaluating the pros of cons of nonchange, asking open-ended questions, using reflective listening, exploring valued goals, highlighting paradoxical statements or behaviors, and reinforcing prochange talk.

Brief MI interventions have been shown to enhance outcome in CBT. Much of the research on MI has been in the areas of addictions and health behaviors (e.g., medication compliance, exercise, diet), although investigators have begun to study MI in the treatment of other conditions, such as depression and anxiety disorders. For example, Westra and Dozois (2006) demonstrated that individuals who received three sessions of MI prior to group CBT for a primary anxiety disorder were more likely to report greater optimism regarding change, increased homework compliance, and greater reductions in target symptoms compared with individuals who did not receive the pretreatment intervention. Brief motivational interventions have been associated with greater treatment compliance, more positive attitudes toward change, and greater willingness to work on problematic behavior in clients with a wide range of problems (Arkowitz, Westra, Miller, & Rollnick, 2008).

In addition to using motivational enhancement interventions as preludes to CBT, clinicians are encouraged to continually assess and address motivation to change throughout therapy (Miller & Rollnick, 2002). With the understanding that readiness and motivation to change fluctuate over the course of treatment, it is important for therapists to remain highly attentive and responsive to the motivational issues and subtle forms of resistance throughout therapy. Several tools have been developed to monitor motivation (Cockell, Geller, & Linden, 2002; Miller & Tonigan, 1996). Also, the regular administration of simple Likert scales (e.g., How important is it for you to change this behavior? How confident are you that you could make a change? How important is _____ to you now?) creates an opportunity to directly address concerns about change. Although more research is needed, MI may enhance relapse prevention and may be administered to clients in booster sessions following completion of CBT as a way of maintaining treatment gains.

Acceptance and Mindfulness-Based Interventions

Perhaps the most striking similarity among the "newer generation" cognitive and behavioral therapies (e.g., DBT, ACT, MBCT) has been the inclusion of mindfulness and acceptance-based interventions (Martin, 1997).

As previously noted, one of the factors contributing to poor treatment response is the inability to tolerate the unpleasant, intense, and negative emotions that often emerge in therapy. For example, clients who have difficulty regulating their emotions (e.g., clients with anger management problems, intense anxiety responses, borderline personality disorder) may avoid or only partially respond to action-oriented treatments or to sessions involving exposure techniques.

Acceptance and mindfulness-based interventions are based on two guiding principles: (a) Psychological distress is maintained by efforts to avoid or suppress emotional experiencing, and (b) we cannot change or respond effectively to what we first do not accept or acknowledge. Such approaches strive to decrease experiential avoidance while fostering an attitude of openness, curiosity, and acceptance of one's internal world. These interventions are particularly useful for clients who have traditionally not responded favorably to contemporary CBT protocols. Like motivational interviewing/enhancement strategies, these interventions can be used as preludes or adjuncts to CBT and as relapse prevention methods. Research shows promising results for acceptance and mindfulness interventions for clients with depression (Segal et al., 2002), eating disorders (Telch, Agras, & Linehan, 2001), substance abuse (Hayes, Wilson, et al., 2004), borderline personality disorder (Linehan, 1993a), schizophrenia (Bach & Hayes, 2002), and GAD (Roemer & Orsillo, 2007).

Acceptance, which Linehan (1993b) irreverently described as "the only way out of hell" (p. 102), has become an essential and well-established component of many mainstream therapies. Essentially, acceptance is the ability to take a "non-evaluative posture toward living with oneself and the world, characterized by compassion, kindness, openness, present-centeredness, and willingness" (Eifert & Forsyth, 2005, p. 70). The goal of adopting an "accepting posture" is to facilitate awareness of internal events "without unnecessary attempts to change their frequency or form" (Hayes et al., 2006, p. 7). In other words, the ability to nonjudgmentally view experience without having to act on it tends to decrease distress while enhancing one's awareness and understanding of one's thoughts, emotions, and sensations. Acceptance can be facilitated by the active teaching of concepts and skills. Clients are taught that pain is a natural and difficult part of life, and that pain intensifies and ultimately develops into suffering when it is coupled with nonacceptance. To radically accept something means to let go of it or accept the situation as it currently exists (Linehan, 1993b).

Mindfulness-based approaches have also received increased attention in recent years as an effective intervention for numerous emotional, psychological, and physical disorders (see Baer, 2003, for a review). Although recognized as the cornerstone of Buddhist practice for centuries, mindfulness has become an essential and valuable component of psychotherapy (Martin, 1997). Williams, Teasdale, Segal, and Kabat-Zinn (2007) defined *mindful-*

ness as "the awareness that emerges through paying attention on purpose, in the present moment, and non-judgmentally to things as they are" (p. 47). Mindfulness is the process of focusing attention and becoming fully aware of reality without judgment or attempts to change or modify the experience.

The inclusion of mindfulness training in CBT marks an important shift in treatment focus. Although CBT seeks to identify and modify the content of one's thoughts, mindfulness cultivates awareness of the inherent process that characterizes one's style of thinking. In effect, mindfulness allows an individual to develop a nonreactive and nonjudgmental relationship with his or her thoughts and emotions by fostering a passive awareness of the various problematic responses and styles of thinking that contribute to emotional suffering. The ability to observe a distressing thought or emotion without immediately responding to it creates an opportunity for individuals to consider more alternative solutions. Through guided mindfulness practices (e.g., breathing meditations, the body scan, mindful eating), clients learn to gradually detach themselves and take a step back from intense emotions and impulsive urges.

Some promising empirical data show that mindfulness-based interventions are beneficial for clients with chronic pain (Kabat-Zinn, Lipworth, Burney, & Sellers, 1986), panic symptoms and GAD (Kabat-Zinn et al., 1992), social phobia (Bögels, Sijbers, & Voncken, 2006), and problem gambling (Toneatto, Vettese, & Nguyen, 2007). Segal et al. (2002) developed MBCT as a relapse-prevention strategy for clients with recurrent episodes of major depression. MBCT integrates mindfulness training with traditional components of CT in an effort to increase awareness of maladaptive patterns of negative, hopeless, and ruminative thinking that typically precedes and is thought to contribute to a major depressive relapse (Teasdale et al., 2000; Teasdale, Segal, & Williams, 1995). To date, research has shown that clients receiving MBCT are less likely to relapse compared with those who received treatment as usual (Kenny & Williams, 2007; Ma & Teasdale, 2004).

Enhancing Emotion Regulation

As previously noted, resistance, ambivalence, and poor clinical outcome may be related to a more pervasive inability to tolerate and regulate intense emotions. In therapy, clients often block, minimize, or distract from emotions that they experience as overwhelming, unbearable, or frustrating. However, the identification and experience of emotions is a critical part of cognitive and behavioral techniques. If clients show difficulty identifying and managing strong emotional states, strategies aimed at these skills may be useful. In an effort to address these concerns, investigators have developed and incorporated innovative emotion regulation interventions into existing cognitive and behavioral approaches with promising results. For example, *unified* protocols that aim to treat a number of emotional disorders, including anxiety and depression, emphasize emotion regulation as an essential feature of treatment (e.g., Barlow, Allen, & Choate, 2004). CBT protocols for clients with eating disorders have recently been modified to include modules on "mood intolerance" (Fairburn, Cooper, & Shafran, 2003) and a more pronounced focus on identifying and accepting affective experiences (Corstorphine, 2006). Adding emotion-focused or emotion regulation strategies to CBT has demonstrated positive outcomes for anxious children (Suveg, Kendall, Comer, & Robin, 2006), PTSD related to childhood abuse (Cloitre, Koenen, Cohen, & Han, 2002), and couples therapy (Kirby & Baucom, 2007). For clients with treatment-resistant anxiety disorders, Mennin (2006) proposed an integrated emotion regulation model that includes elements of emotion-focused therapy, CBT, mindfulness, and specific skills training. Some of the commonly used tools and strategies that are particularly relevant to and compatible with contemporary CBT protocols are as follows:

1. *Explore the function and expression of emotions.* One way to reduce fear and apprehension surrounding intense emotions is to help clients develop a greater understanding of the expression, function, and purpose of emotions. Working with clients to discover the adaptive and maladaptive aspects of emotions helps them to explore and transform negative affect through a process of awareness, understanding, and, ultimately, acceptance. Many CBT exercises can easily be adapted to facilitate such exploration. For example, clients can use daily monitoring forms to more accurately label internal emotional states, evaluate the pros and cons of acting on or suppressing emotions, and use mindfulness skills to observe and describe emotions. In DBT, clients learn to distinguish between emotional mind, rational mind, and wise mind. While originally conceptualized as a tool to help clients with borderline personality disorder, this skill has been adapted for use with clients with OCD (Wilhelm & Steketee, 2006) and would likely be helpful for clients with other emotion regulation problems.

2. *Distinguish between primary and secondary emotions.* Helping clients develop an understanding of the relationship between primary and secondary emotions can increase their ability to evaluate their responses in a more adaptive, less impulsive manner. *Primary emotions* are fundamentally adaptive in nature and are described as automatic and direct processes that are associated with a specific action tendency. Fear, for example, is often an adaptive primary emotional response to a life-threatening situation, involving activation of the flight or fight response. Primary emotions may become maladaptive, however, when they become embroiled in overlearned

responses (Elliott, Watson, Goldman, & Greenberg, 2004), such as the intense fear of benign social situations experienced by people with social phobia. In contrast, *secondary emotions* are defined as reactions to primary emotional responses or as "emotions about emotions" (e.g., feeling shame in response to feeling anger). Secondary emotional processes serve to obscure and replace the original emotion, thereby producing actions that are typically inappropriate and unhelpful for the context.

3. *Integrate experiential exercises.* Exercises for enhancing emotion regulation in session range from writing and drawing activities (Corstorphine, 2006) to two-chair work (L. Greenberg, 2002). Depending on the therapist's level of comfort and the client's degree of willingness, these strategies can be helpful ways of working with clients to reduce the impact of emotional difficulties that often interfere with effective therapy. Such exercises can be particularly anxiety provoking for clients and may not be appropriate until clients develop basic emotion regulation skills.

Specific Skills Training Approaches

Clients who have multiple or complex clinical presentations may benefit more from CBT when specific skills training interventions are added. As previously discussed, limited social skills, pervasive difficulties acting assertively, an inability to self-soothe, and poor impulse control are examples of skill deficits that commonly interfere with effective treatment. Helping clients develop a broader repertoire of coping skills may increase their sense of agency and confidence and allow them to respond more effectively to standard treatment. Typically, skills groups include training in assertiveness, emotion regulation, and interpersonal effectiveness. Such approaches have been successfully used as stand-alone or adjunctive interventions for clients with a wide range of psychological illnesses including schizophrenia, substance use disorders, major depression, and social phobia (Corrigan, 1991; Dilk & Bond, 1996; Herbert et al., 2005; Roder et al., 2002).

Along these lines, components of interpersonal psychotherapy (IPT) have been adopted and integrated into CBT approaches to maximize clinical outcome (Borkovec, Newman, & Castonguay, 2003; Nevonen & Broberg, 2006; Scapillato & Manassis, 2002). Although originally designed as an individual-based, short-term (e.g., 12–16 sessions) intervention for depression (Klerman, Weissman, Rounsaville, & Chevron, 1984), modified group-based IPT protocols have been successfully used in the treatment of adolescent depression (Mufson & Sills, 2006), bulimia nervosa (Fairburn, 1993), binge eating disorder (Wilfley et al., 2003), substance abuse, and anxiety disorders

(Bleiberg, & Markowitz, 2005; Scapillato & Manassis, 2002). On the basis of the premise that symptoms exist and are maintained within a transactional interpersonal context, IPT strives to reduce psychological distress and problematic behavior by attending to the following key areas: interpersonal disputes, role transitions, responses to grief, and interpersonal deficits (Weissman, Markowitz, & Klerman, 2000). Given that interpersonal difficulties (e.g., poor communication skills, inability to assert needs, ongoing conflict) often interfere with treatment gains both during active treatment and in the posttherapy phase, IPT-informed interventions added to, or sequenced with, standard CBT may serve to enhance retention and augment clinical change. Whether used as an adjunctive group-based approach or added as a component of relapse prevention, an IPT framework could serve to promote effective communication, assertiveness training, and conflict resolution skills.

Supplementing CBT with skills training may be especially important for clients with comorbid Axis II disorders (Linehan 1993a). In addition to pervasive and complex symptom presentations, Stanley et al. (2001) argued that the treatment of clients with personality disorders is complicated by the presence of "entrenched skill deficits" that affect numerous areas of functioning. To effectively address these issues, the authors proposed a two-pronged approach that combines insight oriented/problem-identification interventions with "deficit compensation" (p. 326). Though a detailed description of skills training for specific populations is beyond the scope of this chapter, Stanley et al. (2001) proposed several viable ways of using skills-based interventions for various Axis I and Axis II disorders.

Addressing Perfectionism

Elevated levels of perfectionism have been identified in anxiety disorders (Antony, Purdon, Huta, & Swinson, 1998), eating disorders (Bastiani, Rao, Weltzin, & Kaye, 1995), and depression (e.g., Flett, Hewitt, Blankstein, & Mosher, 1995). Some studies have suggested that perfectionism predicts symptom change in the treatment of depression (Hawley, Ho, Zuroff, & 2006) and elevated perfectionism can interfere with the outcome of CBT (e.g., Blatt et al., 1995). Studies suggested that standard CBT leads to changes in perfectionism. For example, Ashbaugh et al. (2007) found that CBT for social phobia led to reductions in perfectionism scores, though not as low as levels reported by a community sample. More recent studies examining the effect of a CBT intervention directly targeting perfectionism are also encouraging (Pleva & Wade, 2007; Riley, Lee, Cooper, Fairburn, & Shafran, 2007), suggesting that adding treatment sessions specifically focused on perfectionism may be useful for clients whose perfectionistic tendencies appear to interfere with treatment.

MODIFYING THERAPIST VARIABLES FOR TREATMENT-RESISTANT CLIENTS

A number of therapist variables may negatively influence outcome of CBTs. Without basic therapeutic variables in place, such as a working alliance, therapist empathy, and basic therapist skill, even a well-validated treatment such as CBT will likely encounter roadblocks. The sections that follow review several therapist variables that may have an impact on success when working with nonresponsive clients.

Working Alliance

It is broadly believed that the therapeutic alliance has a significant effect on the progress and outcome of treatment. Research on CBT has suggested that a positive alliance is correlated with positive outcomes (e.g., Castonguay et al., 1996). The relationship between alliance and outcome is consistent even when therapist competence is controlled (Trepka, Rees, Shapiro, Hardy, & Barkham, 2004). This relationship is not always straightforward, however, with some studies suggesting that changes in symptoms may contribute to a better therapeutic alliance, rather than vice versa (Feeley, DeRubeis, & Gelfand, 1999). Therapeutic alliance has also been shown to mediate the relationship between interpersonal style and therapy outcome (Saatsi, Hardy, & Cahill, 2007), suggesting that a strong alliance may enhance treatment outcome for clients with avoidant or insecure interpersonal styles. More recent research examining outcomes of CBT for depression has suggested that the therapeutic alliance affects levels of perfectionism, which in turn affect rate of change in depressive symptoms (Hawley et al., 2006). Thus, a strong therapeutic alliance has a number of important relationships with outcome in CBT.

If clients are not responding to CBT interventions, it is useful to examine the working relationship between client and therapist. The therapeutic alliance involves not only a bond between client and therapist but also mutually agreed upon goals for therapy. It is helpful to review the therapy goals to ensure that they are reasonable, meaningful, and important to the client, rather than reflecting goals held only by the therapist and not shared by the client. Research has suggested that indications of collaboration between therapist and client had a positive predictive relationship with alliance ratings in CBT for children (Creed & Kendall, 2005).

Therapists can work to improve the bond between therapist and client. This can include emphasizing warmth, interest, and alertness during therapy sessions, providing evidence that the therapist is competent, and ensuring that honesty and mutual respect are present (Ackerman & Hilsenroth, 2003). A study of therapy sessions rated as demonstrating a "high alliance" versus a "low alliance" found that high alliance sessions were characterized by encouragement of discussion of therapy process, client progress, and client goals (Watson & McMullen, 2005).

Modifying Therapist Expectations

In addition to examining client goals to ensure they are reasonable and meaningful, it can also be helpful to examine therapist expectations of the client. At times, therapists may need to temper their expectations for a particular client, especially one who is not responding to standard CBT strategies. Although it is reasonable for therapists to have basic expectations for what the client will contribute to the therapeutic relationship, exceedingly high expectations will not be helpful for either the therapist or client. As noted earlier, many clients have ambivalent and complex feelings about making necessary changes in therapy. The use and impact of motivational enhancement strategies was reviewed earlier in this chapter; the importance of remembering and validating a client's stage of readiness for change is an important therapist variable to consider. Sometimes the simple act of relaxing expectations for oneself and for the client can provide an atmosphere wherein small changes can occur more easily, even if larger charges are yet to come. Indeed, a recent study suggested that when client motivation was low, greater therapist adherence to the treatment protocol predicted worse outcome of CBT for panic disorder (Huppert, Barlow, Gorman, Shear, & Woods, 2006). These results can be interpreted to suggest that therapist flexibility (especially with clients with low motivation) may be a more helpful stance than rigidly adhering to one's protocol and expectations.

Similarly, therapists' attributions for failures in therapy should be examined. Research has suggested that when therapists perceive that treatment noncompliance is due to stable and controllable factors, they are less helpful and understanding (Forsyth, 2007). This study also suggested that diagnostic status had an effect on therapist views of noncompliance, with therapists being more understanding when the diagnosis was major depressive disorder versus borderline personality disorder.

Therapy-Interfering Behaviors

A *therapy-interfering behavior* is any behavior that disrupts the process or outcome of therapy. Most often such behaviors are examined as arising from the client (e.g., being argumentative, missing sessions). However, therapists may also be guilty of various therapy-interfering behaviors, and the therapist's conscious or nonconscious use of these behaviors may negatively hinder outcome. Examples of therapy-interfering behaviors by therapists include coming late for sessions, being distracted during sessions, allowing differing viewpoints or beliefs between client and therapist to affect the alliance, or allowing personal feelings to affect the work of therapy. Research has suggested that such variables can have a negative impact on outcome. For example, in a study using a cognitive–behavioral analysis system of psychotherapy for chronically depressed individuals (McCullough, 2000), variables such as therapy caseload (which is likely related to therapist burnout) predicted outcome (Vocisano et al., 2004). Similarly, therapy cases with poor outcome show evidence of negative interactional processes between therapist and client, compared with cases with good outcomes (Henry, Strupp, & Schacht, 1990).

Therapists should be mindful of any therapy-interfering behaviors that may be occurring. If such behaviors are identified but difficult to manage, consultation or supervision may be appropriate.

CONCLUSION

Treatment-refractory cases in CBT reveal a great deal about the complex and nonlinear process of change. A substantial number of clients fail or only partially respond to standard CBT protocols. In an effort to develop a more comprehensive and dynamic clinical framework and to effectively treat a greater number of individuals, cognitive–behavioral therapists are striving to advance, modify, and augment contemporary treatment approaches. The aim of this chapter was to provide an overview of several of the innovative ways investigators have attempted to meet these objectives, and to use the existing research literature to make further suggestions. As research in this area accumulates, preliminary evidence suggests that individually tailored and integrative approaches with regard to treatment delivery are beneficial for difficult-to-treat cases. The emphasis on greater collaboration, flexibility, and acceptance-based approaches offers clinicians a dynamic array of tools for motivating, challenging, and managing complex clients.

REFERENCES

Abramowitz, J. S., Foa, E. B., & Franklin, M. E. (2003). Exposure and ritual prevention for obsessive–compulsive disorder: Effects of intensive versus twice-weekly sessions. *Journal of Consulting and Clinical Psychology, 71,* 394–398.

Abramowitz, J. S., Franklin, M. E., Schwartz, S. A., & Furr, J. M. (2003). Symptom presentation and outcome of cognitive–behavioral therapy for obsessive–compulsive disorder. *Journal of Consulting and Clinical Psychology, 71,* 1049–1057.

Ackerman, S. J., & Hilsenroth, M. J. (2003). A review of therapist characteristics and techniques positively impacting the therapeutic alliance. *Clinical Psychology Review, 23,* 1–33.

Addis, M. E., & Jacobson, N. S. (2000). A closer look at the treatment rationale and homework compliance in cognitive–behavioral therapy. *Cognitive Therapy and Research, 24*, 313–326.

Anderson, S., & Morris, J. (2006). Cognitive behavior therapy for people with Asperger syndrome. *Behavioural and Cognitive Psychotherapy, 34*, 293–303.

Antony, M. M., Ledley, D. R., & Heimberg, R. G. (Eds.). (2005). *Improving outcomes and preventing relapse in cognitive behavioral therapy*. New York: Guilford Press.

Antony, M. M., Purdon, C. L., Huta, V., & Swinson, R. P. (1998). Dimensions of perfectionism across the anxiety disorders. *Behaviour Research and Therapy, 36*, 1143–1154.

Arkowitz, H., Westra, H. A., Miller, W. R., & Rollnick, S. (2008). *Motivational interviewing in the treatment of psychological problems*. New York: Guilford Press.

Ashbaugh, A., Antony, M. M., Liss, A., Summerfeldt, L. J., McCabe, R. E., & Swinson, R. P. (2007). Changes in perfectionism following cognitive–behavioral treatment for social phobia. *Depression and Anxiety, 24*, 169–177.

Bach, P. B., & Hayes, S. C. (2002). The use of acceptance and commitment therapy to present the re-hospitalization of psychotic patients: A randomized controlled trial. *Journal of Consulting and Clinical Psychology, 70*, 1129–1139.

Baer, R. A. (2003). Mindfulness training as a clinical intervention: A conceptual and empirical review. *Clinical Psychology: Science and Practice, 10*, 125–143.

Barkham, M., Rees, A., Stiles, W. B., Shapiro, D. A., Hardy, G. E., & Reynolds, S. (1996). Dose-effect relations in time-limited psychotherapy for depression. *Journal of Consulting and Clinical Psychology, 64*, 927–935.

Barlow, D. H., Allen, L. B., & Choate, M. L. (2004). Towards a unified treatment for emotional disorders. *Behavior Therapy, 35*, 205–230.

Bastiani, A. M., Rao, R., Weltzin, T., & Kaye, W. H. (1995). Perfectionism in anorexia nervosa. *International Journal of Eating Disorders, 17*, 147–152.

Bieling, P. J., McCabe, R. E., & Antony, M. M. (2006). *Cognitive behavioral therapy in groups*. New York: Guilford Press.

Blatt, S. J., Quinlan, D. M., Pilkonis, P., & Shea, T. (1995). The effects of need for approval and perfectionism on the brief treatment of depression. *Journal of Consulting and Clinical Psychology, 63*, 125–132.

Bleiberg, K. L., & Markowitz, J. C. (2005). A pilot study of interpersonal psychotherapy for posttraumatic stress disorder. *The American Journal of Psychiatry, 162*, 181–183.

Bögels, S. M., Sijbers, G. F. V. M., & Voncken, M. (2006). Mindfulness and task concentration training for social phobia: A pilot study. *Journal of Cognitive Psychotherapy, 20*, 33–44.

Borkovec, T. D., Newman, M. G., & Castonguay, L. G. (2003). Cognitive–behavioral therapy for generalized anxiety disorder with integrations from interpersonal and experiential therapies. *CNS Spectrums, 8*, 382–389.

Borkovec, T. D., & Roemer, L. (1995). Perceived functions of worry among generalized anxiety disorder subjects: Distraction from more emotionally distressing topics? *Journal of Behavior Therapy and Experimental Psychiatry, 26*, 25–30.

Bowen, R., South, M., Fischer, D., & Looman T. (1994). Depression, mastery and number of group sessions attended predict the outcome of patients with panic and agoraphobia in a behavioural/medication program. *Canadian Journal of Psychiatry, 39,* 283–288.

Brown, E. J., Heimberg, R. G., & Juster, H. R. (1995). Social phobia subtype and avoidant personality disorder: Effect on severity of social phobia, impairment, and outcome of cognitive–behavioral treatment. *Behavior Therapy, 26,* 467–486.

Brown, T. A., Antony, M. M., & Barlow, D. H. (1995). Diagnostic comorbidity in panic disorder: Effect on treatment outcome and course of comorbid diagnoses following treatment. *Journal of Consulting and Clinical Psychology, 63,* 408–418.

Byerly, M., Fisher, R., Carmody, T., & Rush, J. A. (2005). A trial of compliance therapy in outpatients with schizophrenia or schizoaffective disorder. *Journal of Clinical Psychiatry, 66,* 997–1001.

Castonguay, L. G., Goldfried, M. R., Wiser, S., Raue, P. J., & Hayes, A. M. (1996). Predicting the effect of cognitive therapy for depression: A study of unique and common factors. *Journal of Consulting and Clinical Psychology, 64,* 497–504.

Chambless, D. L., Tran, G. Q., & Glass, C. R. (1997). Predictors of response to cognitive–behavioral group therapy for social phobia. *Journal of Anxiety Disorders, 11,* 221–240.

Cloitre, M., Koenen, K. C., Cohen, L. R., & Han, H. (2002). Skills training in affective and interpersonal regulation followed by exposure: A phase-based treatment for PTSD related to childhood abuse. *Journal of Consulting and Clinical Psychology, 70,* 1067–1074.

Cockell, S. J., Geller, J., & Linden, W. (2002). The development of a decisional balance scale for anorexia nervosa. *European Eating Disorders Review, 10,* 359–375.

Corrigan, P. W. (1991). Social skills training in adult psychiatric populations: A meta-analysis. *Journal of Behavior Therapy and Experimental Psychiatry, 22,* 203–210.

Corstorphine, E. (2006). Cognitive–emotional–behavioural therapy for the eating disorders: Working with beliefs about emotions. *European Eating Disorders Review, 14,* 448–461.

Craske, M. G., Farchione, T. J., Allen, L. B., Barrios, V., Stoyanova, M., & Rose, R. (2007). Cognitive behavioral therapy for panic disorder and comorbidity: More of the same or less of more? *Behaviour Research and Therapy, 45,* 1095–1109.

Craske, M. G., Roy-Bryne, P., Stein, M. B., Sullivan, G., Hazlett-Steves, H., Brystritsky, A., & Sherbourne C. (2006). CBT intensity and outcome for panic disorder in a primary care setting. *Behavior Therapy, 37,* 112–119.

Creed, T., & Kendall, P. (2005). Therapist alliance-building behavior within a cognitive–behavioral treatment for anxiety in youth. *Journal of Consulting and Clinical Psychology, 73,* 498–505.

Dilk, M. N., & Bond, G. R. (1996). Meta-analytic evaluation of skills-training research for individuals with severe mental illness. *Journal of Consulting and Clinical Psychology, 64,* 1337–1346.

Eifert, G. H., & Forsyth, J. P. (2005). *Acceptance and commitment therapy for anxiety disorders.* Oakland, CA: New Harbinger.

Elliott, R., Watson, J. C., Goldman, R. N., & Greenberg, L. S. (2004). *Learning emotion-focused therapy: The process-experiential approach to change.* Washington, DC: American Psychological Association.

Fairburn C. G. (1993). Interpersonal psychotherapy for bulimia nervosa. In G. L. Klerman & M. M. Weissman (Eds.), *New applications of interpersonal psychotherapy* (pp. 355–378). Washington, DC: American Psychiatric Press.

Fairburn, C. G., Cooper, Z., & Shafran, R. (2003). Cognitive behavior therapy for eating disorders: A "transdiagnostic" theory and treatment. *Behaviour Research and Therapy, 41,* 509–528.

Feely, M., DeRubeis, R. J., & Gelfand, L. A. (1999). The temporal relation of adherence and alliance to symptom change in cognitive therapy for depression. *Journal of Consulting and Clinical Psychology, 67,* 578–582.

Flett, G. L., Hewitt, P. L., Blankstein, K. R., & Mosher, S. W. (1995). Perfectionism, life events, and depressive symptoms: A test of a diathesis-stress model. *Current Psychology, 14,* 112–137.

Foa, E. B., Abramowitz, J. S., Franklin, M. E., & Kozak, M. J. (1999). Feared consequences, fixity of belief, and treatment outcome in OCD. *Behavior Therapy, 30,* 717–724.

Forsyth, A. (2007). The effects of diagnosis and non-compliance attributions on therapeutic alliance processes in adult acute psychiatric settings. *Journal of Psychiatric and Mental Health Nursing, 14,* 33–40.

Freeman, A., & McCloskey, R. D. (2003). Impediments to effective psychotherapy. In R. L. Leahy (Ed.), *Roadblocks in cognitive–behavioral therapy: Transforming challenges into opportunities for change* (pp. 24–48). New York: Guilford Press.

Goldapple, K., Segal, Z., Garson, C., Lau, M., Bieling, P., Kennedy, S., & Mayberg, H. (2004). Modulation of cortical-limbic pathways in major depression. *Archives of General Psychiatry, 61,* 34–41.

Greenberg, L. (2002). *Emotion-focused therapy: Coaching clients to work through their feelings.* Washington, DC: American Psychological Association.

Greenberg, R. P., Constantino, M. J., & Bruce, N. (2006). Are patient expectations still relevant for psychotherapy process and outcome? *Clinical Psychology Review, 26,* 657–678.

Haaga, D. A., DeRubeis, R. J., Stewart, B. L., & Beck, A. T. (1991). Relationship of intelligence with cognitive therapy outcome. *Behaviour Research and Therapy, 29,* 277–281.

Hamilton, K. E., & Dobson, K. S. (2002). Cognitive therapy of depression: Pretreatment client predictors of outcome. *Clinical Psychology Review, 22,* 875–893.

Hansen, N. B., & Lambert, M. J. (2003). An evaluation of the dose–response relationship in naturalistic treatment settings using survival analysis. *Mental Health Services Research, 5,* 1–12.

Hawley, L. L., Ho, R. M., Zuroff, D. C., & Blatt, S. J. (2006). The relationship of perfectionism, depression and therapeutic alliance during treatment for depression: Latent difference score analysis. *Journal of Consulting and Clinical Psychology, 74,* 930–942.

Hayes, S. C., Follette, V. M., & Linehan, M. M. (2004). *Mindfulness and acceptance: Expanding the cognitive–behavioral tradition.* New York: Guilford Press.

Hayes, S. C., Luoma, J. B., Bond, F. W., Masuda, A., & Lillis, J. (2006). Acceptance and commitment therapy: Model, processes and outcomes. *Behaviour Research and Therapy, 44,* 1–25.

Hayes, S. C., Wilson, K. G., Gifford, E. V., Bissett, R., Piasecki, M., Batten, S. V., et al. (2004). A preliminary trial of twelve-step facilitation and acceptance and commitment therapy with poly substance-abusing methadone-maintained opiate addicts. *Behavior Therapy, 35,* 667–688.

Henry, W. P., Strupp, H. H., & Schacht, T. E. (1990). Patient and therapist introject, interpersonal process, and differential psychotherapy outcome. *Journal of Consulting and Clinical Psychology, 58,* 768–774.

Herbert, J. D., Gaudiano, B. A., Rheingold, A. A., Myers, V. H., Dalrymple, K., & Nolan, E. M. (2005). Social skills training augments the effectiveness of cognitive behavioral group therapy for social anxiety disorder. *Behavior Therapy, 36,* 125–138.

Himle, J., Rassi, S., Haghighatgou, H., Krone, K., Nesse, R., & Ableson, J. (2001). Group behavioral therapy of obsessive–compulsive disorder: Seven- versus twelve-week outcomes. *Depression and Anxiety, 13,* 161–165.

Hinton, D. E., Safren, S. A., Pollack, M. H., & Tran, M. (2006). Cognitive–behavior therapy for Vietnamese refugees with PTSD and comorbid panic attacks. *Cognitive and Behavioral Practice, 13,* 271–281.

Hirschfeld, R. M. A. (1999). Personality disorders and depression: Comorbidity. *Depression and Anxiety, 10,* 142–146.

Howard, K. I., Kopta, S. M., Krause, M. S., & Orlinsky, D. E. (1986). The dose–effect relationship in psychotherapy. *American Psychologist, 41,* 159–164.

Huppert, J. D., Barlow, D. H., Gorman, J. M., Shear, K. M., & Woods, S. W. (2006). The interaction of motivation and therapist adherence predicts outcome in cognitive behavioral therapy for panic disorder: Preliminary findings. *Cognitive and Behavioral Practice, 13,* 198–204.

Joormann, J., Kosfelder, J., & Schulte, D. (2005). The impact of comorbidity of depression on the course of anxiety treatments. *Cognitive Therapy and Research, 29,* 569–591.

Kabat-Zinn, J., Lipworth, L., Burney, R., & Sellers, W. (1986). Four-year follow up of a meditation based program for the self-regulation of chronic pain: Treatment outcomes and compliance. *Journal of Behavioral Medicine, 8,* 163–190.

Kabat-Zinn, J., Massiou, A. O., Kristeller, J., Peterson, L. G., Fletcher, K. E., Pbert, L., et al. (1992). Effectiveness of a meditation-based stress reduction program in the treatment of anxiety disorders. *The American Journal of Psychiatry, 149,* 936–943.

Karatzias, A., Power, K., McGoldreick, T., Brown, K., Buchanan, R., Sharp, D., & Swanson, V. (2007). Predicting treatment outcome on three measures for posttraumatic stress disorder. *European Archives of Psychiatry and Clinical Neuroscience, 257,* 40–46.

Kashdan, T. B., Barrios, V., Forsyth, J. P., & Steger, M. P. (2006). Experiential avoidance as a generalized psychological vulnerability: Comparisons with coping and emotion regulation strategies. *Behaviour Research and Therapy, 44,* 1301–1320.

Kenny, M. A., & Williams, J. M. G. (2007). Treatment resistant depressed patients show a good response to mindfulness-based cognitive therapy. *Behaviour Research and Therapy, 45,* 617–625.

Kirby, J. S., & Baucom, D. H. (2007). Treating emotion dysregulation in a couples context: A pilot study of a couples skills group intervention. *Journal of Marital and Family Therapy, 33,* 375–391.

Klerman, G. L., Weissman, M. M., Rounsaville, B. J., & Chevron, E. S. (1984). *Interpersonal psychotherapy of depression.* New York: Basic Books.

Kraft, S., Puschner, B., & Kordy, H. (2006). Treatment intensity and regularity in early outpatient psychotherapy and its relation to outcome. *Clinical Psychology and Psychotherapy, 13,* 397–404.

Linehan, M. M. (1993a). *Cognitive behavioral treatment of borderline personality disorder.* New York: Guilford Press.

Linehan, M. M. (1993b). *Skills training manual for treating borderline personality disorder.* New York: Guilford Press.

Ma, S. H., & Teasdale, J. D. (2004). Mindfulness-based cognitive therapy for depression: Replication and exploration of differential relapse prevention effects. *Journal of Consulting and Clinical Psychology, 72,* 31–40.

Martin, J. R. (1997). Mindfulness: A proposed common factor. *Journal of Psychotherapy Integration, 7,* 291–312.

McCullough, J. P. (2000). *Treatment for chronic depression: Cognitive–behavioral analysis system of psychotherapy.* New York: Guilford Press.

McLean P. D., Woody, S., Taylor, S., & Koch, W. J. (1998). Comorbid panic disorder and major depression: Implications for cognitive–behavioral therapy. *Journal of Consulting and Clinical Psychology, 66,* 240–247.

Meehan, K. G., Loeb, K. L., Roberto, C. A., & Attia, E. (2006). Mood change during weight restoration in patients with anorexia nervosa. *International Journal of Eating Disorders, 39,* 587–589.

Mennin, D. S. (2006). Emotion regulation therapy: An integrative approach to treatment-resistant anxiety disorders. *Journal of Contemporary Psychotherapy, 36,* 95–105.

Mennin, D. S., Heimberg, R. G., Turk, C. L., & Fresco, D. M. (2005). Preliminary evidence for an emotion dysregulation model of generalized anxiety disorder. *Behaviour Research and Therapy, 43,* 1281–1310.

Miller, W. R., & Rollnick, S. (2002). *Motivational interviewing: Preparing people for change* (2nd ed.). New York: Guilford Press.

Miller, W. R., & Tonigan, J. S. (1996). Assessing drinkers' motivation to change: The Stages of Change Readiness and Treatment Eagerness Scale (SOCRATES). *Psychology of Addictive Behaviors, 10,* 81–89.

Moorey, S. (1996). When bad things happen to rational people: Cognitive therapy in adverse life circumstances. In P. M. Salkovskis (Ed.), *Frontiers of cognitive therapy* (pp. 450–469). New York: Guilford Press.

Mörtberg, E., Berglund, G., & Sundin, Ö. (2005). Intensive cognitive behavioral group treatment for social phobia: A pilot study. *Cognitive Behaviour Therapy, 34,* 41–49.

Mufson, L., & Sills, R. (2006). Interpersonal psychotherapy for depressed adolescents (IPT-A): An overview. *Nordic Journal of Psychiatry, 60,* 431–437.

Neimeyer, R. A., & Feixas, G. (1990). The role of homework and skill acquisition in the outcome of group cognitive therapy for depression. *Behavior Therapy, 21,* 281–292.

Nevonen, L., & Broberg, A. (2006). A comparison of sequenced individual and group psychotherapy for patients with bulimia nervosa. *International Journal of Eating Disorders, 39,* 117–127.

O'Leary, D., & Costello, F. (2001). Personality and outcome in depression: An 18 month prospective follow-up study. *Journal of Affective Disorders, 63,* 67–78.

Persons, J. B., Burns, D. D., & Perloff, J. M. (1988). Predictors of dropout and outcome in cognitive therapy for depression in a private practice setting. *Cognitive Therapy and Research, 12,* 557–575.

Pleva, J., & Wade, T. D. (2007). Guided self-help versus pure self-help for perfectionism: A randomised controlled trial. *Behaviour Research and Therapy, 45,* 849–861.

Prochaska, J. O., & DiClemente, C. C. (1992). The transtheoretical approach. In J. C. Norcross & M. R. Goldfried (Eds.), *Handbook of psychotherapy integration* (pp. 300–334). New York: Basic Books.

Reardon, M. L., Cukrowicz, K. C., Reeves, M. D., & Joiner, T. E. J. (2002). Duration and regularity of therapy attendance as predictors of treatment outcome in an adult outpatient population. *Psychotherapy Research, 12,* 273–285.

Rhéaume, J., Freeston, M. H., Léger, E., & Ladouceur, R. (1998). Bad luck: An underestimated factor in the development of obsessive–compulsive disorder. *Clinical Psychology and Psychotherapy, 5,* 1–12.

Riley, C., Lee, M., Cooper, Z., Fairburn, C. G., & Shafran, R. (2007). A randomised controlled trial of cognitive–behaviour therapy for clinical perfectionism: A preliminary study. *Behaviour Research and Therapy, 45,* 2221–2231.

Roder, V., Brenner, H. D., Muller, D., Lachler, M., Zorn, P., Reisch, T., et al. (2002). Development of specific social skills training programmes for schizophrenia patients: Results of a multicentre study. *Acta Psychiatrica Scandinavica, 105,* 363–371.

Roemer, L., & Orsillo, S. M. (2007). An open trial of an acceptance-based behavior therapy for generalized anxiety disorder. *Behavior Therapy, 38,* 72–85.

Rosqvist, J., Egan, D., Manzo, P., Baer, L., Jenike, M., & Willis, B. S. (2001). Home-based behavior therapy for obsessive–compulsive disorder: A case-series with data. *Journal of Anxiety Disorders, 15,* 395–400.

Rowa, K., Antony, M. M., Summerfeldt, L. J., Purdon C., Young L., & Swinson, R. P. (2007). Office-based vs. home-based behavioral treatment for obsessive–compulsive disorder: A preliminary study. *Behaviour Research and Therapy, 45,* 1883–1892.

Saatsi, S., Hardy, G. E., & Cahill, J. (2007). Predictors of outcome and completion status in cognitive therapy for depression. *Psychotherapy Research, 17,* 185–195.

Safran, J. D., & Segal, Z. V. (1990). Refining strategies for research on self-representations in emotional disorders. *Cognitive Therapy and Research, 14,*143–160.

Scapillato, D., & Manassis, K. (2002). Cognitive–behavioral/interpersonal group treatment for anxious adolescents. *Journal of the American Academy of Child & Adolescent Psychiatry, 41,* 739–741.

Segal, Z. V., Williams, J. M. G., & Teasdale, J. T. (2002). *Mindfulness-based cognitive therapy for depression: A new approach to preventing relapse.* New York: Guilford Press.

Stanley, B., Bundy, E., & Beberman, R. (2001). Skills training as an adjunctive treatment for personality disorders. *Journal of Psychiatric Practice, 7,* 324–335.

Storch, E. A., Geffken, G. R., Merlo, L. J., Mann, G., Duke, D., Munson, M., et al. (2007). Family-based cognitive–behavioral therapy for pediatric obsessive–compulsive disorder: Comparison of intensive and weekly approaches. *Journal of the American Academy of Child & Adolescent Psychiatry, 46,* 469–478.

Suveg, C., Kendall, P. C., Comer, J. S., & Robin, J. (2006). Emotion-focused cognitive–behavioral therapy for anxious youth: A multiple-baseline evaluation. *Journal of Contemporary Psychotherapy, 36,* 77–85.

Taylor, S., Koch, W. J., Fecteau, G., Fedoroff, I. C., Thordasrson, D. S., & Nicki, R. M. (2001). Posttraumatic stress disorder arising after road traffic collisions: Patterns of response to cognitive–behavioral therapy. *Journal of Consulting and Clinical Psychology, 63,* 541–551.

Teasdale, J. D., Segal, Z., & Williams, M. G. (1995). How does cognitive therapy prevent depressive relapse and why should attentional control (mindfulness) training help? *Behaviour Research and Therapy, 33,* 25–39.

Teasdale, J. D., Segal, Z. V., Williams, J. M. G., Ridgeway, V. A., Soulsby, J. M., & Lau, M. A. (2000). Prevention of relapse/recurrence in major depression by mindfulness-based cognitive therapy. *Journal of Consulting and Clinical Psychology, 68,* 615–623.

Telch, C. F., Agras, W. S., & Linehan, M. M. (2001). Dialectical behavior therapy for binge eating disorder. *Journal of Consulting and Clinical Psychology, 69,* 1061–1065.

Toneatto, T., Vettese, L., & Nguyen, L. (2007). The role of mindfulness in the cognitive–behavioral treatment of problem gambling. *Journal of Gambling, 19,* 91–100.

Trepka, C., Rees, A., Shapiro, D. A., Hardy, G. E., & Barkham, M. (2004). Therapist competence and outcome of cognitive therapy for depression. *Cognitive Therapy and Research, 28,* 143–157.

Tsao, J. C., Mystkowski, J. L., Zucker, B. G., & Craske, M. G. (2005). Impact of cognitive–behavioral therapy for panic disorder on comorbidity: A controlled investigation. *Behaviour Research and Therapy, 43*, 959–970.

Vitousek, K., & Watson, S. (1998). Enhancing motivation for change in treatment resistant eating disorders. *Clinical Psychology Review, 18*, 391–420.

Vocisano, C., Arnow, B., Blalock, J. A., Vivian, D., Manber, R., & Rush, A. J. (2004). Therapist variables that predict symptom change in psychotherapy with chronically depressed outpatients. *Psychotherapy: Theory, Research, Practice, Training, 41*, 255–265.

Watson, J. C., & McMullen, E. J. (2005). An examination of therapist and client behavior in high- and low-alliance sessions in cognitive–behavioral therapy and process experiential therapy. *Psychotherapy: Theory, Research, Practice, and Training, 42*, 297–310.

Weissman, M. M., Markowitz, J. C., & Klerman, G. L. (2000). *Comprehensive guide to interpersonal psychotherapy.* New York: Basic Books.

Westen, D., & Morrisson, K. (2001). A multidimensional meta-analysis of treatments for depression, panic, and generalized anxiety disorder: An empirical examination of the status of empirically supported therapies. *Journal of Consulting and Clinical Psychology, 69*, 875–899.

Westra, H. A., & Dozois, D. J. A., (2006). Preparing clients for cognitive behavior therapy: A randomized pilot study of motivational interviewing for anxiety. *Cognitive Therapy and Research, 30*, 481–498.

Westra, H. A., Dozois, D. J. A., & Marcus, M. (2007). Expectancy, homework compliance, and initial change in cognitive–behavioral therapy for anxiety. *Journal of Consulting and Clinical Psychology, 75*, 363–373.

Wilfley, D. E., Agras, W. S., Telch, C. F., Rossiter, E. M., Schneider, J. A., Cole, A. G., et al. (1993). Group cognitive–behavioral therapy and group interpersonal psychotherapy for the nonpurging bulimic individual: A controlled comparison. *Journal of Consulting and Clinical Psychology, 61*, 296–305.

Wilhelm, S., & Steketee, G. S. (2006). *Cognitive therapy for obsessive–compulsive disorder: A guide for professionals.* Oakland: CA: New Harbinger.

Williams, M., Teasdale, J., Segal, Z., & Kabat-Zinn, J. (2007). *The mindful way through depression: Freeing yourself from chronic unhappiness.* New York: Guilford Press.

Wonderlich, S., & Mitchel, J. E. (2001). The role of personality in the onset of eating disorders and treatment implications [Special issue]. *Psychiatric Clinics of North America, 24*, 249–258.

II

TREATING REFRACTORY CASES IN SPECIFIC DIAGNOSTIC POPULATIONS AND CLINICAL PROBLEMS

3

PANIC WITH AGORAPHOBIA

MELISSA M. MAGARO AND MICHELLE G. CRASKE

Considerable research has informed current conceptualizations of panic disorder and agoraphobia. Research has also supported the use of cognitive–behavioral therapy (CBT) as a highly efficacious treatment for panic disorder (Barlow, 2002; Barlow, Gorman, Shear, & Woods, 2000; Craske & Barlow, 2001; Gould, Otto, & Pollack, 1995). Despite the well-established efficacy of CBT, some clients do not respond well to treatment. Therefore, it is critical to identify the factors that lead to poor treatment response and to reflect on ways to tailor treatment protocols to address such elements. This chapter includes a clinical description of panic disorder and agoraphobia and a cognitive–behavioral conceptualization of the problem, as well as descriptions of effective treatment, identification of factors associated with poor response, and a Conclusion section that includes suggestions for future directions.

SIGNIFICANCE OF PANIC DISORDER

Evidence from epidemiological studies has suggested that between 2% and 6% of the general population will experience panic disorder at some point in their lives (Kessler, Berglund, Demler, Jin, & Walters, 2005). Furthermore, the consequences of an episode of panic disorder can be debilitating given the distress and/or avoidance or agoraphobia that arises from the fear of future attacks (Hansson, 2002; Lochner et al., 2003). Lifestyle changes, such as less frequent social interaction, inability to be away from familiar places such as home or work, and avoidance of day-to-day activities like grocery shopping or driving a motor vehicle, can quickly limit the functioning of an individual with panic disorder and create substantial distress. The fear and accompanying behavioral avoidance associated with this disorder can significantly affect the lives of friends and family as well. The impact on functioning is clear when examining the economic burden of panic disorder (Katon et al., 1996; Klerman, 1991; Siegel, Jones, & Wilson, 1990). Although a single episode of panic disorder or agoraphobia can cause considerable interference and distress, the conditions tend to be chronic. Left untreated, about one third of cases fully remit without relapse (Katschnig & Amering, 1998; Roy-Byrne & Cowley, 1995).

PRESENTING FEATURES AND DSM CRITERIA

Panic attacks, as defined in the *Diagnostic and Statistical Manual of Mental Disorders* (*DSM–IV–TR*; 4th ed., text rev.; American Psychiatric Association, 2000), are episodes of intense fear or dread accompanied by physical symptoms such as pounding heart, shortness of breath, numbness or tingling sensations, dizziness or lightheadedness, hot flushes, or chills. Additionally, cognitive symptoms may occur in the midst of a panic attack, such as fears of fainting, dying, or going crazy. In contrast to episodes of anxious mood, which might last hours or days, panic attacks are discrete episodes of heightened arousal. The onset of an attack may be sudden and unexpected, and the anxiety generally peaks within 10 to 15 minutes. The presence of recurrent unexpected attacks is a diagnostic criterion for panic disorder. As such, if an individual is experiencing panic attacks exclusively in "expected" situations such as social settings, then further exploration of differential diagnoses would be required because panic disorder may not be appropriate despite the presence of recurrent panic attacks. This latter point raises an important point regarding the distinction between panic attacks and panic disorder.

Although panic attacks are a central and necessary feature of panic disorder, the *DSM–IV–TR* does not recognize panic attacks as an Axis I disorder. Thus, panic attacks are not in and of themselves considered a psychological disorder. Panic attacks occur in approximately 3% to 5% of the general population who do not meet criteria for panic disorder (Norton, Cox, & Schwartz, 1992) and are common in the context of other anxiety disorders. For a diagnosis of panic disorder to be considered, one must experience at least 1 month of persistent worry about future attacks, concerns about their consequences, or significant behavior change in response to the attacks (American Psychiatric Association, 1994). To return to the example mentioned earlier, in which an individual experiences panic attacks exclusively in the context of social situations, worry about being judged negatively for having a panic attack in public would not fit the criteria for panic disorder. Rather, it is fear of the fear that distinguishes someone with panic disorder from someone with an anxiety or mood disorder who also panics.

Significant behavioral change may help distinguish someone as panic disordered. This situational avoidance or endurance of anxiety-provoking situations with extreme distress is referred to as *agoraphobia*. Situations in which the individual feels that escape will be difficult or that help will not be available in the event of a panic attack are often avoided. Typical examples of agoraphobia include avoidance of shopping malls, open spaces, movie theaters, traveling by plane or bus, crowded venues, or being alone. Agoraphobia does not always accompany panic disorder, but individuals with agoraphobia who seek treatment nearly always report a history of panic that contributed to their avoidance (Goisman, Warshaw, Peterson, & Rogers, 1994; Wittchen, Reed, & Kessler, 1998). Estimates of the prevalence of agoraphobia without panic disorder are low, ranging from .8% for 1-year prevalence to 1.4% for lifetime prevalence (Kessler et al., 2005).

COGNITIVE–BEHAVIORAL THERAPY FOR PANIC DISORDER

Current conceptualizations view panic disorder as an acquired fear of bodily sensations (such as pounding heart or shortness of breath). This fear can lead to behavioral changes in the service of avoiding situations that may trigger feared sensations, a phenomenon also known as agoraphobia. CBT for panic disorder is aimed at reducing fear in response to physiological sensations typical of panic attacks; this is achieved through both cognitive restructuring (Arntz & van den Hout, 1996; Beck & Zebb, 1994; Öst & Westling, 1995; Stanley et al., 1996) and exposure (Barlow, 2002; Barlow, Brown, & Craske, 1994; Craske, Lang, Aikens, & Mystkowski, 2005). Generally early in treatment, the CBT therapist will provide psychoeducation regarding panic attacks and anxiety in general. This education may include information regarding the symptoms experienced during panic attacks (e.g., correcting misbeliefs that clients are having a heart attack when in fact they are experiencing heart palpitations in the context of a panic attack). The therapist and client also discuss the ways in which the cycle of panic is maintained, highlighting the roles of cognitions about anxiety symptoms and behavioral avoidance. The cognitive element involves identifying misappraisals of physical symptoms (e.g., "If I feel dizzy, I'm going to faint") and restructuring those cognitions to generate more realistic alternatives grounded in the data (e.g., "I have felt dizzy before but never fainted").

Once cognitive restructuring has been introduced, the client begins to engage in systematic exposure. Exposure exercises are designed to provide exposure to feared sensations (interoceptive exposure) and to real-life situations that bring about feared sensations (in vivo exposures). Interoceptive exposure can be achieved in a variety of ways, including spinning to induce dizziness, hyperventilating to create shortness of breath, or staring into a mirror to bring about feelings of unreality. When the client experiences feelings similar to those of panic, the therapist encourages him or her to use the coping skills learned in order to maintain in the situation and not escape the sensation. Deliberately inducing a sensation that the client would normally avoid provides the opportunity to test the accuracy of cognitions (e.g., "If I don't calm down, I'm going to lose it"). In addition, clients learn that sensations are not dangerous and that intense feelings can be tolerated. In vivo exposure targets the same kind of learning in situations typically avoided; that is, through repeated exposure, clients learn that they can tolerate the physical sensations in particular situations and that those sensations are not harmful.

EFFICACY OF COGNITIVE–BEHAVIORAL THERAPY FOR PANIC DISORDER

Research on the efficacy of CBT for panic disorder is particularly well developed. Clinical trials have consistently supported the use of CBT as an effective first-line treatment for panic disorder (e.g., Barlow, Gorman, Shear, & Woods, 2000; Craske, Brown, & Barlow, 1991; Craske et al., 2007; Margraf, Barlow, Clark, & Telch, 1993; Öst, Westling, & Hellström, 1993; Otto, Smits, & Reese, 2004). Gould, Otto, and Pollack (1995) conducted a large-scale meta-analysis of effectiveness trials, comparing CBT, pharmacological treatment, and combination treatment for panic disorder. CBT yielded the highest mean effect size ($d = .68$) compared with pharmacological treatments ($d = .47$) and the combination of the two ($d = .56$).

Cognitive–behavioral interventions included in the meta-analysis were cognitive restructuring, interoceptive exposure, in vivo exposure, flooding, and/or relaxation exercises. In a 2-year cross-sectional follow-up, 80% of patients remained panic free (Craske et al., 1991). Within CBT, those treatments that included both cognitive restructuring and exposure yielded the highest effect sizes ($ES = .88$). Group therapy contexts have had similar success (Galassi, Quercioli, Charismas, Niccolai, & Barciulli, 2007).

Some researchers have highlighted the lack of studies examining longer term outcomes (greater than 2 years) to assess maintenance of gains and potential relapse of panic symptoms. Kenardy, Robinson, and Dob (2005) conducted a long-term follow-up of individuals who received CBT as part of a randomized controlled trial. Patients were reassessed between 6 and 8 years following treatment termination. When considering the percentage of people who remained panic free after treatment, the long-term follow-up data (57%) were similar to those of the 6-month follow-up (65%).

To complement the wealth of efficacy trials, there are a growing number of effectiveness trials that further support the use of CBT as a first-line treatment for panic. Wade, Treat, and Stuart (1998) transported a 15-session manualized CBT treatment to a community mental health center and found short- and long-term (1-year follow-up) treatment gains similar to those of clinical trials (Stuart, Treat, & Wade, 2000). Penava, Otto, Maki, and Pollack (1998) focused on rates of improvement in patients receiving CBT for panic in an outpatient setting. The authors found the greatest reduction in symptoms in the first third of the 12-week manualized treatment. These findings challenge previous research that has suggested that CBT produces gains slowly over time, often following treatment termination. Our own work demonstrates the effectiveness of condensed CBT when delivered to patients within primary care clinics in combination with recommendations regarding medications (Roy-Byrne et al., 2005). It is interesting that the positive benefits in terms of symptom status and quality of life 1 year later were more directly attributable to CBT than to medications (Craske, Golinelli, et al., 2005). Furthermore, the greater the number of CBT sessions and follow-up phone contacts, the more positive the results (Craske et al., 2006).

It should be noted that results regarding both efficacy and effectiveness vary dramatically on the basis of the method of assessment. One important distinction is cross-sectional assessment (e.g., panic frequency over the past month) versus longitudinal methodology (e.g., need for further treatment). Cross-sectional assessment provides a snapshot of the client's symptomatology and/or functioning at the time of the follow-up visit, often focusing on the previous month. In contrast, longitudinal methods allow for examination of the follow-up interval as a whole and provide information about course of the disorder and treatment gains. To illustrate the potential discrepancies between cross-sectional versus longitudinal assessment, Brown and Barlow (1995) used both methods and found that 74% of patients were classified as panic free at the 24-month follow-up when using a cross-sectional approach, and 56% had reached high end-state functioning (which is a proxy for "cured"). In contrast, when using more stringent longitudinal methods (e.g., requiring that patients had both reached a high end-state functioning status and had sought no further treatment), only 48% of patients met criteria.

FACTORS ASSOCIATED WITH POOR RESPONSE

Although the data support CBT as an efficacious and effective treatment for panic disorder, clearly treatment response rates have indicated that for a percentage of individuals panic does not remit following treatment and for others relapse occurs in the long term. As such, it is critical to understand what factors are associated with poor response to improve therapeutic approaches and adapt treatments for diverse populations.

Comorbidity of Mood Disorders

A host of studies have demonstrated that the majority of individuals with a *DSM–IV* (American Psychiatric Association, 1994) anxiety disorder also have at least one additional disorder (Brown & Barlow, 1992; Sanderson, Di Nardo, Rapee, & Barlow, 1990). Clark (1989) found that 67% of individuals with panic or panic with agoraphobia had a past or present diagnosis of major depression. Brown, Antony, and Barlow (1995) found that 51% of those enrolled in a treatment study for panic disorder had a comorbid diagnosis, most often other anxiety disorders, such as GAD or social phobia, and mood disorders. The role of comorbidity in treatment outcome has gained attention from researchers in the past decade. Early work on the role of comorbidity in treatment outcome for panic came primarily from pharmacological treatment studies (Mennin & Heimberg, 2000), and such results do not seem appropriately generalizable to psychotherapeutic outcome studies; nor do those findings further our understanding of factors that may impact such outcomes.

Despite the growing body of literature examining comorbidity in relation to treatment outcome beyond psychotropic approaches, the results remain equivocal. Brown, Antony, and Barlow (1995) found that individuals with comorbid mood disorder at pretreatment were less likely to be panic free or achieve high end-state functioning at posttreatment than those without a comorbid mood disorder. However, there were no significant differences at 3-month follow-up between those with comorbid depression and those without. Tsao, Lewin, and Craske (1998) found that individuals with comorbidity at pretreatment showed a trend for reduced likelihood of high outcome at posttreatment. Other investigators have similarly found that individuals with concurrent diagnoses at pretreatment showed less favorable treatment response than did those who did not have comorbid conditions (Grunhaus, Pande, Brown, & Greden, 1994; O'Rourke, Fahy, Brophy, & Prescott, 1996; Reif, Trenkamp, Auer, & Fichter, 2000).

In contrast, other studies have found that individuals with comorbid depression and those without responded similarly to CBT approaches. Laberge, Gauthier, Cote, Plamondon, and Cormier (1993) found no differences in treatment outcome between those with and without comorbid depression diagnoses. Likewise, when examining end-state functioning following CBT, McLean, Woody, Taylor, and Koch (1998) found that pretreatment comorbid depression did not significantly predict treatment outcome.

Comorbidity, as a generic term referring to the co-occurrence of disorders, does not address the issue of primary versus secondary diagnoses. *Primary diagnosis* generally refers to the most clinically significant diagnosis, although sometimes it is used to denote the diagnosis that occurred first chronologically. The issue of primary versus secondary diagnoses is relevant to this discussion because it has been suggested that the distinction may moderate the relationship between depression and treatment outcome. When examining the effects of history of comorbid depression, Maddock and Blacker (1991) treated 20 outpatients with panic disorder with a symptom-focused approach. The researchers found that outcome did not differ significantly between those with no history of depression and those with a history of secondary depression, although individuals with a history of primary depression showed the worst outcomes.

Thus, the literature is equivocal as to whether depression has an adverse effect on treatment outcome for panic disorder. As such, questions remain regarding how to manage comorbid depression. Some studies (Craske et al., 2007; Tsao, Mystkowski, Zucker, & Craske, 2002, 2005) have suggested that no adaptation is necessary when working with comorbid disorders because targeted CBT will be equally effective with or without the presence of other disorders. Furthermore, according to these studies, comorbid conditions actually improve following targeted panic disorder treatment. Other studies suggest that depression needs to be addressed in the context of treatment. Marks (1987) suggested that depression may create motivation issues that may impede exposure exercises. Further, Telch (1988) theorized that negative cognitive schemas typical of mood disorders may interfere with new learning and discount treatment gains. Attention should be given to such factors. Pharmacologically, clinicians may consider the addition of antidepressants to the treatment plan to address comorbid depression. Given the high efficacy rates of CBT for panic disorder, Laberge, Gauthier, Cote, Plamondon, and Cormier (1992) recommended that psychotherapy be tried before pharmacological interventions if the panic disorder is primary to the depressive disorder. Medication may be considered when suicidality is present or the client is in need of immediate relief.

Axis II Comorbidity

Although researchers long ago realized the importance of screening for comorbid diagnoses in addition to the target disorders in treatment studies, to date, few studies have included Axis II diagnoses in their comprehensive diagnostic screening procedures. This may be because of the limited availability of reliable and valid methods of assessment. The available options range from self-report questionnaires to structured clinical interviews; questionnaires are used much more frequently, despite criticism that these inventories are not independent from illness severity (Marchesi, Cantoni, Fontò, Giannelli, & Maggini, 2005). It has been suggested that one weakness of the extant assessment measures is the inability to differentiate abnormal personality traits from clinically significant personality disorders (Noyes, Reich, Suelzer, & Christiansen, 1991). Indeed, Mennin and Heimberg (2000) suggested that some of the traits detected on personality assessment may be capturing abnormal personality traits associated with or a consequence of panic disorder as opposed to true Axis II symptomatology. Of those that have examined personality disorders, the results are not convergent. Chambless, Renneberg, Goldstein, and Gracely (1992) used Versions I and II of the Millon Clinical Multiaxial Inventory with a sample of 165 agoraphobic outpatients and found that 90% of the sample met criteria for at least one Axis II disorder, the most common being avoidant and dependent personality disorder. Such findings extend to traits, as individuals with panic disorder tend to have an increased rate of avoidant, dependent, histrionic, and borderline traits (Mavissakalian & Hamann, 1986). Thus, comorbidity with personality disorder and/or traits is common in anxiety disorders, especially panic disorder and agoraphobia. This raises the question of how personality disorders affect treatment outcome. Dreesen, Arntz, Luttels, and Sallaerts (1994), in a prospective outcome study, screened for personality disorders using the Structured Clinical Interview Schedule for Personality Disorders (SCID-II) prior to CBT treatment for panic disorder. They found that at pretreatment, comorbid Axis II disorders were associated with more severe Axis I psychopathology, specifically panic disorder symptoms and impairment, yet therapeutic change paralleled that in those individuals without personality disorder diagnoses. The authors suggested that although individuals with comorbid Axis II disorders may not reach the same end-state level of functioning, the change scores indicate that the rates of improvement and trajectories are similar. One way in which personality disorders may diminish treatment gains is through poor therapeutic process. Dreesen and Arntz (1999) examined the relationship between therapist-reported dysfunctional process in treating anxiety disorders and independent diagnostic ratings of personality disorders using the SCID-II. They found that independent ratings of symptomatology were only weakly associated with therapist-reported complications, whereas therapist-rated symptomatology was highly correlated with therapist-reported complications. This suggests that perceptions of personality may be influencing therapists' experience with such clients. The authors cited this as further support that personality disorders do not interfere with or diminish the potential benefits of CBT for Axis I disorders, specifically anxiety disorders.

In contrast, other studies have demonstrated that personality disorders and traits are associated with poor treatment response. Hoffart and Hedley (1997) conducted a 6-week intervention study comparing cognitive therapy with guided-mastery therapy (i.e., self-efficacy-based exposure therapy). They found that the number of dependent personality traits at pretreatment was significantly correlated with less improvement at the 1-year follow-up. Similarly, Marchand, Goyer, Dupuis, and Mainguy (1998) found that individuals with personality disorder diagnoses improved less and more slowly in a CBT study for panic disorder with agoraphobia than their "no personality disorder" counterparts. Although the authors highlighted the marked improvements in all groups from pretest to posttest and 3-month follow-ups, the personality disorder group stopped improving posttreatment, whereas the "no personality disorder" group continued to improve beyond the posttreatment assessment.

Although there are mixed findings regarding the effect of comorbid personality disorders on treatment outcome, it is necessary for clinicians to be aware of potential adjustments that are necessary when working with these clients. For instance, clients may exhibit decreased motivation, especially with regard to exposure and between-session homework. Such factors may account for the slowed progress of clients with comorbid Axis II symptomatology that has been found. Given that numerous studies have found change rates and trajectories to parallel those of clients without comorbidity, treatment length may need to be increased to allow such clients to reach the same end-state functioning as their noncomorbid counterparts. Finally, because few treatment outcome studies comprehensively screen for personality disorders and even fewer have the statistical power to examine specific personality disorders, further research is needed to better understand what specific disorders are associated with poor outcome and therefore might benefit from tailored approaches.

Medical Comorbidity

Studies have suggested that severity of medical comorbidity may adversely affect treatment outcomes for major depression (Iosifescu et al., 2003; Oslin et al., 2002). There is also evidence that anxiety disorders are elevated in populations with medical comorbidity. For example, the prevalence of panic disorder among patients with major medical illness is 4.3% (Löwe et al., 2003), and panic disorder or panic symptoms are present in 9.4% of primary care medical patients (Roy-Byrne et al., 2005). Some examples of medical conditions that have a high comorbidity with panic disorder include respiratory disease, cardiac disease, vestibular dysfunction, and hyperthyroidism/hypothyroidism. Roy-Byrne, Russo, Cowley, and Katon (2003) found that when comparing usual care with pharmacological treatment with Paxil, patients who showed consistent response to treatment (defined as positive response at the majority of follow-up interviews over a 1-year period) had significantly fewer comorbid medical conditions, hospitalizations, and emergency room visits. These data raise the question of whether comorbid medical disorders might adversely affect treatment response similar to that seen in studies of depression. Roy-Byrne et al. (2005) conducted the first study examining the effects of comorbid medical conditions on the treatment of anxiety disorders with CBT. The study was conducted in a primary care setting in which outpatients received up to six sessions of CBT and medication recommendations for panic disorder. Similar to past research, the investigators found that individuals with a greater medical burden displayed greater psychiatric illness (as measured by symptoms and impairment) at baseline. Nonetheless, the response to CBT was comparable for those with greater severity of medical illness and those with less or no medical comorbidity. On the other hand, although the overall trajectories of both groups were parallel, the group with greater severity of medical conditions at baseline did not achieve the same end-state functioning as those with less severe medical comorbidity. The authors suggested that extending treatments to increase therapeutic dose for individuals with medical comorbidity may show more comparable outcomes for both groups.

When working with medical comorbidity, we recommend that clinicians work closely with physicians and inquire regarding potential contraindications of exposures to interoceptive and external cues given the specific medical condition. Medical "clearance" prior to onset of exposure therapy is a good standard of practice but is especially important in working with medical comorbidity. Furthermore, in the context of CBT, it is important to help clients learn to articulate the differences between medical symptoms and nonmedical symptoms, and possibly utilize ongoing monitoring of relevant health indices (e.g., blood pressure or heart rate monitors) during exposure therapy. Cognitively, it is important to engage in problem solving around real medical issues as a way of decatastrophizing such feared events and increasing coping skills.

Comorbidity of Substance Abuse and Dependence

As mentioned previously, estimates of the prevalence of panic disorder in the general population range between 2% and 6% (Kessler et al., 2005), but within a population of individuals with alcohol dependence, those estimates increase dramatically, ranging from 5% to 42% (Kushner, Sher, & Beitman, 1990). Comorbidity with alcoholism occurs in approximately 15% to 21% of individuals with a diagnosed anxiety disorder (Bibb & Chambless, 1986; Thyer, 1986). Although the rates of comorbid anxiety and alcohol disorders are high, very few studies have examined the direction of the relationship between the two. Kushner et al.'s (1990) review yielded mixed results, with some studies reporting the onset of the anxiety disorder prior to the substance disorder, some reporting the opposite direction, and still others reporting concurrent onset. Lehman, Brown, and Barlow (1998) suggested that the high comorbidity may be due to self-medication as a means of reducing anxiety, whereas others have suggested that substances like tobacco (Breslau & Klein, 1999) and stimulants (Cox, Norton, Dorward, & Fergusson, 1989) may precipitate panic attacks. In line with this hypothesis, a reduction in alcohol use would be expected as clients gain coping skills for managing panic and anxiety. Unfortunately, the majority of research studies exclude individuals with comorbid substance disorder, although one series of case studies (Lehman, Brown, & Barlow, 1998) found that CBT for panic did reduce alcohol consumption. In the absence of clear research-based guidelines, it has been suggested that clinicians should strive to understand which disorder is primary and treat that first; therefore, if substance disorder is primary, it would be treated first while delaying treatment of the panic disorder (Marshall, 1997). Further research on the effects of comorbidity on treatment is desperately needed given the common co-occurrence of anxiety and substance disorders.

Treatment Compliance

One of the basic tenets of CBT is new learning and acquisition of new skills through experience, most often achieved through homework. Although homework may be one of the most distinct features of CBT compared with other forms of psychotherapy, and a feature that is presumed to be critical to therapeutic change, the relationship between homework compliance and treatment outcome remains unclear. Edelman and Chambless (1993) found equivocal results when comparing protocols with no homework to those with homework components. Other researchers have found homework compliance to be a significant predictor of outcome (Barlow, O'Brien, & Last, 1984; Edelman & Chambless, 1993; Michelson, Mavissakalian, Marchione, Dancu, & Greenwald, 1986), whereas others have found no relationship (Mavissakalian & Michelson, 1983). The divergent results may be explained by the operationalization of *compliance*, which could refer to quantity or quality. Schmidt and Woolaway-Bickle (2000) addressed this very question within a 12-session group CBT protocol for panic disorder. The investigators found that client-reported compliance was not associated with outcome, yet therapist-reported compliance was associated with positive changes in outcome measures. In addition, they found that the combination of independent evaluators and therapists to assess quality of homework compliance resulted in quality becoming an even better predictor of outcome. Quality of homework was assessed using various predetermined criteria, for example, whether a specific task was identified, whether the exposure evoked moderate levels of anxiety/fear, whether the participant remained in the situation until fear subsided, and whether coping strategies where identified and used. Thus, poor quality of homework may be a barrier to success with CBT.

Consequently, understanding what factors are associated with homework compliance is useful. Conoley, Padula, Payton, and Daniels (1994) found, not surprisingly, that task difficulty was negatively correlated with homework compliance, keeping in mind that the therapeutically indicated tasks (e.g., facing feared sensations and situations) are sufficiently difficult for the client. In many cases clients have avoided the tasks all together, sometimes for years prior to treatment, and as such therapists must be mindful of this potential barrier. Detweiler and Whisman (1999) suggested that progression from less difficult to more difficult tasks might improve compliance by improving self-efficacy. Fortunately, the standard practice of developing a fear hierarchy and making progression contingent on success fits nicely with this model. Furthermore, conducting in-session exposures prior to assignment of similar out-of-session exposures may also increase compliance by allowing the client to experience success with the task. This also allows the therapist to provide guidance during the exposure itself, including highlighting the rationale for exposure. It is interesting that therapist empathy has not been found to be predictive of compliance (Burns & Nolen-Hoeksema, 1991).

Safety-Seeking Behaviors and Safety Signals

Broadly defined, *safety-seeking behaviors* are actions that one engages in to gain a sense of safety or security in the face of perceived danger. Lohr, Olatunji, and Sawchuk (2007) divided these behaviors into three categories: (a) behavioral avoidance of situations, (b) escape from anxiety-provoking situations, and (c) behaviors in situations aimed at preventing the onset of aversive events. From a cognitive–behavioral perspective, all three categories of safety-seeking contribute to the maintenance of anxiety. This may occur by interrupting the habituation to feared stimuli (Rachman, 1984) and/or by interfering with the learning process of corrective information (Salkovskis, 1991). In a review of behavioral treatment for panic disorder with agoraphobia, Steketee and Shapiro (1995) noted that one of the strongest predictors of poor outcome was severe avoidance behavior. Avoidance is a natural response to fear because it serves to prevent the onset of a perceived or expected aversive event, but when it becomes the only means of coping with fear or anxiety, it is problematic. Thus, safety-seeking behaviors, such as avoidance, are activated in response to perceived threat or danger signals.

A *safety signal* indicates the offset of an aversive event or predicts the absence of onset of an aversive event. Safety signals may include external environments (e.g., one's car) or internal feelings (e.g., the deceleration of heart rate could signal safety). Powerful external safety signals for individuals who panic include home, hospitals, and, in contemporary times, cell phones (Rachman, 1983), as well as trusted persons (Carter, Hollon, Carson, & Shelton, 1995; Rachman, 1993). There has been much research on safety signals, both experimentally and clinically, and humans and animals consistently seek out safety in the presence of danger cues that signal a potential threat (Baum, 1986; Jacobs & LoLordo, 1976; Rachman, 1984; Woody & Rachman, 1994). Although it can be argued that safety signals may aid clients in approaching feared situations, overreliance can be problematic. For instance, always having a particular individual present during exposure may contribute to the maintenance of catastrophic beliefs when feared outcomes do not occur (Salkovskis, Clark, & Gelder, 1996). Individuals who serve as safety signals may facilitate escape from anxiety-provoking situations (Rachman, 1984). Safety signals in various forms may prevent corrective learning (Salkovskis, 1991) and interfere with exposure therapy (Salkovskis, Clark, Hackmann, Wells, & Gelder, 1999). Even the perception of the availability of safety signals has been shown to be detrimental to outcomes from exposure therapy (Powers, Smits, & Telch, 2004). More specifically, according to current models of CBT for anxiety, exposure to feared situations allows clients to gather evidence to disconfirm their threat-laden beliefs in a given situation (which could be the belief that a particular negative outcome will occur or the belief that they will not be able to cope with fear itself). This corrective learning then alters their perception of that situation in the future. When safety signals are present, such as carrying medication or having a trusted friend present during exposure, clients often attribute the absence of feared outcomes or their ability to cope to the presence of the safety signal, as if the safety signal has prevented the feared catastrophe. Thus, they may view the exposure as a "near miss," which in turn maintains anxiety in the long term. Similarly, avoidance and escape may be viewed as means of preventing feared outcomes and interrupt corrective learning.

Medication as a safety signal warrants special attention given that many clients are concurrently taking medication for anxiety while in CBT. Selective serotonin reuptake inhibitors and serotonin–norepinephrine reuptake inhibitors are commonly prescribed medications that are taken daily for the treatment of anxiety disorders, whereas benzodiazepines are fast-acting medications that are generally prescribed on an as needed basis. The latter is of interest in the context of safety signals because clients may develop a reliance on the availability of the medication as a way to feel safe in feared situations. The knowledge alone that the drug is available may be enough to reduce fear and anxiety and thereby interfere with learning. Therefore, it is critical for clinicians to check in regularly about the presence or use of medications, especially during exposure, and to incorporate exposure without medication into the fear hierarchy. In other words, when medications are used as safety signals, it is essential that their use be weaned throughout exposure therapy.

CASE EXAMPLE

Norma, a 41-year-old woman, sought treatment for panic disorder with severe agoraphobia that she had been experiencing for approximately 9 years. Norma had quit school 7 years prior because of panic disorder. She was divorced and currently lived with a male friend, Stuart, who supported her financially; she had no children. At the time of intake, Norma reported that she was experiencing on average one full-symptom panic attack per day. During those attacks, she generally experienced trembling or shaking, feelings of unreality, sweating, and dizziness in addition to fearing that she might do something uncontrolled or die. She explained that she worried every waking hour about having another attack and that she feared she would go crazy as a result of the attacks. Her agoraphobic avoidance was extreme; Norma reported that she could not be at home alone and that she would not leave the house without Stuart. Also, she avoided substances, activities, and places that evoked physiological sensations related to her panic attacks, including caffeine, exercise, hot and cold places, sex, and crowded places. Stuart always accompanied Norma to her weekly clinic appointments and remained in the waiting room during her sessions. She also reported that Stuart carried Ativan for her in case she had an attack. She explained that she would be housebound if it were not for Stuart. Although Stuart clearly was Norma's primary safety signal, Norma also carried her cellular phone with her at all times in case she lost sight of him while in public. The Ativan she carried "just in case" she had an attack was also a safety signal.

Norma reported having had a traumatic experience of being hospitalized previously and enduring intense pain while being treated. It remained unclear as to whether this hospitalization was due to strictly medical conditions or was psychosomatic in nature. Nonetheless, she feared that a panic attack in public that required calling 911 would place her once again in the hospital and that she would be administered chemicals that would permanently affect her physically (e.g., she might go blind). She reported that she did not believe that she could endure such an experience again. This experience and subsequent beliefs complicated her presentation because she feared not only the sensations of panic attacks but also the possibility that panic attacks could become so severe that she would require hospitalization, which would then lead to even greater fears of being physically harmed. Despite the unusual nature of these cognitions, there was no evidence that Norma was delusional.

In addition, Norma viewed the world as a generally bad and dangerous place and cited examples like the hospital incident as evidence supporting such beliefs. These thoughts were consistent with her comorbid diagnosis of recurrent major depressive disorder. Norma had lost almost 10 pounds in the 2 months prior to baseline in addition to experiencing hypersomnia, difficulty concentrating, and suicidal ideation (without plan or intent).

From a traditional cognitive–behavioral perspective, Norma's panic disorder and agoraphobia were treated through the use of breathing retraining, cognitive restructuring, and exposure therapy. Perhaps the most problematic feature of her presentation was the comorbid major depression. The hopeless nature of Norma's depression decreased her motivation to attend therapy and her ability to complete between-session homework, in addition to negatively affecting her beliefs regarding treatment effectiveness. Furthermore, when Norma did successfully complete homework assignments, especially exposures, throughout the week, her tendency was to discount or minimize her accomplishments. These depressive cognitions disrupted the cycle of reinforcement that is expected during exposure therapy wherein a client engages in a feared behavior, feels a sense of accomplishment, and is reinforced to engage in further behaviors.

One strategy to address her comorbid depression was to help her understand the contributory role that her behavioral choices regarding avoidance had on her depression and to emphasize that exposure practices, much like behavioral activation, would likely serve to lift mood. As Norma engaged in behavioral exposure exercises, it was important to process experiences in order to identify and address any depressive cognitions that might interfere with the reinforcement of behavioral changes. For instance, when Norma experienced anxiety or difficulty during exposure, she tended to interpret this as confirmation of her negative core beliefs regarding her inability to "get better" or the dangerousness of the outside world. Furthermore, when she experienced success, she would discount the exposure by saying something such as, "Most people are able to leave their house without panicking." Cognitive restructuring was aimed at helping Norma to develop alternative interpretations that valued her accomplishments relative to her own levels of fear and avoidance.

Consistent with the data on improvements in comorbid conditions, the therapist working with Norma continued to focus on her primary and most severe diagnosis, which was the panic disorder, while incorporating the depression into the conceptualization of the cycle of panic for the client in addition to encouraging generalization of the strategies for coping with anxiety to instances of depressed mood. Norma's therapist addressed her medication options prior to treatment, but because of her negative hospitalization experience, Norma did not wish to take any psychotropic medications. Although antidepressants certainly would not have guaranteed success, they might have helped elevate Norma's mood and perhaps improve her outcome.

Another issue to tackle in treatment was Norma's interpersonal dependency on her live-in friend, Stuart. Conceptualized as a safety signal, Norma's relationship with Stuart had to be addressed in therapy for her to make treatment gains. Norma reported that she felt safe and secure if Stuart was in sight but became anxious and fearful in his absence. Furthermore, Norma believed that the horrible events she feared (e.g., dying) had been prevented by his mere presence. Thus, by continuing to rely on Stuart as a safety signal, Norma would not learn that feared catastrophes do not occur when she was alone either at home or in public. She had to first understand how Stuart contributed to the maintenance of her anxiety and that she and the therapist could work together to decrease the use of safety signals, in this case spending time independent of Stuart, to test her hypothesis that feared events might occur without Stuart.

It would have been helpful to include Stuart in treatment to educate him about the role that he was playing and to explain the rationale for asking him to decrease behaviors that helped the client feel at ease. However, he was unwilling to be involved. Oatley and Hodgson (1987) suggested that integration of spouses or partners into CBT helps reinforce positive behaviors in addition to increasing adherence to exposure exercises. Some time ago, we found that including the significant other in all aspects of treatment resulted in greater improvement over a 2-year follow-up in comparison with excluding unwilling partners (Cerny, Barlow, Craske, & Hamadi, 1987). In a review of the literature, Byrne, Carr, and Clark (2004) found that couples-based treatments (which consisted of partner-assisted exposure and martial therapy) were as effective as individual-based CBT. Furthermore, maintenance of treatment gains may be enhanced in couples-focused treatments because the partner encourages and supports continued exposure to feared situations. As Norma became comfortable with the therapist, concerns arose about the therapist becoming a new safety signal. To address these, the therapist and Norma performed in-session exposures that involved walking out of sight of the therapist for varying amounts of time. It is important that Norma was encouraged to practice every exposure that she experienced under the guidance of the therapist when she was alone.

Even without Stuart's direct involvement, Norma made some gains. For instance, at the outset of treatment Stuart would wait outside the therapy room at Norma's request, and by the end of treatment he would remain in the waiting room on another floor of the building or even leave the building during her sessions. The therapist was mindful of secondary gains that may have been reinforcing Norma's behavior, such as being able to spend the majority of her time with her best friend, and was conscious of this potential barrier. Thus, items were built into the hierarchy, such as driving alone, so that Norma would feel intrinsic reinforcement from accomplishments that did not involve Stuart. Norma was able to slowly increase the physical proximity from Stuart, although these gains seemed to plateau when she reached a point at which she believed that she could drive to sessions alone. However, Stuart did not support this exercise and thus would not allow Norma to borrow his car for such purposes. This again speaks to the potential value of involving significant others in the therapy. If significant others are not able or willing to participate, the client should be encouraged to build an independent lifestyle.

Another blockade to her progress occurred when she experienced a traumatic event during an exposure. As she was leaving her house to go for an exposure walk, her dog ran into the street and was killed by oncoming traffic. This unexpected event heightened Norma's anxiety and activated depressive cognitions around leaving the house; she did not wish to engage in future exposures. The therapist expressed empathy toward the loss and eventually helped Norma to return to regular exposures by returning to lower level exposures on her hierarchy and working from there. Although the client's response to the event was understandable, it was critical to help her understand how escape and avoidance maintain avoidance by eliminating the opportunity for new learning to occur.

At posttreatment, Norma had made modest improvement, but she continued to rely on Stuart to function on a day-to-day basis. She exemplifies many of the factors that can interfere with treatment outcomes, including comorbid depression, severe avoidance, reliance on safety signals, and varying levels of compliance. Norma's case study also highlights the value of longer therapy, which may have addressed the complexities of her presentation and helped her achieve her goals of independence.

CONCLUSION

CBT continues to be considered the first-line treatment for panic disorder and agoraphobia. Although CBT has been shown to be both efficacious and effective in treating the fear and anxiety associated with panic, there remains a subset of individuals who are nonresponders. It is important to understand what factors are associated with nonresponse and how to address such factors clinically.

Comorbidity of psychological disorders, treatment compliance, and safety-seeking behaviors have been discussed as variables that may negatively impact treatment outcome, yet other factors remain virtually unexamined. For instance, there is a paucity of research examining the association between cultural factors and treatment outcome. Furthermore, some research has suggested that African American individuals experience a high comorbidity of panic disorder and isolated sleep paralysis (Bell et al., 1984; Paradis, Friedman, & Hatch, 1997), although little is known about how such comorbidity may impact treatment response. To understand relevant factors, studies must be comprehensive and theoretically driven in choosing pretreatment and follow-up assessment measures. In addition to exploring other factors that might contribute to poor outcome, future research should aim to move beyond identification of factors and explore how such factors affect treatment response. For instance, it remains unclear whether the process of therapy is different for individuals with comorbid diagnoses than for individuals without diagnoses.

REFERENCES

American Psychiatric Association. (1994). *Diagnostic and statistical manual of mental disorders* (4th ed.). Washington, DC: Author.

American Psychiatric Association. (2000). *Diagnostic and statistical manual of mental disorders* (4th ed., text rev.). Washington, DC: Author.

Arntz, A., & van den Hout, M. (1996). Psychological treatments of panic disorder without agoraphobia: Cognitive therapy versus applied relaxation. *Behaviour Research and Therapy, 34,* 113–121.

Barlow, D. H. (2002). *Anxiety and its disorders: The nature and treatment of anxiety and panic* (2nd ed.). New York: Guilford Press.

Barlow, D. H., Brown, T. A., & Craske, M. G. (1994). Definitions of panic attacks and panic disorder in the *DSM–IV*: Implications for research. *Journal of Abnormal Psychology, 103,* 553–564.

Barlow, D. H., Gorman, J. M., Shear, M. K., & Woods, S. W. (2000). Cognitive–behavioral therapy, imipramine, or their combination for panic disorder: A randomized controlled trial. *JAMA, 283,* 2529–2536.

Barlow, D. H., O'Brien, G. T., & Last, C. G. (1984). Couples treatment of agoraphobia. *Behavior Therapy, 15,* 41–58.

Baum, M. (1986). An animal model for agoraphobia using a safety-signal analysis. *Behaviour Research and Therapy, 24,* 87–89.

Beck, J. G., & Zebb, B. J. (1994). Behavioral assessment and treatment of panic disorder: Current status, future directions. *Behavior Therapy, 25,* 581–611.

Bell, C. C., Shakoor, B., Thompson, B., Dew, D., Hughley, E., Mays, R., et al. (1984). Prevalence of isolated sleep paralysis in black subjects. *Journal of the National Medical Association, 76,* 501–508.

Bibb, J. L., & Chambless, D. L. (1986). Alcohol use and abuse among diagnosed agoraphobics. *Behaviour Research and Therapy, 24,* 49–58.

Breslau, N., & Klein, D. F. (1999). Smoking and panic attacks: An epidemiologic investigation. *Archives of General Psychiatry, 56,* 1141–1147.

Brown, T. A., Antony, M. M., & Barlow, D. H. (1995). Diagnostic comorbidity in panic disorder: Effect on treatment outcome and course of comorbid diagnoses following treatment. *Journal of Consulting and Clinical Psychology, 63,* 408–418.

Brown, T. A., & Barlow, D. H. (1992). Comorbidity among anxiety disorders: Implications for treatment and *DSM–IV*. *Journal of Consulting and Clinical Psychology, 60,* 835–840.

Brown, T. A., & Barlow, D. H. (1995). Long-term outcome in cognitive–behavioral treatment of panic disorder: Clinical predictors and alternative strategies for assessment. *Journal of Consulting and Clinical Psychology, 63,* 754–765.

Burns, D. D., & Nolen-Hoeksema, S. (1991). Coping styles, homework assignments and the effectiveness of cognitive behavioral therapy. *Journal of Consulting and Clinical Psychology, 59,* 305–311.

Byrne, D., Carr, A., & Clark, M. (2004). The efficacy of couples-based interventions for panic disorder with agoraphobia. *Journal of Family Therapy, 26,* 105–125.

Carter, M. M., Hollon, S. D., Carson, R., & Shelton, R. C. (1995). Effects of a safe person on induced distress following a biological challenge in panic disorder with agoraphobia. *Journal of Abnormal Psychology, 104,* 156–163.

Cerny, J. A., Barlow, D. H., Craske, M. G., & Himadi, W. G. (1987). Couples treatment of agoraphobia: A two-year follow-up. *Behavior Therapy, 18,* 401–415.

Chambless, D. L., Renneberg, B., Goldstein, A., & Gracely, E. J. (1992). MCMI-diagnosed personality disorders among agoraphobic outpatients: Prevalence and relationship to severity and treatment outcome. *Journal of Anxiety Disorders, 6,* 193–211.

Clark, D. M. (1989). *Anxiety states: Panic and generalized anxiety.* New York: Oxford University Press.

Conoley, C. W., Padula, M. A., Payton, D. S., & Daniels, J. A. (1994). Predictors of client implementation of counselor recommendations: Match with problem, difficulty level, and building on client strengths. *Journal of Counseling Psychology, 41,* 3–7.

Cox, B. J., Norton, G. R., Dorward, J., & Fergusson, P. A. (1989). The relationship between panic attacks and chemical dependencies. *Addictive Behaviors, 14,* 53–60.

Craske, M. G., & Barlow, D. H. (2001). Panic disorder and agoraphobia. In D. H. Barlow (Ed.), *Clinical handbook of psychological disorders: A step-by-step treatment manual* (3rd ed., pp. 1–59). New York: Guilford Press.

Craske, M. G., Brown, T. A., & Barlow, D. H. (1991). Behavioral treatment of panic disorder: A two-year follow-up study. *Behaviour Research and Therapy, 22,* 289–304.

Craske, M. G., Farchione, T. J., Allen, L. B., Barrios, V., Stoyanova M., Rose, R., et al. (2007). Cognitive behavioral therapy for panic disorder and comorbidity: More of the same or less of more? *Behaviour Research and Therapy, 45,* 1095–1109.

Craske, M. G., Golinelli, D., Stein, M. B., Roy-Byrne, P., Bystritsky, A., & Sherbourne, C. (2005). Does the addition of cognitive behavioral therapy improve panic disorder treatment outcome relative to medication alone in the primary-care setting? *Psychological Medicine, 35,* 1645–1654.

Craske, M. G., Lang, A. J., Aikins, D., & Mystkowski, J. (2005). Cognitive behavioral therapy for nocturnal panic. *Behavior Therapy, 36,* 43–54.

Craske, M. G., Roy-Byrne, P., Stein, M. B., Sullivan, G., Hazlett-Stevens, H., Bystritsky, A., et al. (2006). CBT intensity and outcome for panic disorder in a primary care setting. *Behavior Therapy, 37,* 112–119.

Detweiler, J. B., & Whisman, M. A. (1999). The role of homework assignments in cognitive therapy for depression: Potential methods for enhancing adherence. *Clinical Psychological Science, 6,* 267–282.

Dreesen, L., & Arntz, A. (1999). Personality disorders have no excessively negative impact on therapist-rated therapy process in the cognitive and behavioral treatment of Axis I anxiety disorders. *Clinical Psychology and Psychotherapy, 6,* 384–394.

Dreesen, L., Arntz, A., Luttels, C., & Sallaerts, S. (1994). Personality disorders do not influence the results of cognitive behavior therapies for anxiety disorders. *Comprehensive Psychiatry, 35,* 265–274.

Edelman, R. E., & Chambless, D. L. (1993). Compliance during session and homework in exposure-based treatment of agoraphobia. *Behavior Research Therapy, 31,* 767–773.

Galassi, F., Quercioli, S., Charismas, D., Niccolai, V., & Barciulli, E. (2007). Cognitive–behavioral group treatment for panic disorder with agoraphobia. *Journal of Clinical Psychology, 63,* 409–416.

Goisman, R. M., Warshaw, M. G., Peterson, L. G., & Rogers, M. P. (1994). Panic, agoraphobia, and panic disorder with agoraphobia: Data from a multicenter anxiety disorders study. *The Journal of Nervous and Mental Disease, 182,* 72–79.

Gould, R. A., Otto, M. W., & Pollack, M. H. (1995). A meta-analysis of treatment outcome for panic disorder. *Clinical Psychology Review, 15,* 819–844.

Grunhaus, L., Pande, A. C., Brown, M. B., & Greden, J. F. (1994). Clinical characteristics of patients with concurrent major depressive disorder and panic disorder. *The American Journal of Psychiatry, 151,* 541–546.

Hansson, L. (2002). Quality of life in depression and anxiety. *International Review of Psychiatry, 14,* 185–189.

Hoffart, A., & Hedley, L. M. (1997). Personality traits among panic disorder with agoraphobia patients before and after symptom-focused treatment. *Journal of Anxiety Disorders, 6,* 77–87.

Iosifescu, D. V., Nierenberg, A. A., Alpert, J. E., Smith, M., Bitran, S., Dording, C., et al. (2003). The impact of medical comorbidity on acute treatment in major depressive disorder. *The American Journal of Psychiatry, 160,* 2122–2127.

Jacobs, W. J., & LoLordo, V. M. (1977). The sensory basis of avoidance responding in the rat: Relative dominance of auditory or visual warning signals and safety signals. *Learning and Motivation, 8,* 448–466.

Katon, W., Russo, J., Sherbourne, C., Stein, M. B., Craske, M., Fan, M., et al. (2006). Incremental cost-effectiveness of a collaborative care intervention for panic disorder. *Psychological Medicine, 36,* 353–363.

Katschnig, H., & Amering, M. (1998). The long-term course of panic disorder and its predictors. *Journal of Clinical Psychopharmacology, 18*(Suppl. 2), 6S–11S.

Kenardy, J., Robinson, S., & Dob, R. (2005). Cognitive behaviour therapy for panic disorder: Long-term follow-up. *Cognitive Behaviour Therapy, 34,* 75–78.

Kessler, R. C., Berglund, P., Demler, O., Jin, R., & Walters, E. E. (2005). Lifetime prevalence and age-of-onset distributions of DSM–IV disorders in the national comorbidity survey replication. *Archives of General Psychiatry, 62,* 593–602.

Klerman, G. L. (1991). Panic disorder: Strategies for long-term treatment. *Journal of Clinical Psychiatry, 52,* 3–5.

Kushner, M. G., Sher, K. J., & Beitman, B. D. (1990). The relation between alcohol problems and the anxiety disorders. *The American Journal of Psychiatry, 147,* 685–695.

Laberge, B., Gauthier, J., Cote, G., Plamondon, J., & Cormier, H. J. (1992). The treatment of coexisting panic and depression: A review of the literature. *Journal of Anxiety Disorders, 6,* 169–180.

Laberge, B., Gauthier, J. G., Cote, G., Plamondon, J., & Cormier, H. J. (1993). Cognitive behavioral therapy of panic disorder with secondary major depression: A preliminary investigation. *Journal of Consulting and Clinical Psychology, 61,* 1028–1037.

Lehman, C. L., Brown, T. A., & Barlow, D. H. (1998). Effects of cognitive–behavioral treatment for panic disorder with agoraphobia on concurrent alcohol abuse. *Behavior Therapy, 29,* 423–433.

Lochner, C., Mogotsi, M., du Toit, P. L., Kaminer, D., Niehaus, D. J., & Stein, D. J. (2003). Quality of life in anxiety disorders: A comparison of obsessive–compulsive disorder, social anxiety disorder, and panic disorder. *Psychopathology, 36*, 255–262.

Lohr, J. M., Olatunji, B. O., & Sawchuk, C. N. (2007). A functional analysis of danger and safety signals in anxiety disorders. *Clinical Psychology Review, 27*, 114–126.

Löwe, B., Grafe, K., Kroenke, K., Zipfel, S., Quenter, A., Wild, B., et al. (2003). Predictors of psychiatric comorbidity in medical outpatients. *Psychosomatic Medicine, 65*, 764–770.

Maddock, R. J., & Blacker, K. H. (1991). Response to treatment in panic disorder with associated depression. *Psychopathology, 24*, 1–6.

Marchand, A., Goyer, L. R., Dupuis, G., & Mainguy, N. (1998). Personality disorders and the outcome of cognitive–behavioural treatment of panic disorder with agoraphobia. *Canadian Journal of Behavioural Science, 30*, 14–23.

Marchesi, C., Cantoni, A., Fontò, S., Giannelli, M. R., & Maggini, C. (2005). The effect of pharmacotherapy on personality disorders in panic disorder: A one-year naturalistic study. *Journal of Affective Disorders, 89*, 189–194.

Margraf, J., Barlow, D. H., Clark, D. M., & Telch, M. J. (1993). Psychological treatment of panic: Work in progress on outcome, active ingredients, and follow-up. *Behaviour Research and Therapy, 31*, 1–8.

Marks, I. M. (1987). Behavioral aspects of panic disorder. *The American Journal of Psychiatry, 144*, 1160–1165.

Marshall, J. R. (1997). Alcohol and substance abuse in panic disorder. *Journal of Clinical Psychiatry, 58*, 46–50.

Mavissakalian, M., & Hamann, M. S. (1986). *DSM–III* personality disorder in agoraphobia. *Comprehensive Psychiatry, 27*, 471–479.

Mavissakalian, M., & Michelson, L. (1983). Self-directed in vivo exposure practice in behavioral and pharmacological treatments of agoraphobia. *Behavior Therapy, 14*, 506–519.

McLean, P. D., Woody, S., Taylor, S., & Koch, W. J. (1998). Comorbid panic disorder and major depression: Implications for cognitive–behavioral therapy. *Journal of Consulting and Clinical Psychology, 66*, 240–247.

Mennin, D. S., & Heimberg, R. G. (2000). The impact of comorbid mood and personality disorders in the cognitive–behavioral treatment of panic disorder. *Clinical Psychology Review, 20*, 339–357.

Michelson, L., Mavissakalian, M., Marchione, K., Dancu, C., & Greenwald, M. (1986). The role of self-directed in vivo exposure in cognitive, behavioral, and psychophysiological treatments of agoraphobia. *Behavior Therapy, 17*, 91–108.

Norton, G. R., Cox, B. J., & Schwartz, M. A. (1992). Critical analysis of the *DSM–III–R* classification of panic disorder: A survey of current opinions. *Journal of Anxiety Disorders, 6*, 159–167.

Noyes, R., Reich, J. H., Suelzer, M., & Christiansen, J. (1991). Personality traits associated with panic disorder: Change associated with treatment. *Comprehensive Psychiatry, 32*, 283–294.

Oatley, K., & Hodgson, D. (1987). Influence of husbands on the outcome of their agoraphobic wives' therapy. *The British Journal of Psychiatry, 150,* 380–386.

O'Rourke, D., Fahy, T. J., Brophy, J., & Prescott, P. (1996). The Galway study of panic disorder III: Outcome at 5 to 6 years. *The British Journal of Psychiatry, 168,* 462–469.

Oslin, D. W., Datto, C. J., Kallan, M. J., Katz, I. R., Edell, W. S., & TenHave, T. (2002). Association between medical comorbidity and treatment outcomes in late-life depression. *Journal of American Geriatric Society, 50,* 823–828.

Öst, L., & Westling, B. E. (1995). Applied relaxation vs. cognitive behavior therapy in the treatment of panic disorder. *Behaviour Research and Therapy, 33,* 145–158.

Öst, L., Westling, B. E., & Hellström, K. (1993). Applied relaxation, exposure in vivo and cognitive methods in the treatment of panic disorder with agoraphobia. *Behaviour Research and Therapy, 31,* 383–394.

Otto, M. W., Smits, J. A. J., & Reese, H. E. (2004). Cognitive–behavioral therapy for the treatment of anxiety disorders. *Journal of Clinical Psychiatry, 65*(Suppl. 5), 34–41.

Paradis, C. M., Friedman, S., & Hatch, M. (1997). Isolated sleep paralysis in African Americans with panic disorder. *Cultural Diversity and Mental Health, 3,* 69–76.

Penava, S. J., Otto, M. W., Maki, K. M., & Pollack, M. H. (1998). Rate of improvement during cognitive–behavioral group treatment for panic disorder. *Behaviour Research and Therapy, 36,* 665–673.

Powers, M. B., Smits, J. A. J., & Telch, M. J. (2004). Disentangling the effects of safety behavior utilization and safety-behavior availability during exposure based treatments: A placebo-controlled trial. *Journal of Consulting and Clinical Psychology, 72,* 448–454.

Rachman, S. (1983). The modification of agoraphobic behaviour: Fresh possibilities. *Behaviour Research and Therapy, 21,* 567–574.

Rachman, S. (1984). Agoraphobia: A safety-signal perspective. *Behaviour Research and Therapy, 22,* 59–70.

Rachman, S. (1993). A critique of cognitive therapy for anxiety disorders. *Journal of Behavior Therapy and Experimental Psychiatry, 24,* 279–288.

Reif, W., Trenkamp, S., Auer, C., & Fichter, M. M. (2000). Cognitive behavior therapy in panic disorder and comorbid major depression. *Psychotherapy and Psychosomatics, 69,* 70–78.

Roy-Byrne, P., & Cowley, D. S. (1995). Course and outcome of panic disorder: A review of recent follow-up studies. *Anxiety, 1,* 151–160.

Roy-Byrne, P., Russo, J., Cowley, D. S., & Katon, W. J. (2003). Unemployment and emergency room visits predict prior treatment outcome in primary care panic disorder. *Journal of Clinical Psychiatry, 64,* 383–389.

Roy-Byrne, P., Stein, M. B., Russo, J., Craske, M., Katon, W., Sullivan, G., et al. (2005). Medical illness and response to treatment in primary care panic disorder. *General Hospital Psychiatry, 27,* 237–243.

Salkovskis, P. M. (1991). The importance of behaviour in the maintenance of anxiety and panic: A cognitive account. *Behavioural Psychotherapy, 19*, 6–19.

Salkovskis, P. M., Clark, D. M., & Gelder, M. G. (1996). Cognition–behaviour links in the persistence of panic. *Behaviour Research and Therapy, 34*, 453–458.

Salkovskis, P. M., Clark, D. M., Hackmann, A., Wells, A., & Gelder, M. G. (1999). An experimental investigation of the role of safety-seeking behaviours in the maintenance of panic disorder with agoraphobia. *Behaviour Research and Therapy, 27*, 559–574.

Sanderson, W. C., DiNardo, P. A., Rapee, R. M., & Barlow, D. H. (1990). Syndrome comorbidity in patients diagnosed with a *DSM–III–R* anxiety disorder. *Journal of Abnormal Psychology, 99*, 308–312.

Schmidt, N. B., & Woolaway-Bickle, K. (2000). The effects of treatment compliance on outcome in cognitive–behavioral therapy for panic disorder: Quality versus quantity. *Journal of Consulting and Clinical Psychology, 68*, 13–18.

Siegel, L., Jones, W. C., & Wilson, J. O. (1990). Economic and life consequences experienced by a group of individuals with panic disorder. *Journal of Anxiety Disorders, 4*, 201–211.

Stanley, M. A., Beck, J. G., Averill, P. M., Baldwin, L. E., Deagle, E. A., & Stadler, J. G. (1996). Patterns of change during cognitive behavioral treatment for panic disorder. *The Journal of Nervous and Mental Disease, 184*, 567–572.

Steketee, G., & Shapiro, L. J. (1995). Predicting behavioral treatment outcome for agoraphobia and obsessive compulsive disorder. *Clinical Psychology Review, 15*, 317–346.

Stuart, G. L., Treat, T. A., & Wade, W. A. (2000). Effectiveness of an empirically based treatment for panic disorder delivered in a service clinic setting: 1-year follow-up. *Journal of Consulting and Clinical Psychology, 68*, 506–512.

Telch, M. J. (1988). *Combined pharmacological and psychological treatments for panic sufferers.* Hillsdale, NJ: Erlbaum.

Thyer, B. A. (1986). Alcohol abuse among clinically anxious patients. *Behaviour Research and Therapy, 24*, 357–359.

Tsao, J. C. I., Lewin, M. R., & Craske, M. G. (1998). The effects of cognitive–behavior therapy for panic disorder on comorbid conditions. *Journal of Anxiety Disorders, 12*, 357–371.

Tsao, J. C. I., Mystkowski, J. L., Zucker, B. G., & Craske, M. G. (2002). Effects of cognitive–behavioral therapy for panic disorder on comorbid conditions: Replication and extension. *Behavior Therapy, 33*, 493–509.

Tsao, J. C. I., Mystkowski, J. L., Zucker, B. G., & Craske, M. G. (2005). Impact of cognitive–behavioral therapy for panic disorder on comorbidity: A controlled investigation. *Behaviour Research and Therapy, 43*, 958–970.

Wade, W. A., Treat, T. A., & Stuart, G. L. (1998). Transporting an empirically supported treatment for panic disorder to a service clinic setting: A benchmarking strategy. *Journal of Consulting and Clinical Psychology, 66*, 231–239.

Wittchen, H., Reed, V., & Kessler, R. C. (1998). The relationship of agoraphobia and panic in a community sample of adolescents and young adults. *Archives of General Psychiatry, 55,* 1017–1024.

Woody, S., & Rachman, S. (1994). Generalized anxiety disorder (GAD) as an unsuccessful search for safety. *Clinical Psychology Review, 14,* 743–753.

4

SOCIAL ANXIETY DISORDER

ANNA ROSENBERG, DEBORAH ROTH LEDLEY,
AND RICHARD G. HEIMBERG

Social anxiety disorder (also known as *social phobia*) is a highly prevalent and impairing disorder characterized by "a marked or persistent fear of social or performance situations" (American Psychiatric Association, 1994, p. 411). Such situations span the range from the near-ubiquitous fear of public speaking to initiating and maintaining conversations, performing activities in front of other people (e.g., writing, eating, drinking), speaking with authority figures, or making requests of others (e.g., asking others to change their behavior, asking for a raise at work; Holt, Heimberg, Hope, & Liebowitz, 1992). The core fear of individuals with social anxiety disorder is that they will do or say something in these situations that will elicit negative evaluation from others.

Individuals with social anxiety disorder typically experience substantial physiological arousal (e.g., blushing, shaking, sweating), often reporting panic attacks in social situations (Jack, Heimberg, & Mennin, 1999). They also worry that these symptoms will be visible to others and lead these other persons to assume that they are extremely anxious to the exclusion of more benign interpretations (Roth, Antony, & Swinson, 2001). This preference for unfavorable explanations represents a general pattern of negative, catastrophic thinking. In addition, individuals with social anxiety are more likely to notice negative social cues and dismiss positive ones in social situations (Veljaca & Rapee, 1998). Their behavior reflects various degrees of avoidance of social situations, including subtle avoidance, such as going to a party but only talking to familiar persons. They may also engage in safety behaviors, such as wearing makeup to hide blushing or holding on to a podium to prevent their hands from trembling (Wells et al., 1995).

Individuals with social anxiety disorder who fear numerous social and performance situations are referred to as having the *generalized* type of social anxiety disorder, whereas persons with more limited fears (e.g., only public speaking) are said to have *nongeneralized* social anxiety disorder. Generalized social anxiety disorder is associated with more severe social anxiety symptoms and greater impairment than nongeneralized social anxiety disorder (Heimberg, Holt, Schneier, Spitzer, & Liebowitz, 1993).

Recent epidemiological data from the National Comorbidity Survey Replication (NCS-R; Kessler, Berglund, et al., 2005) show that anxiety disorders are the most prevalent class of psychiatric disorders, with 31.2% of the population meeting criteria for at least one anxiety disorder at some time in their lives and 18.7% of the population meeting criteria for at least one anxiety disorder in the previous year. Social anxiety disorder is the most prevalent anxiety disorder, with 12.1% meeting criteria for the disorder at some time in their lives and 6.8% meeting criteria in the past year (Kessler, Berglund, et al., 2005; Kessler, Chiu, Demler, Merikangas, & Walters, 2005).

Social anxiety disorder is associated with a high degree of Axis I comorbidity. In the original NCS, 81% of individuals with social anxiety disorder met criteria for at least one other psychiatric disorder (Magee, Eaton, Wittchen, McGonagle, & Kessler, 1996), most typically another anxiety disorder. In fact, 56.9% of individuals with social anxiety disorder met criteria for at least one other anxiety disorder. In the NCS-R, the occurrence of social anxiety disorder was significantly related to the occurrence of panic disorder, agoraphobia, specific phobia, posttraumatic stress disorder, and separation anxiety disorder (Kessler, Chiu, et al., 2005).

Anxiety disorders have an earlier age of onset than many other psychiatric disorders (Kessler, Berglund, et al., 2005). The median age of onset for social anxiety disorder is 13, and disorders commonly comorbid with it tend to have a later age of onset (e.g., age 20 for substance use, age 30 for mood disorders). Social anxiety disorder may be a risk factor for the later development of other disorders (Magee et al., 1996; Schneier, Johnson, Hornig, Liebowitz, & Weissman, 1992).

Data from epidemiological studies have suggested that social anxiety disorder is more common in women than in men (Magee et al., 1996), but in clinical samples, men slightly outnumber women (Chapman, Mannuzza, & Fyer, 1995; Stein, 1997). It has been postulated that it is more costly for men than for women to go untreated because men are typically expected to be more outgoing and assertive in both their personal and professional lives (Weinstock, 1999).

It is not surprising that individuals with social anxiety disorder experience impairment across numerous domains. Compared with individuals without the disorder, individuals with social anxiety disorder have lower levels of educational attainment, lower income, and higher rates of unemployment (Magee et al., 1996). Clinicians who work with this population often notice that their patients are grossly underemployed given their intelligence and abilities. As an example, a patient with severe social anxiety disorder whom we treated worked as a paralegal rather than attending law school despite having credentials that would have garnered him entrance to the top law schools in the country. The patient avoided applying because he greatly feared being called on in class and could not imagine doing trial work when he eventually graduated. It is also not surprising that social anxiety disorder is associated with impairments in the social realm. Individuals with the disorder are less likely to be married than people without the disorder (Schneier et al., 1992) and to suffer impairment in both their romantic relationships and their friendships (Schneier et al., 1994; Whisman, Sheldon, & Goernig, 2000).

DESCRIPTION OF EFFECTIVE TREATMENTS FOR SOCIAL ANXIETY DISORDER

Psychotherapy

The most commonly studied psychotherapy for social anxiety disorder is cognitive–behavioral therapy (CBT). CBT protocols for social anxiety typically include psychoeducation, imaginal and in vivo exposure to feared social situations, and cognitive restructuring (CR). In the sections that follow, we describe these techniques, as well as two other variants of CBT: social skills training (SST), and progressive muscle relaxation and applied relaxation.

Psychoeducation

CBT for social anxiety disorder usually includes two to four sessions devoted to psychoeducation. The purpose of these sessions is twofold. It allows the therapist to educate the patient about social anxiety disorder, including its etiology, maintenance, and presentation, and to introduce the cognitive–behavioral model. Additionally, these sessions offer time for the therapist and patient to establish rapport, creating a foundation for collaborative work before diving into next steps of treatment, which can be challenging and anxiety-provoking for patients. During psychoeducation sessions, therapists typically share numerous vignettes describing individuals with social anxiety disorder, providing patients with the opportunity to compare and contrast their own experiences with those of others.

Exposure

Exposure treatment consists of imagined (*imaginal exposure*) or actual (*in vivo exposure*) confrontation of social and/or performance situations that the patient fears and/or avoids. Prior to beginning exposure treatment, the therapist works with the patient to create a hierarchy of feared situations, rank ordered from least to most anxiety provoking. This hierarchy then serves as a road map for the treatment, beginning with less anxiety-provoking situations and progressing to the higher rated items. Often, exposure to a feared situation first occurs during a treatment session. The patient then completes a similar in vivo exposure for homework to facilitate generalization to the "real world." There has been limited research regarding imaginal exposure for social anxiety disorder, but there is consistent support for the efficacy of in vivo exposure (Al-Kubaisy et al., 1992; Newman, Hofmann, Trabert, Roth, & Taylor, 1994; Turner, Beidel, & Jacob, 1994).

Exposure-based treatments were originally developed on the basis of traditional notions of the processes of habituation and extinction. However, recent research in animal experimental psychology has suggested that these processes do not produce unlearning or relearning in the classical sense but rather appear to produce new learning that competes, more or less successfully, with the old (Bouton, 2002). Important theoretical work (Foa & Kozak, 1986) has suggested that anxiety reduction is best achieved when the fear system is fully engaged (as indexed by increased physiological arousal) and in the presence of disconfirmatory information. To maximize the effectiveness of exposure interventions, all relevant safety behaviors should be identified in advance and prevented (Wells et al., 1995), and patients should be instructed to maintain attention on the situation (Wells & Papageorgiou, 1998).

Cognitive Restructuring

CR refers to the identification of automatic thoughts, recognizing the thinking errors in them, and challenging automatic thoughts with potential alternatives. The goal of CR is for the patient to view the world in a less biased way and to be less likely to reflexively expect negative outcomes. As an example, an individual with social anxiety disorder might notice that the women at the table adjacent to him in a coffee shop are laughing. He might assume that the women are laughing at him, perhaps because he is having coffee alone. He might immediately have the thought, "They think I am a loser" or "They think I have no friends." CR involves helping the patient to recognize that there are errors in his thinking and to consider alternative interpretations (e.g., "They are laughing at a joke that one woman told to the other").

Combined Cognitive Restructuring and Exposure

As we noted earlier, most treatment protocols for social anxiety disorder combine CR and exposure. In the sections that follow, we review two examples of such treatments. Heimberg and Becker's (2002) cognitive–behavioral group therapy (CBGT), along with its more recent adaptation to individual treatment (Hope, Heimberg, Juster, & Turk, 2000; Hope, Heimberg, & Turk, 2006), is the most researched protocol for social anxiety disorder. We also review Clark's (2001) cognitive therapy (CT), another CBT that has garnered impressive results.

Heimberg's Cognitive–Behavioral Group Therapy and Individual Cognitive–Behavioral Therapy. Heimberg's CBGT typically consists of a group of five to six patients and two therapists (Heimberg & Becker, 2002). The protocol is usually carried out in 12 weekly sessions, each lasting 2.5 hours. Over the first two sessions, patients are educated about the nature of social anxiety according to the cognitive–behavioral model (Rapee & Heimberg, 1997). Next, patients learn and practice CR techniques. Therapists work with patients to create a fear and avoidance hierarchy on which each patient lists his or her feared situations in ascending order. Target situations, from easiest to hardest, are initially tackled though in-session exposures. The exposures are structured and include pre- and postexposure CR. This structure ensures that patients have an opportunity to gather unbiased information to challenge their faulty beliefs about themselves and others in social situations. There are many other benefits to conducting exposures in a group setting, including practicing social interactions in a safe environment, getting feedback from group members, and learning from other patients' experiences. Patients complete in vivo exposures between sessions. CBGT has consistently been found to be efficacious when compared with a control psychotherapy (educational supportive group therapy) and pill placebo (Heimberg et al., 1990; Heimberg et al., 1998; Liebowitz et al., 1999) and has recently been shown to be more efficacious than meditation-based stress reduction (Koszycki, Benger, Shlik, & Bradwejn, 2007).

Heimberg and colleagues have adapted CBGT to an individual format (Hope et al., 2000, 2006). Although there are many advantages to group therapy, it is not always feasible in general practice. Furthermore, some patients with social anxiety disorder are reluctant to engage in group treatment. For these reasons, having an effective individual treatment available is of the utmost importance. Heimberg's individual CBT involves 16 one-hour weekly sessions conducted over 16 to 20 weeks. Individual therapy comprises the same components as CBGT, including psychoeducation, CR, and in-session and in vivo exposure. Ledley et al. (in press) demonstrated that this individualized CBT is as efficacious as the group package.

Clark's Cognitive Therapy. Clark's CT is based on the premise that safety behaviors and self-focused attention maintain social anxiety (D. M. Clark, 2001). *Safety behaviors* are actions meant to mask the outwardly visible signs of anxiety (e.g., blushing) or to otherwise protect the person from threat of social humiliation or embarrassment. The problem is that safety behaviors can "backfire" because they are often more noticeable and unusual than the anxiety symptoms they are meant to mask (e.g., wearing very heavy makeup or a turtleneck in the heat of summer to hide blushing). Furthermore, safety behaviors heighten self-focused attention, increasing the likelihood that patients will miss out on important social cues.

In Clark's CT, the therapist works with the patient to construct a unique model of social anxiety specifying the way self-focused attention and safety behaviors maintain social anxiety. The focus of therapy involves dropping safety behaviors and shifting one's attention from an internal focus on the self onto external stimuli in the social world. Patients engage in "behavioral experiments" to test their biased views. This treatment has also shown substantial efficacy (D. M. Clark et al., 2003, 2006).

Social Skills Training

SST is based on the assertion that individuals with social anxiety disorder lack adequate social skills. Their anxiety results from the negative responses of others that result, in turn, from their poor skills. In SST, the therapist first models appropriate behavior, such as eye contact. Then, the patient practices the skills in "behavior rehearsals," receiving corrective feedback and social reinforcement along the way. Afterward, the patient practices newly learned behavior in his or her daily life. In the past, SST has been used as a treatment for social anxiety disorder on its own, but there is little empirical support for doing so (Ponniah & Hollon, 2007). For some time, however, it has been included as a component of broader treatment packages that include CR and/or exposure (e.g., Davidson et al., 2004; Turner, Beidel, Cooley-Quille, Woody, & Messer, 1994). Limited evidence has suggested that SST may be a helpful addition to CBGT for at least some patients (Herbert et al., 2005).

Progressive Muscle Relaxation and Applied Relaxation

The goal of relaxation training is to reduce the physiological arousal that is a common aspect of the anxiety response. *Progressive muscle relaxation* involves alternating tightening and releasing each muscle group. On its own, progressive muscle relaxation has been shown to have minimal effects (e.g., Alström, Norlund, Persson, Hårding, & Ljungqvist, 1984) and has been used as a control condition in studies of other treatments of social anxiety disorder (e.g., Al-Kubaisy et al., 1992). However, *applied relaxation*, which combines gradual exposure to feared situations with progressive muscle relaxation (Öst, 1987), may be useful in the treatment of social anxiety disorder. Individuals are instructed to recognize physiological symptoms associated with anxiety. Progressive muscle relaxation is then applied to nonanxiety-provoking situations and through graduated exposure to anxiety-provoking situations at the first sign of physiological arousal. Applied relaxation has been studied as a treatment for social anxiety disorder, with data suggesting that it is efficacious as a primary treatment and when combined with other CBT techniques (e.g., Bögels, 2006; D. M. Clark et al., 2006). No study has compared applied relaxation with exposure alone to determine whether the inclusion of relaxation enhances treatment efficacy.

Pharmacotherapy

Medications are also frequently used to treat social anxiety disorder. Selective serotonin reuptake inhibitors (SSRIs), such as paroxetine, sertraline, fluvoxamine, fluoxetine, citalopram, and escitalopram, and the serotonin–norepinephrine reuptake inhibitor (SNRI) venlafaxine are considered the first-line pharmacological treatments for social anxiety disorder (Blackmore, Erwin, Heimberg, Magee, & Fresco, in press; Blanco et al., 2003; Ledley & Heimberg, 2005). These medications have demonstrated efficacy in placebo-controlled trials and have more favorable side-effects profiles than other available medications for social anxiety disorder. Fluoxetine is the only SSRI that has had mixed results in controlled trials, with two studies failing to find a difference between fluoxetine and placebo (D. M. Clark et al., 2003; Kobak, Greist, Jefferson, & Katzelnick, 2002) and one study finding fluoxetine to be superior to placebo (Davidson et al., 2004).

Monoamine oxidase inhibitors (MAOIs) are another class of drugs that has been used in the treatment of social anxiety disorder. MAOIs, such as phenelzine sulfate, have been found to be efficacious (Blanco et al., 2003). However, the dietary restrictions necessary to protect against serious medical side effects (i.e., rapidly escalating blood pressure and related effects when one ingests food, beverages, or medications containing the amino acid tyramine) have made the traditional MAOIs a less preferred treatment choice since the appearance of the SSRIs. A subset of MAOIs, the reversible MAOIs (e.g., brofaramine, moclobemide), do not have the serious side effects and dietary restrictions of the traditional MAOIs. However, the efficacy of moclobemide has been questioned (Noyes et al., 1997; Oosterbaan, van Balkom, Spinhoven, van Oppen, & van Dyck, 2001; Schneier et al., 1998; cf. Versiani et al., 1992), and brofaromine is no longer in worldwide production.

Benzodiazepines, such as clonazepam and alprazolam, are another class of drugs frequently used in the treatment of anxiety disorders. Results are mixed for this drug class, with several studies finding clonazepam to be efficacious in the treatment of social anxiety disorder (Davidson et al., 1993; Otto et al., 2000) and one study finding no difference between alprazolam and placebo (Gelernter et al., 1991). The use of benzodiazepines has several other drawbacks, including their potential lack of efficacy for comorbid mood disorders and potential rebound of anxiety after withdrawal. Benzodiazepines also have the potential of abuse and are thus not recommended for individuals with substance abuse histories.

Other medications used in the treatment of social anxiety disorder include the anticonvulsants gabapentin and pregabalin, the asipirone buspirone, and beta-adrenergic blockers such as atenolol. Gabapentin and buspirone seem to only be efficacious at larger doses (Pande et al., 1999; Schneier et al., 1993). Beta-adrenergic blockers may only be efficacious on an as-needed basis for performance anxiety, like one might experience when playing a musical instrument in front of an audience (Turner, Beidel, & Jacob, 1994).

Few studies have directly compared medications with each other, and those that have done so have not been conclusive. One study comparing escitalopram at different dosages with paroxetine and placebo found no differences between the active treatments at Week 12, but at Week 24 the highest dose of escitalopram (20 mg) was superior to paroxetine (20 mg) on some measures of social anxiety (Lader, Stender, Burger, & Nil, 2004). Another study found venlafaxine and paroxetine to both be superior to placebo but not different from each other (Liebowitz, Gelenberg, & Munjack, 2005). Further research on the comparative efficacy of medications for social anxiety disorder would be helpful.

COMPARISON AND COMBINATION OF COGNITIVE–BEHAVIORAL THERAPY AND MEDICATION

A limited number of studies have examined the differential efficacy of CBT and medication. Three of these studies found CBT to be more effective than medications; however, the medications used in two of these studies, buspirone and atenolol, have not been shown to be superior to placebo (D. B. Clark & Agras, 1991; D. M. Clark et al., 2003; Turner, Beidel, & Jacob, 1994). The third study used fluoxetine, which, as noted earlier, has mixed evidence for its efficacy in social anxiety disorder. Another study found little difference between CBGT and the benzodiazepine clonazepam (Otto et al., 2000). Heimberg et al. (1998) examined the differential efficacy of CBGT and the MAOI phenelzine, a medication considered by some to be the best established pharmacological treatment for social anxiety (Blanco et al., 2003). The large multisite study compared the two active treatments with each other and with two placebo control conditions, a pill placebo, and an educational supportive group treatment. At the end of 12 weeks, CBGT and phenelzine were both superior to the control conditions but did not differ from each other. Patients receiving phenelzine made quicker gains, whereas patients in the CBGT group were more likely to retain gains at follow-up (Liebowitz et al., 1999).

Studies of the combination of CBT and medication have yielded mixed results. Falloon, Lloyd, and Harpin (1981) did not find additive effects when administering the beta-adrenergic blocker propranolol to patients receiving SST. Heimberg (2003) found the combination of CBGT and phenelzine to be superior to placebo but not consistently superior to phenelzine alone. Davidson et al. (2004) found no differences among group CBT, fluoxetine, and combined treatment. Another study examining sertraline, exposure, and combined treatment found all active treatments to be superior to placebo after 12 weeks (Blomhoff et al., 2001). At 24 weeks, active treatments did not differ from each other, but only sertraline (alone or in combination with exposure) was superior to placebo. However, at 1-year follow-up, only patients who received exposure continued to improve, whereas patients receiving sertraline alone or combined treatment showed a degree of deterioration (Haug et al., 2003). Future studies should examine whether different approaches to combining CBT and medication yield differential outcomes. In all of these studies, CBT and medication were administered concurrently. It is possible that combined treatments more consistently yield superior results when CBT and medication are administered sequentially instead of concurrently. Our group has recently completed such a study in which all patients receive 12 weeks of paroxetine, followed by random assignment of medication responders to continued medication alone or continued medication plus CBT.

META-ANALYSES

A number of meta-analyses have examined the efficacy of CBT for social anxiety disorder. In the meta-analysis by Feske and Chambless (1995), the within-group effect sizes for exposure versus CR plus exposure were similar at posttreatment and follow-up. The controlled (i.e., in comparison with a control condition) effect size for exposure was significantly greater than the controlled effect size for CR plus exposure, although this finding was not replicated in the other meta-analyses reported in this section. A greater number of sessions of exposure was associated with better outcome.

Taylor (1996) examined the efficacy of various CBTs, including exposure, CR, CR plus exposure, SST, as well as placebo (including pill placebo and attention placebo) and wait-list control conditions. All active treatments had similar effect sizes, significantly larger than wait-list controls, but only the combination of CR plus exposure had a significantly larger effect size than placebo controls. There were no differences among the active treatments in effect size at follow-up and no differences between group and individual treatment.

Gould, Buckminster, Pollack, Otto, and Yap (1997) conducted a meta-analysis of CBT and pharmacotherapy. They found no differences in outcome between CBT, pharmacotherapy, and combined treatment for social anxiety disorder, nor did they find any differences in attrition. Gains resulting from CBT were maintained during follow-up, but there were so few follow-up evaluations of medication treatments that the differential long-term efficacy of CBT versus medication could not be well evaluated. Studies of exposure alone, CR plus exposure, and SSRIs had large effect sizes, whereas studies of CR alone, SST alone, MAOIs, and benzodiazepines had moderate effect sizes. Beta blockers and buspirone were less effective than placebo. A limitation of their conclusions is that only one to three studies were available for each drug class other than the MAOIs ($n = 5$). Like Taylor (1996), Gould et al. (1997) found no differences between group and individual treatment.

Fedoroff and Taylor (2001) examined benzodiazepines, SSRIs, MAOIs, exposure, CR, CR plus exposure, SST, applied relaxation, wait-list control, pill placebo, and attention placebo. Benzodiazepines and SSRIs were superior to the three control treatments and applied relaxation when self-report measures were examined. Also for self-report measures, benzodiazepines were superior to MAOIs, CR, CR plus exposure, and SST. CR plus exposure was superior to applied relaxation and to attention placebo and wait-list controls. There were no other differences among the psychological treatments.

FACTORS THAT LEAD TO POOR TREATMENT RESPONSE

Several factors may be related to poor treatment response. These involve the diagnostic aspects of clinical presentation, including subtype of social anxiety disorder and comorbidity with other disorders. Other variations in presentation, such as overvalued ideation, anger, trauma history, and the significance of a socially traumatic event in the maintenance of the disorder, may also influence treatment response but have been less widely researched. Treatment expectancy, homework compliance, and ambivalence regarding change are other factors that have been identified as related to poor treatment response.

Diagnostic Aspects of Clinical Presentation

Individuals with generalized social anxiety disorder are less likely to reach high end-state functioning with treatment than individuals with nongeneralized social anxiety disorder. This is likely because patients with generalized social anxiety begin treatment with more severe symptoms than patients with nongeneralized social anxiety disorder. Although both groups make similar gains during treatment, differences in pretreatment severity account for more residual symptoms posttreatment. Elsewhere, we have suggested that longer or more intense treatment of individuals with generalized social anxiety disorder can result in end-state functioning comparable with that observed after treatment in individuals with nongeneralized social anxiety disorder (see Brown, Heimberg, & Juster, 1995).

The presence of avoidant personality disorder (APD) has been identified as another moderator of treatment response. About 60% of individuals with generalized social anxiety disorder are diagnosed with APD. Some studies have found treatment to be less effective for individuals with comorbid APD (e.g., Chambless, Tran, & Glass, 1997; Feske, Perry, Chambless, Renneberg, & Goldstein, 1996), whereas others have not found the presence of APD to affect treatment outcome (e.g., Brown et al., 1995; Hope, Herbert, & White, 1995). Some researchers consider APD to be a more severe variant of social anxiety disorder (Heimberg, 1996) and have noted that it remits with standard treatment for social anxiety disorder. For example, Brown et al. (1995) found that 47% of patients with social anxiety disorder and comorbid APD no longer met criteria for APD after CBT for social anxiety disorder.

Depression has also been identified as a risk factor for poor treatment response. Chambless et al. (1997) found pretreatment depression to be a robust predictor of treatment outcome. In their study, individuals with higher levels of pretreatment depression made fewer gains than those with lower levels of depression. Similarly, Ledley et al. (2005) reported that in the Davidson et al. (2004) trial comparing fluoxetine, CBT, and their combination, patients with higher levels of pretreatment depression demonstrated higher levels of social anxiety before treatment, changed less over the course of treatment, were more likely to be classified as nonresponders, and were more likely to drop out of treatment, regardless of treatment condition, than patients who were less depressed. However, when Erwin, Heimberg, Juster, and Mindlin (2002) examined comorbid depressive disorder as a moderator of treatment outcome, they found that patients with social anxiety disorder and comorbid depression made gains similar to those made by patients with social anxiety disorder alone or with only comorbid anxiety disorders. Nevertheless, individuals with greater pretreatment depression finished treatment with greater residual social anxiety posttreatment. Of note, they were no longer more depressed than patients without comorbid depression before treatment.

Comorbid substance abuse has recently been identified as a factor that may complicate the treatment of social anxiety disorder. Alcohol use disorders and social anxiety disorder co-occur at a particularly high rate, with nearly half of individuals with a lifetime diagnosis of social anxiety disorder meeting criteria for a lifetime diagnosis of an alcohol use disorder (Grant et al., 2005). In addition, socially anxious patients with a lifetime history of an alcohol use disorder are more likely to have greater symptoms of social anxiety and greater impairment in interpersonal functioning (Schneier, Martin, Liebowitz, Gorman, & Fyer, 1989). A recent case study examined supplementing CBT for social anxiety disorder with motivation enhancement therapy for the alcohol use disorder (Buckner, Ledley, Heimberg, & Schmidt, 2008). Motivation enhancement therapy is a four-session intervention that combines motivational interviewing with feedback regarding the patient's drinking behavior. The results of the case study indicated significant improvement in both social anxiety disorder and the alcohol use disorder.

Other Variations in Presentation

Overvalued ideation, or an inability to adopt an alternative perspective, has been shown to be predictive of poor outcome in the treatment of anxiety disorders, most notably obsessive–compulsive disorder (see Veale, 2007). Although overvalued ideation has not been examined specifically in patients with social anxiety disorder, our clinical experience has suggested that it can be problematic here too. Such rigidity may make it more difficult for a patient to accept and commit to therapy. Additionally, the practice of in-session exposures may be less effective if a patient is unable or unwilling to suspend disbelief and role-play through the exposure.

In one study, we examined how patient anger affected treatment outcome. Individuals who experienced anger more frequently, were more quick tempered, and were more likely to perceive unfair treatment by others were less likely to stay in treatment for the full 12-session course of CBGT (Erwin, Heimberg, Schneier, & Liebowitz, 2003). Among those who completed treatment, patients who experienced more extreme anger and who were more likely to inhibit their anger made less treatment gains than less angry patients.

Several studies have indicated that a history of childhood abuse may influence and complicate the presentation of an anxiety disorder. For example, panic disorder patients with histories of childhood trauma have an earlier onset of the disorder (Kipper et al., 2007) and are more likely to have comorbid depression and a history of suicide attempts (Friedman et al., 2002). Research examining differentiation in presentation and response to treatment among social anxiety disorder patients with histories of trauma is currently unavailable, but our clinical experience has suggested a more complicated presentation for patients with a history of childhood trauma.

Preliminary research has suggested that some individuals with social anxiety disorder may have posttraumatic stress disorder (PTSD)–like reactions to socially traumatic events to which they attribute the onset or exacerbation of their social anxiety. Erwin, Heimberg, Marx, and Franklin (2006) found that over 95% of their sample of patients with social anxiety disorder reported experiencing such an event, and 78% of this group found these experiences significant enough to have at least some reexperiencing, avoidance, or hyperarousal symptoms associated with the event for more than 3 months. These results suggest that it would be fruitful to examine the efficacy of prolonged exposure to these socially traumatic experiences as part of the treatment of a substantial number of socially anxious patients.

A preliminary study recently examined another technique to directly address memories of unpleasant social experiences among patients with social anxiety (Wild, Hackmann, & Clark, 2008). In one session lasting approximately 1.5 hours, patients were instructed in CR and a process called memory rescripting. During memory rescripting, patients imagined the event at the age it had occurred, then imagined it at their current age watching their younger self and intervening if they wished, and finally imagined it as their younger self with the adult self in the room, intervening as before. In the control condition, a therapist encouraged the patient to talk about the early memory and the image associated with it, providing supportive listening and reflection without challenging the patient. Individuals who received the rescripting session were less likely to fully believe the encapsulated belief represented in the memory, were less distressed by the memory, and gave lower anxiety ratings when visualizing feared social situations than control participants.

Motivation, Treatment Expectancy, and Homework Compliance

Patients often have mixed reactions to treatment. Ambivalence regarding change and poor motivation are additional factors that can lead to poor treatment response across a variety of disorders. Motivation for change has been found to be a predictor of outcome in the treatment of generalized anxiety disorder (Dugas et al., 2003). The impact of motivation for change on treatment outcome is an area for future research in social anxiety disorder, but our clinical experience has suggested it as an important moderator. A recent pilot study with a mixed group of patients with panic disorder, social anxiety disorder, and generalized anxiety disorder examined the benefit of adding three sessions of motivational interviewing prior to group CBT (Westra & Dozois, 2006). Individuals who received motivational interviewing, compared with those who received no pretreatment intervention, showed an increase in positive expectancy for anxiety change before CBT, had greater homework compliance during treatment, and were more likely to be responders to treatment after the course of CBT.

Several studies have examined the effects of treatment expectancy and homework compliance on outcome. In two studies, patients who found treatment to be credible and expected treatment gains did better than those who held more negative expectations regarding treatment (Chambless et al., 1997; Safren, Heimberg, & Juster, 1997). Homework compliance has also been related to treatment gains. Individuals who are more compliant have been found to make greater gains than less compliant individuals both immediately following treatment (Leung & Heimberg, 1996) and at a 6-month follow-up (Edelman & Chambless, 1995). However, Woody and Adessky (2002) did not find support for this relationship.

To summarize, treatment expectancy and homework compliance have been found to be positively related to treatment outcome. On the other hand, mixed findings have been obtained when social anxiety disorder subtype, APD, and pretreatment depression were examined as predictors of outcome. Each of these features is related to greater severity of social anxiety, which may be the causal factor here. Because individuals with generalized social anxiety disorder, APD, and depression have more severe social anxiety symptoms at pretreatment, they continue to score higher on measures of social anxiety posttreatment even when they have made gains of magnitude similar to those made by individuals without these features. It is possible that individuals with these complex presentations may benefit from longer or more intensive treatment. Comorbid substance abuse, anger, overvalued ideation, ambivalence toward change, trauma history, and PTSD-like reactions to socially stressful events are factors that may influence treatment response but require further research.

CASE EXAMPLE

Evan was a 40-year-old Caucasian gay man who presented for CBT for social anxiety disorder. He had been anxious for as long as he could remember. He recalled having grown up with a highly critical mother who often belittled him in social situations. Evan recounted stories of family get-togethers at which his mother would kick him under the table to indicate that he should stop talking, or stop eating, or sit up straighter.

From a very young age, Evan recognized that he was gay, which his mother found unacceptable. Evan explained that his mother clearly favored his siblings, who were all heterosexual, outgoing, and successful in their professional lives. He reported that his sexual orientation also affected his relationships with peers when he was growing up. As a school-age child, Evan wanted to spend his play time with girls. However, the girls rejected him (because he was a boy), and the boys teased him for being feminine. This left Evan feeling rejected and socially isolated. By the time he got to high school and college, Evan mostly kept to himself.

Despite his difficulties in the social domain, Evan did reasonably well in school and college. Upon graduating, he moved across the country to gain some distance from his family. He worked for 20 years in computer services. Most recently, he worked at a computer help center where all of his interactions with clients were online. Online interactions were much easier for him than face-to-face or phone interactions. Evan worked in a large room with other colleagues and became casual friends with a few, but he rarely got together with friends outside of work. He dated occasionally, but had never had a long-term relationship.

Evan's social anxiety disorder primarily led to distress and impairment in the social realm; he felt quite comfortable and competent in the workplace. At his assessment, he explained that his major concern was with his body weight and shape. He worried that other men would judge him negatively because he was not "young, thin and toned." In the vicious cycle that so often affects patients with anxiety disorders, Evan refused to go to the gym because he feared that people would judge the weight that he lifted and his physique negatively. As such, he was slightly overweight when he presented for treatment. Evan feared the time when he would have to reveal his body to his dating partner, and so steadfastly refused to date until he became more fit and attractive. Another reason that Evan found dating situations difficult was that he feared eating in front of other people. He worried that he might spill something, and he also felt concerned that people would judge him badly for eating at all since he perceived himself to be so grossly overweight and unattractive.

Evan also described the more typical concerns of socially anxious individuals, worrying that he would say the wrong thing or not know what to say in social interactions. He stated that he was "terrible" at initiating conversations. He said that he felt slightly more at ease if someone else started the conversation, but he then often ended conversations abruptly because he was worried he would run out of things to say.

Two years ago, Evan decided to move back to his hometown. He moved back in with his parents to save money so that he could afford to go back to school. He decided that he wanted to pursue a law degree and work to further gay rights. In the past 2 years, however, he had done little to accomplish these goals. He so feared being rejected by law schools that he had not yet applied—or even taken his law school admissions test. As already noted, Evan also avoided dating, as well as less formal social interactions. As the 2 years passed, Evan's social anxiety intensified, and he also developed major depressive disorder.

Evan struggled a fair bit when he started CBT for social anxiety disorder. One possible explanation for this was his significant comorbid depression. Early on in treatment, Evan did not complete reading assignments for homework because he was "too tired." A few weeks into treatment, he reported that he was unable to do any self-monitoring homework because simply recording how anxious and depressed he felt each day made him feel more anxious and depressed. When it came time to do CR homework, Evan got "stuck" again, stating that "there is no other way to possibly look at my horrible situation." This ongoing difficulty with homework concerned his therapist because, as was noted earlier, homework compliance has been shown to be predictive of treatment outcome among patients with social anxiety disorder.

During treatment sessions, it was even more evident that Evan was having a difficult time seeing his situation from a different perspective. Evan spent much of his sessions debating the utility of the treatment with his therapist. He simply refused to consider that he could view himself or the world around him in a different way.

Evan completed six treatment sessions. He was very receptive to the psychoeducational material and found it helpful to recognize how early difficulties with his mother and his peers might have contributed to the development of his social anxiety. He had much more difficulty with CR. At Session

6, he told his therapist that he doubted that the treatment was going to work for him because he did not "buy" the idea of CR. His therapist encouraged him to complete three more treatment sessions, during which he would begin doing exposures, and for them to then reevaluate his progress and his feelings about therapy at Session 10. His therapist explained that some patients find exposures to be the most effective way to challenge faulty beliefs because exposures involve gathering direct evidence to counter them, as opposed to "talking it through," as is the case with CR. Evan agreed to this plan but then e-mailed his therapist when he got home and said he would not be coming back for additional treatment.

Evan and his therapist had one final session to discuss what he had gained from treatment and to suggest referrals for other kinds of therapy that might be more appealing to Evan at this point. Two months later, Evan recontacted his therapist and asked whether he could resume CBT. In the interim, he had pursued supportive psychotherapy. He had found it very useful to talk about his upbringing and to process his day-to-day frustrations about how stagnant his life had become. Yet, he came to recognize that he needed treatment that focused on his social anxiety and the consequent depression, loneliness, and stagnation that he experienced.

After a session to catch up and regroup, Evan's therapist decided to move ahead with exposures rather than continue with sessions focused on CR. Although Evan seemed slightly more open to CR than he had been in the past, his therapist hypothesized that he might gain more from the cognitive work that occurs prior to and following each exposure. The first exposure was a casual conversation with a male role-player. Evan's automatic thoughts prior to the exposure fell into two categories—negative thoughts about his shape and weight (e.g., "He'll think I'm a fat slob") and negative thoughts about his ability to carry on a conversation (e.g., "I won't know what to say," "There will be long pauses"). Evan was able to carry on a 5-minute conversation with the role-player. There was a slight pause at one point, but Evan moved the conversation on to a different topic. Following the conversation, Evan had the opportunity to ask the role-player about his impressions. The role-player explained that he enjoyed talking with Evan and thought he was brave to be considering a career change in his 40s. He also noted that he thought Evan would be doing very important and much-needed work. During the postprocessing of the exposure, Evan was surprised that the conversation went as well as it did. When he was asked what he had learned, he said, "I can't believe he cared about what I said, instead of what I looked like." His therapist pointed out that he had made a cognitive shift over the course of the exposure: He came to view himself and the social world in a different way than he had expected (at least during this one interaction). This single exposure experience helped Evan to be slightly more open to the idea that he could make significant changes in his life if he fully engaged in treatment.

As Evan progressed with treatment, he would occasionally come back to his earlier argumentative stance. This would typically occur when his therapist encouraged him to move up the hierarchy to an increasingly difficult exposure, particularly one that would take place in the "real world" outside of the session. Evan would initially resist and argue that the treatment was not working. In these instances, his therapist would review with him all of the gains he had made to date and would remind him how each new hierarchy item had seemed insurmountable until he tried it and then practiced it repeatedly. As the weeks passed and Evan became more active in his world, he started to report that his depression was lifting. He was able to go to the gym, he went on a few dates (and ate during them), and he also held some informational interviews with lawyers to see whether he indeed wanted to pursue this new career path.

CBT for social anxiety disorder typically lasts for 16 to 20 sessions. Evan completed 30 sessions. Because his beliefs were so rigid, his therapist felt it was necessary to do more than the usual number of in-session exposures. Even when Evan became more willing to do exposures on his own for homework, he would often come away from these experiences having made negative interpretations. In-session exposures afforded his therapist the opportunity to lead him through the postprocessing and help Evan arrive at an unbiased interpretation of how he had done. Some sessions were also dedicated to helping Evan with his uncertainty about his career path. His therapist used a cognitive–behavioral approach to help him with this crucial issue.

After 30 sessions, Evan had made remarkable gains. He no longer met criteria for social anxiety disorder or depression. He had started to exercise, lost some weight, and felt less concerned that people would judge him on the basis of his appearance. He felt comfortable with the idea that some people would judge him negatively in this respect but no longer felt that it was important to impress these "shallow" (in his words) people. Although it is difficult to be certain in the context of an individual case, we attribute much of his improvement to his increasing willingness over the course of treatment to entertain alternative viewpoints to his own maladaptive and flawed ones. As he became more willing to do so, he "listened to" the evidence that in-session and in vivo exposures brought to bear on his beliefs, and he became less argumentative with the therapist and more flexible in his own thinking.

After much deliberation, Evan decided to return to his work in the computer field, rather than starting law school. He continued to feel passionate about advancing gay rights, and with social anxiety now less of an issue, he decided to volunteer at a center for gay youth. In his 1st week there, he was amazed at how comfortable he felt talking with the young people, as well as with the other volunteers who were closer to his own age. He began to go out on the weekends with friends from the youth center and from the gym. After working for a few months, Evan was also able to get his own apartment in the heart of the city, opening up opportunities to meet new people. As is so often the case in the treatment of persons with social anxiety disorder, each new success brought about additional challenges; some brought on increased anxiety, but as Evan faced each one, his sense of social competence and his essential value as a human being grew larger.

CONCLUSIONS AND FUTURE DIRECTIONS

Social anxiety disorder affects 12% of the population at some point in their lifetime and frequently results in impairment in both the social and professional domains. Fortunately, several treatments have been found to be efficacious for social anxiety disorder, specifically CBT and pharmacotherapy. The most efficacious forms of CBT include psychoeducation, CR, and exposure and are equally efficacious whether delivered in individual or group format. With regard to pharmacotherapy, SSRIs and the SNRI venlafaxine are the preferred medications because of their efficacy, more benign side-effects profile than the MAOIs, and lower potential for abuse than the benzodiazepines. Fluoxetine is the only SSRI with mixed findings regarding its efficacy in treating social anxiety disorder.

Although CBT has been shown to be consistently efficacious for social anxiety disorder, it does not appear to be equally efficacious for all patients. Rather, factors such as treatment expectancy and homework compliance affect treatment outcome, and it is possible that willingness to engage in homework tasks varies as a function of expectancy. Furthermore, patients with APD, the generalized subtype of social anxiety disorder, or comorbid depression are likely to display greater severity of social anxiety and may require longer and/or more intensive treatment.

Additionally, recent research has suggested that individuals with comorbid substance abuse may benefit from several extra sessions devoted to motivational interviewing and feedback regarding their substance abuse. For patients with salient memories regarding socially traumatic events who may have PTSD-like reactions to these events, amending the standard treatment to focus on these memories may be helpful, either through prolonged exposure or through rescripting of the memory. Through our clinical experience, we have identified other potential moderators of treatment, such as ambivalence regarding change, trauma history, and overvalued ideation. Further research is necessary to examine the influence of these factors on treatment outcome and to determine whether the treatment additions and modifications that they suggest will increase treatment success.

REFERENCES

Al-Kubaisy, T., Marks, I. M., Logsdail, S., Marks, M. P., Lovell, K., Sungur, M., & Araya, R. (1992). Role of exposure homework in phobia reduction: A controlled study. *Behavior Therapy, 23,* 599–621.

Alström, J. E., Nordlund, C. L., Persson, G., Hårding, M., & Ljungqvist, C. (1984). Effects of four treatment methods on social phobia patients not suitable for insight-oriented psychotherapy. *Acta Psychiatrica Scandinavica, 70,* 97–110.

American Psychiatric Association. (1994). *Diagnostic and statistical manual of mental disorders* (4th ed.). Washington, DC: Author.

Blackmore, M. A., Erwin, B. A., Heimberg, R. G., Magee, L., & Fresco, D. M. (in press). Social anxiety disorder and specific phobias. In M. Gelder, N. Andreasen, & J. Lopez-Ibor (Eds.), *The new Oxford textbook of psychiatry* (2nd ed.). London: Oxford University Press.

Blanco, C., Schneier, F. R., Schmidt, A., Blanco-Jerez, C.-R., Marshall, R. D., Sanchez-Lacày, A., & Liebowitz, M. R. (2003). Pharmacological treatment of social anxiety disorder: A meta-analysis. *Depression and Anxiety, 18,* 29–40.

Blomhoff, S., Haug, T. T., Hellstrøm, K., Holme, I., Humble, M., Madsbu, H. P., & Wolde, J. E. (2001). Randomized controlled general practice trial of sertraline, exposure therapy, and combined treatment in generalized social phobia. *The British Journal of Psychiatry, 179,* 23–30.

Bögels, S. M. (2006). Task concentration training versus applied relaxation, in combination with cognitive therapy, for social phobia patients with fear of blushing, trembling, and sweating. *Behaviour Research and Therapy, 44,* 1199–1210.

Bouton, M. E. (2002). Context, ambiguity, and unlearning: Sources of relapse after behavioral extinction. *Biological Psychiatry, 52,* 976–986.

Brown, E. J., Heimberg, R. G., & Juster, H. R. (1995). Social phobia subtype and avoidant personality disorder: Effect on severity of social phobia, impairment, and outcome of cognitive–behavioral treatment. *Behavior Therapy, 26,* 467–486.

Buckner, J., Ledley, D. R., Heimberg, R. G., & Schmidt, N. (2008). Treating comorbid social anxiety and alcohol use disorders: Combining motivation enhancement therapy with cognitive–behavioral therapy. *Clinical Case Studies, 7,* 208–223.

Chambless, D. L., Tran, G. Q., & Glass, C. R. (1997). Predictors of response to cognitive–behavioral group therapy for social phobia. *Journal of Anxiety Disorders, 11,* 221–240.

Chapman, T. F., Mannuzza, S., & Fyer, A. J. (1995). Epidemiology and family studies of social phobia. In R. G. Heimberg, M. R. Liebowitz, D. A. Hope, & F. R. Schneier (Eds.), *Social phobia: Diagnosis, assessment, and treatment* (pp. 21–40). New York: Guilford Press.

Clark, D. B., & Agras, W. S. (1991). The assessment and treatment of performance anxiety in musicians. *The American Journal of Psychiatry, 148,* 598–605.

Clark, D. M. (2001). A cognitive perspective on social phobia. In W. R. Crozier & L. E. Alden (Eds.), *International handbook of social anxiety* (pp. 405–430). Chichester, England: Wiley.

Clark, D. M., Ehlers, A., Hackman, A., McManus, F., Fennell, M., Grey, N., et al. (2006). Cognitive therapy versus exposure plus applied relaxation in social phobia: A randomized controlled trial. *Journal of Consulting and Clinical Psychology, 74,* 568–578.

Clark, D. M., Ehlers, A., McManus, F., Hackmann, A., Fennell, M., Campbell, H., et al. (2003). Cognitive therapy vs. fluoxetine in generalized social phobia: A randomized placebo controlled trial. *Journal of Consulting and Clinical Psychology, 71*, 1058–1067.

Davidson, J. R. T., Foa, E. B., Huppert, J. D., Keefe, F. J., Franklin, M. E., Compton, J. S., et al. (2004). Fluoxetine, comprehensive cognitive behavioral therapy, and placebo in generalized social phobia. *Archives of General Psychiatry, 61*, 1005–1013.

Davidson, J. R. T., Potts, N., Richichi, E., Krishnan, R., Ford, S. M., Smith, R., & Wilson W. H. (1993). Treatment of social phobia with clonazepam and placebo. *Journal of Clinical Psychopharmacology, 13*, 423–428.

Dugas, M. J., Ladouceur, R., Léger, E., Freeston, M., Langlois, F., Provencher, M. D., & Boisvert, J.-M. (2003). Group cognitive–behavioral therapy for generalized anxiety disorder: Treatment outcome and long-term follow up. *Journal of Consulting and Clinical Psychology, 71*, 821–825.

Edelman, R. E., & Chambless, D. L. (1995). Adherence during sessions and homework in cognitive–behavioral group treatment of social phobia. *Behaviour Research and Therapy, 33*, 573–577.

Erwin, B. A., Heimberg, R. G., Juster, H. R., & Mindlin, M. (2002). Comorbid anxiety and mood disorders among persons with social anxiety disorder. *Behaviour Research and Therapy, 40*, 19–35.

Erwin, B. A., Heimberg, R. G., Marx, B. P., & Franklin, M. E. (2006). Traumatic and socially stressful life events among persons with social anxiety disorder. *Journal of Anxiety Disorders, 20*, 896–914.

Erwin, B. A., Heimberg, R. G., Schneier, F. R., & Liebowitz, M. R. (2003). Anger experience and anger expression in social anxiety disorder: Pretreatment profile and predictors of attrition and response to cognitive–behavioral treatment. *Behavior Therapy, 34*, 331–350.

Falloon, I. R. H., Lloyd, G. G., & Harpin, R. E. (1981). The treatment of social phobia: Real-life rehearsal with nonprofessional therapists. *The Journal of Nervous and Mental Disease, 169*, 180–184.

Fedoroff, I. C., & Taylor, S. (2001). Psychological and pharmacological treatments for social anxiety disorder: A meta-analysis. *Journal of Clinical Psychopharmacology, 21*, 311–324.

Feske, U., & Chambless, D. L. (1995). Cognitive behavioral versus exposure only treatment for social phobia: A meta-analysis. *Behavior Therapy, 26*, 695–720.

Feske, U., Perry, K. J., Chambless, D. L., Renneberg, B., & Goldstein, A. (1996). Avoidant personality disorder as a predictor for treatment outcome among generalized social phobics. *Journal of Personality Disorders, 10*, 174–184.

Foa, E. B., & Kozak, M. J. (1986). Emotional processing of fear: Exposure to corrective information. *Psychological Bulletin, 99*, 20–35.

Gelernter, C. S., Uhde, T. W., Cimbolic, P., Arnkoff, D. B., Vittone, B. J., Tancer, M. E., & Bartko, J. J. (1991). Cognitive–behavioral and pharmacological treatments of social phobia: A controlled study. *Archives of General Psychiatry, 48*, 938–945.

Gould, R. A., Buckminster, S., Pollack, M. H., Otto, M., & Yap, L. (1997). Cognitive behavioral and pharmacological treatment for social phobia: A meta-analysis. *Clinical Psychology: Science and Practice, 4,* 291–306.

Grant, B. F., Hasin, D. S., Blanco, C., Stinson, F. S., Chou, S. P., Goldstein, R. B., et al. (2005). The epidemiology of social anxiety disorder in the United States: Results from the National Epidemiologic Survey on Alcohol and Related Conditions. *Journal of Clinical Psychiatry, 66,* 1351–1361.

Haug, T. T., Blomhoff, S., Hellstrøm, K., Holme, I., Humble, M., Madsbu, H. P., & Wold, J. E. (2003). Exposure therapy and sertraline in social phobia: 1-year follow-up of a randomised controlled trial. *The British Journal of Psychiatry, 182,* 312–318.

Heimberg, R. G. (1996). Social phobia, avoidant personality disorder, and the multiaxial conceptualization of interpersonal anxiety. In P. Salkovskis (Ed.), *Trends in cognitive and behavioural therapies* (pp. 43–62). Sussex, England: Wiley.

Heimberg, R. G. (2003, March). *Cognitive–behavioral and psychotherapeutic strategies for social anxiety disorder.* A paper presented at the annual meeting of the Anxiety Disorders Association of America, Toronto, Ontario, Canada.

Heimberg, R. G., & Becker, R. E. (2002). *Cognitive–behavioral group therapy for social phobia: Basic mechanisms and clinical applications.* New York: Guilford Press.

Heimberg, R. G., Dodge, C. S., Hope, D. A., Kennedy, C. R., Zollo, L., & Becker, R. E. (1990). Cognitive–behavioral group treatment of social phobia: Comparison to a credible placebo control. *Cognitive Therapy and Research, 14,* 1–23.

Heimberg, R. G., Holt, C. S., Schneier, F. R., Spitzer, R. L., & Liebowitz, M. R. (1993). The issue of subtypes in the diagnosis of social phobia. *Journal of Anxiety Disorders, 7,* 249–269.

Heimberg, R. G., Liebowitz, M. R., Hope, D. A., Schneier, F. R., Holt, C. S., Welkowitz, L., et al. (1998). Cognitive–behavioral group therapy versus phenelzine in social phobia: 12 week outcome. *Archives of General Psychiatry, 55,* 1133–1141.

Herbert, J. D., Gaudiano, B. A., Rheingold, A. A., Myers, V. H., Dalrymple, K., & Nolan, E. M. (2005). Social skills training augments the effectiveness of cognitive behavioral group therapy for social anxiety disorder. *Behavior Therapy, 36,* 125–138.

Holt, C. S., Heimberg, R. G., Hope, D. A., & Liebowitz, M. R. (1992). Situational domains of social phobia. *Journal of Anxiety Disorders, 6,* 63–77.

Hope, D. A., Heimberg, R. G., Juster, H. R., & Turk, C. L. (2000). *Managing social anxiety: A cognitive–behavioral therapy approach.* New York: Oxford University Press.

Hope, D. A., Heimberg, R. G., & Turk, C. L. (2006). *Therapist guide for managing social anxiety: A cognitive–behavioral therapy approach.* New York: Oxford University Press.

Hope, D. A., Herbert, J. D., & White, C. (1995). Diagnostic subtype, avoidant personality disorder, and efficacy of cognitive behavioral group therapy for social phobia. *Cognitive Therapy and Research, 19,* 285–303.

Jack, M. S., Heimberg, R. G., & Mennin, D. S. (1999). Situational panic attacks: Impact on social phobia with and without panic disorder. *Depression and Anxiety, 10*, 112–118.

Kessler, R. C., Berglund, P., Demler, O., Jin, R., Merikangas, K., & Walters, E. E. (2005). Lifetime prevalence and age-of-onset distributions of *DSM–IV* disorders in the National Comorbidity Survey Replication. *Archives of General Psychiatry, 62*, 593–602.

Kessler, R. C., Chiu, W. T., Demler, O., Merikangas, K., & Walters, E. E. (2005). Prevalence, severity, and comorbidity of 12-month *DSM–IV* disorders in the National Comorbidity Survey Replication. *Archives of General Psychiatry, 62*, 617–627.

Kipper, L., Blaya, C., Wachleski, C., Dornelles, M., Salum, G. A., Heldt, E., & Manfro, G. G. (2007). Trauma and defense style as predictors of pharmacological treatment in panic patients. *European Psychiatry, 22*, 87–91.

Kobak, K. A., Greist, J. H., Jefferson, J. W., & Katzelnick, D. J. (2002). Fluoxetine in social phobia: A double-blind, placebo-controlled pilot study. *Journal of Clinical Psychopharmacology, 22*, 257–262.

Koszycki, D., Benger, M., Shlik, J., & Bradwejn, J. (2007). Randomized trial of a meditation-based stress reduction program and cognitive behavior therapy in generalized social anxiety disorder. *Behaviour Research and Therapy, 45*, 2518–2526.

Lader, M., Stender, K., Burger, V., & Nil, R. (2004). Efficacy and tolerability of escitalopram in 12- and 24-week treatment of social anxiety disorder: Randomised, double-blind, placebo-controlled, fixed-dose study. *Depression and Anxiety, 19*, 241–248.

Ledley, D. R., & Heimberg, R. G. (2005). Social anxiety disorder. In M. M. Antony, D. R. Ledley, & R. G. Heimberg (Eds.), *Improving outcomes and preventing relapse in cognitive–behavioral therapy*. New York: Guilford Press.

Ledley, D. R., Heimberg, R. G., Hope, D. A., Hayes, S. A., Zaider, T. I., Van Dyke, M., et al. (in press). Efficacy of a manualized and workbook-driven individual treatment for social anxiety disorder. *Behavior Therapy*.

Ledley, D. R., Huppert, J. D., Foa, E. B., Davidson, J. R. T., Keefe, F. J., & Potts, N. L. S. (2005). Impact of depressive symptoms on the treatment of generalized social anxiety disorder. *Depression and Anxiety, 22*, 161–167.

Leung, A. W., & Heimberg, R. G. (1996). Homework compliance, perceptions of control, and outcome of cognitive–behavioral treatment of social phobia. *Behaviour Research and Therapy, 34*, 423–432.

Liebowitz, M. R., Gelenberg, A. J., & Munjack, D. (2005). Venlafaxine extended release vs. placebo and paroxetine in social anxiety disorder. *Archives of General Psychiatry, 62*, 190–198.

Liebowitz, M. R., Heimberg, R. G., Schneier, F. R., Hope, D. A., Davies, S., Holt, C. S., et al. (1999). Cognitive–behavioral group therapy versus phenelzine in social phobia: Long-term outcome. *Depression and Anxiety, 10*, 89–98.

Magee, W. J., Eaton, W. W., Wittchen, H.-U., McGonagle, K. A., & Kessler, R. C. (1996). Agoraphobia, simple phobia, and social phobia in the National Comorbidity Survey. *Archives of General Psychiatry, 53,* 159–168.

Newman, M. G., Hofmann, S. G., Trabert, W., Roth, W. T., & Taylor, S. (1994). Does behavioral treatment of social phobia lead to cognitive changes? *Behavior Therapy, 25,* 503–517.

Noyes, R., Moroz, G., Davidson, J. R. T., Liebowitz, M. R., Davidson, A., Siegal, J., et al. (1997). Moclobemide in social phobia: A controlled dose–response trial. *Journal of Clinical Psychopharmacology, 17,* 247–254.

Oosterbaan, D. B., van Balkom, A. J. L. M., Spinhoven, P., van Oppen, P., & van Dyck, R. (2001). Cognitive therapy versus moclobemide in social phobia: A controlled study. *Clinical Psychology and Psychotherapy, 8,* 263–273.

Öst, L. G. (1987). Applied relaxation: Description of a coping technique and review of controlled studies. *Behaviour Research and Therapy, 25,* 397–409.

Otto, M. W., Pollack, M. H., Gould, R. A., Worthington, J. J., McArdle, E. T., Rosenbaum, J. F., & Heimberg, R. G. (2000). A comparison of the efficacy of clonazepam and cognitive–behavioral group therapy for the treatment of social phobia. *Journal of Anxiety Disorders, 14,* 345–358.

Pande, A. C., Davidson, J. R. T., Jefferson, J. W., Janney, C. A., Katzelnick, D. J., Weisler, R. H., et al. (1999). Treatment of social phobia with gabapentin: A placebo-controlled study. *Journal of Clinical Psychopharmacology, 19,* 341–348.

Ponniah, K., & Hollon, S. D. (2007). Empirically supported psychological interventions for social phobia in adults: A qualitative review of randomized controlled trials. *Psychological Medicine, 38,* 3–14.

Rapee, R. M., & Heimberg, R. G. (1997). A cognitive–behavioral model of anxiety in social phobia. *Behaviour Research and Therapy, 35,* 741–756.

Roth, D. A., Antony, M. M., & Swinson, R. P. (2001). Interpretations for anxiety symptoms in social phobia. *Behaviour Research and Therapy, 39,* 129–138.

Safren, S. A., Heimberg, R. G., & Juster, H. R. (1997). Patient expectancies and their relationship to pretreatment symptomatology and outcome of cognitive–behavioral group treatment for social phobia. *Journal of Consulting and Clinical Psychology, 65,* 694–698.

Schneier, F. R., Goetz, D., Campeas, R., Fallon, B., Marshall, R., & Liebowitz, M. R. (1998). Placebo-controlled trial of moclobemide in social phobia. *The British Journal of Psychiatry, 172,* 70–77.

Schneier, F. R., Heckelman, L. R., Garfinkel, R., Campeas, R., Fallon, B. A., Gitow, A., et al. (1994). Functional impairment in social phobia. *Journal of Clinical Psychiatry, 55,* 322–331.

Schneier, F. R., Johnson, J., Hornig, C. D., Liebowitz, M. R., & Weissman, M. M. (1992). Social phobia: Comorbidity and morbidity in an epidemiologic sample. *Archives of General Psychiatry, 49,* 282–288.

Schneier, F. R., Martin, L. Y., Liebowitz, M. R., Gorman, J. M., & Fyer, A. J. (1989). Alcohol abuse in social phobia. *Journal of Anxiety Disorders, 3,* 15–23.

Schneier, F. R., Saoud, J., Campeas, R., Fallon, B. A., Hollander, E., Coplan, J., & Liebowitz, M. R. (1993). Buspirone in social phobia. *Journal of Clinical Psychopharmacology, 13*, 251–256.

Stein, M. B. (1997). Phenomenology and epidemiology of social phobia. *International Clinical Psychopharmacology, 12*(Suppl. 6), S23–S26.

Taylor, S. (1996). Meta-analysis of cognitive–behavioral treatments for social phobia. *Journal of Behavior Therapy and Experimental Psychiatry, 27*, 1–9.

Turner, S. M., Beidel, D. C., Cooley-Quille, M. R., Woody, S. R., & Messer, S. C. (1994). A multi-component behavioral treatment for social phobia: Social effectiveness therapy. *Behaviour Research and Therapy, 32*, 381–390.

Turner, S. M., Beidel, D. C., & Jacob, R. G. (1994). Social phobia: A comparison of behavior therapy and atenolol. *Journal of Consulting and Clinical Psychology, 62*, 350–358.

Veale, D. (2007). Treating obsessive–compulsive disorder in people with poor insight and overvalued ideation. In M. M. Antony, C. Purdon, & L. J. Summerfeldt (Eds.), *Psychological treatment of obsessive–compulsive disorder: Fundamentals and beyond* (pp. 267–280). Washington, DC: American Psychological Association.

Veljaca, K., & Rapee, R. M. (1998). Detection of negative and positive audience behaviours by socially anxious subjects. *Behaviour Research and Therapy, 36*, 311–321.

Versiani, M., Nardi, A. E., Mundim, F. D., Alves, A. A., Liebowitz, M. R., & Amrein, R. (1992). Pharmacotherapy of social phobia: A controlled study of moclobemide and phenelzine. *The British Journal of Psychiatry, 161*, 353–360.

Weinstock, L. S. (1999). Gender differences in the presentation and management of social anxiety disorder. *Journal of Clinical Psychiatry, 60*, 9–13.

Wells, A., Clark, D. M., Salkovskis, P., Ludgate, J., Hackmann, A., & Gelder, M. (1995). Social phobia: The role of in-situation safety behaviors in maintaining anxiety and negative beliefs. *Behavior Therapy, 26*, 153–161.

Wells, A., & Papageorgiou, C. (1998). Social phobia: Effects of external attention in anxiety, negative beliefs, and perspective taking. *Behavior Therapy, 29*, 357–370.

Westra, H. A., & Dozois, D. J. A. (2006). Preparing patients for cognitive behavioural therapy: A randomized pilot study of motivational interviewing for anxiety. *Cognitive Therapy and Research, 30*, 481–498.

Whisman, M., Sheldon, C., & Goernig, P. (2000). Psychiatric disorders and dissatisfaction with social relationships: Does type of relationship matter? *Journal of Abnormal Psychology, 109*, 803–808.

Wild, J., Hackmann, A., & Clark, D. M. (2008). Rescripting early memories linked to negative images in social phobia: A pilot study. *Behavior Therapy, 39*, 47–56.

Woody, S. R., & Adessky, R. S. (2002). Therapeutic alliance, group cohesion, and homework compliance during cognitive–behavioral group treatment of social phobia. *Behavior Therapy, 35*, 5–27.

5

OBSESSIVE–COMPULSIVE DISORDER

DEAN McKAY, STEVEN TAYLOR, AND JONATHAN S. ABRAMOWITZ

The *Diagnostic and Statistical Manual of Mental Disorders* (*DSM–IV–TR*; 4th ed., text rev.; American Psychiatric Association, 2000) defines *obsessive–compulsive disorder* (OCD) according to the presence of obsessions and compulsions. Specifically, *obsessions* are intrusive and unwanted thoughts that, when present, lead to anxiety or distress. *Compulsions* are urges to perform often repetitive behaviors or mental acts (i.e., rituals) intended to reduce or eliminate the distress associated with obsessions. The current diagnostic criteria include an additional specifier of "with poor insight" that is discussed later in this chapter. According to the *DSM*, a diagnosis of OCD is indicated by the presence of either obsessions or compulsions, although in most cases both types of symptoms are present.

Research into the prevalence of OCD has varied, with estimates ranging from 1.1% (Torres et al., 2006) to 3.0% (Bland, Newman, & Orn, 1988). However, the prevalence in the population is generally lower than in outpatient clinical settings, where the disorder has been reported as high as 9.2% (Hantouche, Bouhassira, Lancrenon, & Ravily, 1995). The condition is also frequently marked by comorbid Axis I disorders, particularly other anxiety disorders and mood disorders (Brown, Campbell, Lehman, Grisham, & Mancill, 2001; Denys, Tenney, van Megan, de Gaus, & Westenberg, 2004). Brown et al. (2001) found that in a large sample of clients with anxiety disorders, of 77 individuals with diagnoses of OCD, 41.5% met criteria for a mood disorder and 50.6% met criteria for another anxiety disorder. Denys et al. (2004), in a sample of 420 individuals with OCD, found that 27.1% had a mood disorder and 12.8% had an additional anxiety disorder. Finally, individuals with OCD have a high likelihood of also meeting diagnostic criteria for a personality disorder. Denys et al., for example, found that 20.7% of their OCD sample had a personality disorder in the anxious cluster (Cluster C), 9.7% had a personality disorder in the emotionally expressive cluster (Cluster B), and 1.4% had a personality disorder in the bizarre/eccentric cluster (Cluster A).

Aside from comordibity, OCD is also heterogeneous in terms of the types of obsessions and compulsions that may be present, and most researchers agree that there are dimensions or subtypes of the disorder (McKay et al., 2004). Most of the literature examining dimensions and subtypes of OCD has focused on symptom theme (e.g., washers, checkers), with specific treatment approaches available depending on the pattern of presenting symptoms (Abramowitz, McKay, & Taylor, 2008; Antony, Purdon, & Summerfeldt, 2007). The most consistently identified symptom subtypes include (a) aggressive, sexual, religious, and body-focused obsessions, which are associated with checking or repeating compulsions; (b) obsessions about symmetry and orderliness and ordering or arranging compulsions; (c) obsessions regarding contaminants and corresponding cleaning compulsions; and (d) obsessions and compulsions about the hoarding of objects (Abramowitz, McKay, & Taylor, 2005).

ETIOLOGY OF OBSESSIVE–COMPULSIVE DISORDER

A definitive account of the etiology of OCD is not yet available. There is, however, evidence in support of biological, genetic, and cognitive–behavioral models of onset and maintenance of the disorder. We briefly review these approaches, as well as their influences on empirically supported treatments, in the sections that follow.

Biological Models

A wide range of possible biological models have been proposed, from lesions in specific brain areas to associations with particular blood types (Jenike, 1998). All of these models, however, propose the presence of some physiologic *deficit* that leads to obsessions and compulsions. For example, Jenike (1998) summarized research suggesting that lesions in the hypothalamus are associated with compulsive behavior in rats and described published case reports of individuals whose OCD onset coincided with medical illnesses associated with hypothalamic dysfunction. We have pointed out elsewhere the difficulties with such deficit models in OCD (Taylor, McKay, & Abramowitz, 2005). Specifically, given the heterogeneity of symptom presentation, a single deficit in any area is not adequate in predicting onset and severity of the disorder. Moreover, evidence for any one particular deficit has been inconsistent.

Other dominant biological models of OCD propose the presence of dysfunction, though not necessarily emphasizing deficits, in specific regions of the brain. One in particular is the cortical–striatal hypothesis of OCD, which suggests a *circuitry* model of hyperactivity between specific brain areas that lead to increased anxiety and repetitive behaviors (for detailed discussion, see Rauch & Savage, 2000). Two major systems are implicated in this model: the motor action system and the prefrontal system. Although a single underlying dysfunction is central to the cortical–striatal hypothesis, the same issues apply as with deficit models. First, empirical evidence for the model has been inconsistent, and second, a single dysfunction cannot account for the diverse symptom presentations that characterize OCD.

Pharmacological approaches to the treatment of OCD are associated with the biological view of this disorder, although it was the finding that serotonergic medications (such as clomipramine) were more effective than other tricyclic antidepressant medications (such as imipramine) that led to the first biological dysfunction model of OCD—the serotonin hypothesis (Insel, Mueller, Alterman, Linnoila, & Murphy, 1985). The selective serotonin reuptake inhibitors (SSRIs; e.g., fluoxetine, fluvoxamine) with specific side-effect profiles have shown efficacy in the treatment of OCD relative to placebo (Pato & Zohar, 2001), although there is no clear difference in efficacy among the various SSRIs (Abramowitz, 1997; Flament & Bisserbe, 1997).

Cognitive–Behavioral Models of Etiology

Cognitive–behavioral accounts of the etiology of OCD have been evolving, beginning with purely behavioral descriptions that suggested compulsions arose as a negatively reinforced behavior to alleviate obsessions (for a review, see Clark, 2004). These early accounts were quickly confronted by the problem of obsessions themselves, which are unlike other stimuli that are usually the source of avoidance in negative reinforcement associated with fear learning. Specifically, obsessions are purely internal events and required a different explanatory framework. On the basis of these early observations, the first integrative cognitive–behavioral account came from Rachman and Hodgson (1980), who suggested that OCD is essentially the result of the following cognitive vulnerabilities: dysphoric mood; stress; intolerance of certain thoughts; increased sensitivity to threat; and personality variables, particularly neuroticism, introversion, and elevated emotionality.

Since the time of Rachman and Hodgson (1980), the conceptualization of OCD has centered on how individuals with OCD differ from other people with respect to their reactions to specific thoughts. Unwanted, intrusive thoughts are a common experience in the general population (Freeston, Ladouceur, Thibodeau, & Gagnon, 1991). Individuals with OCD differ in their obsessional experiences from everyday intrusive thoughts in the following ways: (a) higher frequency, (b) higher distress and lower acceptability, (c) guilt provoked by the thought(s), (d) resistance when the thought(s) occur, (e) a sense of loss of control over the thought(s), (f) intrusions appraised as meaningful, (g) substantial time with the thought(s) as focus of consciousness, (h) extensive concern over need to control the thought, and (i) extensive interference with activities (Clark, 2004).

The research described has led to the development of a more comprehensive cognitive model of OCD. This conceptualization suggests that obsessions arise from a specific set of dysfunctional beliefs. These beliefs are activated in response to otherwise normal obsessions. One dysfunctional belief that has received considerable attention is an inflated sense of personal responsibility (Salkovskis, 1985). Several other major dysfunctional beliefs have been hypothesized to increase obsessional problems and associated compulsive behavior. Among these are beliefs such as (a) the overimportance of thoughts (e.g., "My thoughts indicate something significant about me"), (b) the need to control thoughts, (c) overestimation of threat, (d) perfectionism, and (e) intolerance for uncertainty (see Taylor, Abramowitz, & McKay, 2007). Collectively, any of these different dysfunctional beliefs, activated in the presence of an unwanted intrusive thought, could lead to compulsive behavior. Figure 5.1 illustrates the sequence from onset of an intrusive thought through to compulsion and later avoidance behavior to prevent both the onset of obsessions and need to complete rituals.

EMPIRICALLY SUPPORTED PSYCHOLOGICAL TREATMENT OF OBSESSIVE–COMPULSIVE DISORDER

Exposure with response prevention (ERP), which was derived from early behavioral accounts of compulsive rituals, is the most effective treatment for OCD. The essential ingredients of ERP are exposure to stimuli that give rise to obsessional distress and rituals and therapist-assisted resistance of the corresponding rituals. Effective treatment requires clients to continue practicing ERP between sessions. Despite its strong efficacy (Abramowitz, 1996), ERP has some limitations worth noting. First, the intervention is demanding for clients. It is often difficult to ensure that they complete exercises between sessions. Because of the anxiety produced by the exercises, clients are frequently reluctant to practice without the therapist present. Clients also may engage in strategic avoidance between and during sessions. Foa and Kozak (1986) illustrated that clients essentially limit the extent of the range of exposure and engage in planning for undoing the exposure (i.e., in contami-

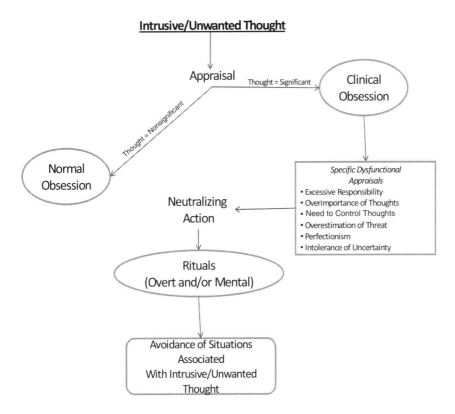

Intrusive/Unwanted Thought

Appraisal

Thought = Significant

Clinical Obsession

Thought = Nonsignificant

Normal Obsession

Neutralizing Action

Specific Dysfunctional Appraisals
- Excessive Responsibility
- Overimportance of Thoughts
- Need to Control Thoughts
- Overestimation of Threat
- Perfectionism
- Intolerance of Uncertainty

Rituals (Overt and/or Mental)

Avoidance of Situations Associated With Intrusive/Unwanted Thought

Figure 5.1. Sequence from intrusive thought to neutralization in normal and clinical obsessions.

nation exposure, cognitively "marking off" the area of exposed skin for later cleaning, as well as avoiding additional contact with the affected area). Another problem involves the "transfer of responsibility" for exposure, essentially attributing any potential negative consequence to the therapist or providing implicit self-directed reassurance. For example, many individuals with OCD have difficulty driving out of concern that they will inadvertently hit a pedestrian. Although this may be a pronounced problem while driving alone, the client could easily transfer responsibility to other passengers, particularly a therapist, reasoning that "my therapist would never let me hit someone without warning me first." This kind of self-directed reassurance typically minimizes the effectiveness of exposure exercises because it limits the activation of key cognitive errors associated with the obsessions.

The various impediments mentioned here represent challenges in treatment, but they can be overcome by creative rearranging of the demands of the activity. For example, in the case of responsibility transfer, it would be reasonable to point out that there are no guarantees and that it is entirely possible that a given feared outcome could happen after completing this exercise. To illustrate, when conducting exposure for contamination fear, the client may assume that the therapist selects areas for purposefully contaminating that are known to be reasonably free of germs. There are several ways this can be overcome. The therapist might ask the client to pick contaminated areas for exposure, decreasing therapist familiarity. The therapist could conduct home-based exposure. These two possibilities limit familiarity, placing the onus on the client to determine the degree of safety and cope with the fact that there are no guarantees. Finally, the therapist could point out flatly that there are no guarantees, noting how illness befalls people all the time despite the fact that their environments are, on average, fairly constant. Aside from these client-related barriers to fully engaging in exposure therapy, many therapists are reluctant to recommend or practice exposure therapy, incorrectly assuming there is great risk to client health by the procedure (Richard & Gloster, 2007).

The practice of ERP includes several different variations. Abramowitz (1996) reviewed all the variants and identified four general approaches: (a) therapist versus self-directed exposure, (b) in vivo versus in imagery, (c) pace of exposure (rapidly confronting the most feared situations versus gradually working through a hierarchy), and (d) degree of response prevention (complete vs. partial). To illustrate, consider a client with concerns over symmetry and orderliness. A therapist may accompany the client in deliberately creating disorder in the environment and request that the client leave the environment in disarray for the foreseeable future (i.e., therapist directed, in vivo, rapid exposure, with complete response prevention). Another therapist might structure treatment for the same client by describing the exercise to be carried out at home after the session; having the client practice the activity by imagining the environment in disarray; and suggesting that when carrying out the exercise independently, the client do so for an area that is of relatively low concern and that it can be reordered after an hour (i.e., self-directed, in imagery, gradual pace, partial response prevention). All kinds of combinations of these four major approaches are possible. Abramowitz (1996) found that although each of the various combinations are generally effective, significantly better outcomes are achieved with therapist-directed exposure and complete response prevention.

Although generally effective, some 25% to 50% of individuals with OCD either refuse or do not show satisfactory outcomes with ERP. Reasons for this include the inherent difficulty of confronting one's own fears and dropping rituals (and client's refusal to do so), the lack of therapist know-how in implementing this treatment, and the lack of emphasis on obsessions in this form of treatment. As a result, cognitive theorists (e.g., Salkovskis, 1985) have developed and begun testing cognitive therapies (CTs) for OCD. These therapies incorporate ERP, yet also emphasize CT aimed at challenging dysfunctional beliefs and appraisals of intrusive thoughts relevant to OCD.

In CT, the role of ERP is primarily as *behavioral experiments* in which confrontation with feared stimuli and ritual abstinence are used to test beliefs that underlie obsessional fear and ritualistic urges. Specifically, behavioral experiments are exercises designed to elicit dysfunctional beliefs associated with intrusive thoughts. To illustrate, if a client believes that thoughts have special importance (overimportance of thoughts), a common exercise used by Dean McKay is to ask the client to deliberately wish for a car in the parking lot to spontaneously burst into flames. When the client observes that the thought did not produce the desired result, the exercise is taken a step further by walking through the parking lot and selecting specific cars that will be the subject of the fiery wish. The next step typically involves moving to ideas that have increasing personal relevance. There are numerous examples of behavioral experiments documented for OCD as well as for other psychological conditions (see Bennett-Levy et al., 2004). Research has suggested that these experiments are critical to the efficacy of CT (Abramowitz, Taylor, & McKay, 2005).

Treatment outcome studies of ERP (in particular) and cognitive–behavioral therapy (CBT; which broadly incorporates ERP and variants of CT) have consistently revealed large effects associated with treatment when compared with placebo, other psychological interventions, and medication (Abramowitz, 1996). However, outcome also varies with presenting symptoms. To illustrate, Abramowitz, Franklin, Schwartz, and Furr (2003) found significant differences in treatment outcome on the basis of major presenting symptom. In this case, individuals with obsessions related to symmetry and ordering, and contamination, showed the best response to treatment, with 76% and 70% showing clinically significant improvement, respectively. Individuals with hoarding showed the poorest response to treatment, with only 31% showing clinically significant improvement. Mataix-Cols, Marks, Greist, Kobak, and Baer (2002) found that different symptom profiles were associated with different levels of compliance and outcome with CBT. This study showed that individuals with symmetry or contamination obsessions were most compliant with, and had the best outcome from, treatment. Clients with poorest compliance and outcome were those with hoarding.

FACTORS LEADING TO POOR TREATMENT RESPONSE

In the sections that follow, we discuss a number of variables that have been associated with poor outcome in CBT for OCD. In the last several years, there has been extensive research on variants of OCD, including symptom presentation, comorbid conditions, overvalued ideation, scrupulosity, and specific therapeutic factors. Each of these factors requires therapists to adjust treatment from typical ERP. In some instances, ERP is not recommended until the complicating factor is addressed. Each of the aforementioned barriers to treatment is discussed here.

Symptom Presentation

As noted earlier, although CBT is efficacious in the treatment of OCD, outcome is moderated by the presenting symptom. As a result, there have been modifications to treatment implementation according to presenting symptoms (Abramowitz, McKay, & Taylor, 2008). The variety of different modifications is extensive and too detailed to provide here. However, one notable exception is with regard to hoarding. Whereas ERP and cognitive strategies developed for OCD have limited effects on hoarding symptoms, treatment approaches emphasizing organization strategies, cognitive interventions for attachment to possessions, decisions regarding the necessity of specific items, and guided practice in discarding materials have shown promise in treating hoarding-related obsessive-compulsive symptoms (Frost & Tolin, 2008).

Comorbid Axis I and Axis II Disorders and Personality Dimensions

On the basis of the epidemiology data described, OCD frequently presents with comorbid mood disorders, particularly major depression. The research on the relation of depression to treatment outcome has been mixed. However, when depression is severe, outcome of OCD treatment is typically poor (e.g., Abramowitz, Franklin, Street, Kozak, & Foa, 2000). Several explanations have been offered to describe this relationship. First, individuals with depression appear to react with very strong emotions when they conduct exposure therapy (Foa, 1979). This emotional reactivity might hinder the natural decrement of distress that is supposed to occur with prolonged and repeated exposure. Second, as a result of the hopelessness, psychomotor retardation, and anhedonia that accompany depression, such individuals might have limited motivation for treatment and therefore not engage in ERP exercises (Abramowitz et al., 2000). Third, individuals with depression show a proneness to misinterpret the significance of intrusive thoughts, leading to especially severe and perhaps treatment-resistant obsessional symptoms.

OCD also frequently co-occurs with Axis II disorders (Denys et al., 2004), most notably those in the anxious cluster (e.g., avoidant personality disorder), although a substantial proportion of individuals with OCD meet criteria for the emotionally expressive, or Cluster B, personality disorders (e.g., histrionic personality disorder). Several studies have examined the relation between personality disorders and OCD treatment outcome. It appears that comorbid conditions from any of the personality clusters impede treatment outcome (Keeley, Storch, Merlo, & Geffken, 2008). What is less clear is whether any particular cluster or specific personality disorder impedes treatment so much that the manner of intervention would require a different approach altogether.

Schizotypal personality disorder and schizotypal traits have received special attention in relation to treatment outcome for OCD, and several authors have noted that the presence of schizotypal personality disorder predicts poorer outcome with CBT (Minichiello, Baer, & Jenike, 1987; Stanley, Turner, & Borden, 1990). Perhaps this is a result of more severe OCD symptoms, which are often present when schizotypal features are apparent (Moritz et al., 2004). McKay and Gruner (2008) have also proposed that the perceptual disturbance and general information processing deficits evident in schizotypy disrupt the processes by which learning occurs in CBT. The fundamental problem lies in the conflict between the demands of CBT, which require the ability to effectively connect the exposure exercises or behavioral experiments with an outcome that differs from the anticipated negative consequence. With disruptions in basic cognitive processes such as those related to schizotypy, there is reduced benefit from therapeutic exercises.

Overvalued Ideation and Poor Insight

The cognitive–behavioral conceptualization of OCD has as its centerpiece the idea that dysfunctional beliefs lead to obsessions and compulsions. Implicit in this model is the assumption that with the right arrangement of disconfirming evidence, these beliefs will become weaker or dissipate altogether. However, the beliefs clients hold regarding their obsessions and the associated dysfunctional beliefs may also be conceptualized as falling along a dimension from obsessional, specifically intrusive thoughts accurately believed to be irrational, to delusional (Kozak & Foa, 1994). Along this dimension are overvalued ideas, in which clients may be convinced that their dysfunctional beliefs are in fact reasonable, and clients may offer various arguments to support their beliefs. To illustrate, consider an individual with contamination fear with overvalued ideation. When presented with ERP exercises that involve touching floors, the person may reply that this is a dangerous activity, arguing that floors are covered with dangerous bacteria. The person might further argue that if others knew this, then no one would complete such an ERP exercise (a global knowledge reason). Overvalued ideas tend to remain stable over time and are associated with poorer treatment outcome (Neziroglu, Stevens, Yaryura-Tobias, & McKay, 2001). One reason for this is that, believing exposure exercises are very dangerous, the individual is unlikely to fully engage and therefore cannot obtain evidence that might disconfirm the strongly held belief.

Scrupulosity

Frequently, clients with OCD present with symptoms that include religious or spiritual components. This can present significant barriers to treatment development as well as implementation. First, with heightened levels of scrupulosity comes an increased risk that ERP-related exercises (e.g., facing thoughts of immoral behavior, reducing prayer rituals) will be perceived as an assault on religion. Second, it can be a challenge for therapists to engineer ERP exercises that are at once likely to be therapeutic and yet not perceived as a violation of the client's religious values or practices. Finally, because social reinforcement of strong religious beliefs is often present in the scrupulous person's environment, it is unlikely that the client will join the therapist in viewing scrupulous symptoms and beliefs as senseless and excessive (i.e., they are overvalued ideas). For example, if a client has extensive checking and washing rituals that he or she reports are tied to religious devotion as part of the Jewish faith, a clinician would be hard pressed to suggest to this client to do any of the following exposure exercises or behavioral experiments: (a) touch or consume even a small amount of pork products (almost certainly offensive to the client), (b) touch areas where there were previously pork products but also highly likely to have been satisfactorily cleaned (problems in balance between treatment appropriate and religious devotion), or (c) engage in behavioral experiments challenging the need to complete ritualistic prayer activities perfectly (the client would find this a sensible activity given the degree of lifestyle devotion to ritual religious activities).

Stimulus–Environment and Stimulus–Outcome Relationships

One of the necessary conditions for the effectiveness of CBT for OCD is the ability to access stimuli that readily provoke obsessions or urges to perform rituals. If we consider the treatment outcome data associated with specific symptoms of OCD (Abramowitz et al., 2003), a common feature among the two groups of symptoms with the best treatment response (i.e., symmetry and ordering, and contamination) is the ease with which clinicians may provoke the obsessions and help the patient stop ritualistic behaviors. Indeed, most contaminants and situations involving asymmetry are tangible and fairly readily found in the environment. Alternatively, hoarding and unacceptable thoughts (which showed modest response, with 46% achieving clinically significant improvement) are often (although not exclusively) associated with more elusive stimuli that might be more difficult to access for exposure exercises. In situations in which fear is provoked primarily by intrusive thoughts and fears of disastrous consequences (as opposed to external triggers), exposure in imagery can be used instead of in vivo. This technique was described in detail by Freeston et al. (1997).

A second important condition is the proximal relation between confrontation with the feared stimulus and the expected feared outcome. Even for symptoms that respond well to treatment (i.e., contamination fear), in some cases the clinical presentation implies a long lag between exposure to the stimulus and feared outcome. For example, Dean McKay treated a client whose primary symptom involved contamination by immoral ideas or people, with the feared negative consequence of decreased functioning at his job and in his family. Exposure to feared stimuli, therefore, would not have a short-term relationship with the feared outcome given that the consequence would accrue slowly over time. Further, the client could easily attribute poor performances to the feared stimuli because these were not closely related in time but were deemed associated nonetheless. One way treatment may be modified involves exposure to environmental stimuli while simultaneously relying on imaginal exposure for the feared consequences. In the example noted previously, the client was exposed to ideas he deemed immoral (i.e., newspaper articles about criminals) while given the instructions to imagine the associated decline in occupational functioning, such as increases in errors and poorer job evaluations. As part of this kind of modified exposure, it is useful to also instruct the client to monitor automatic negative beliefs, particularly those previously identified that are associated with obsessive–compulsive behavior. This, in turn, sets the occasion for directly challenging the dysfunctional beliefs while also allowing the client the opportunity to practice exposure to real stimuli that produce obsessions.

CASE EXAMPLE

Bill was referred for treatment by Dean McKay. At the time of his referral, he was 37 years old and employed as an accountant. He was married and had three children whose ages ranged from 3 to 12 years. He had been married for 14 years. Although he reported that he had a good marriage, his wife was becoming increasingly frustrated with his obsessive–compulsive symptoms. During the initial session, Bill noted that he felt he had always been "a bit obsessional" since childhood, although his parents did not notice, and he hid some of his behaviors from his friends.

Bill presented with several major symptoms of OCD. He had contamination fears due to exposure to blasphemy. He defined *blasphemy* as follows: any occasion in which he passed houses of worship while simultaneously thinking of immoral images or foul language, any time he might think of well-respected famous historical figures in a negative light (i.e., negative thoughts about the political ideation of Gandhi), any time he questioned the comments or ideas of historical writers or scholars (i.e., seeing newsstand tabloids with new Nostradamus predictions and then thinking that Nostradamus was a moron), and any time he was in the presence of someone who committed a blasphemous act, such as cursing. Each day, Bill kept track of his blasphemous encounters and would wash his hands for each encounter. For this task, he defined a "single hand wash" as getting his hands wet, then dried. Therefore, he reasoned, he could wash quickly even though his list of blasphemes was often extensive each day. He also reported significant problems with checking, particularly his water faucets and stove, although he also found himself checking his work more than would be otherwise necessary in his line of work. He also frequently had difficulty driving out of concern that he might have hit pedestrians. Therefore, while driving, he could not tolerate the radio because it would interfere with his concentration. He avoided driving whenever possible because this concern. He also reported that he had numerous lucky numbers (prime numbers, except 13) and unlucky numbers (6, 13, 22). Whenever he had to write these numbers, he did so only in pencil to ensure that they could be erased. Finally, he also expressed concerns with symmetry and ordering. For these symptoms, his concerns were tied to religiosity, as he took orderliness to be a natural modern extension of the saying "Cleanliness is next to godliness."

In addition to these presenting symptoms associated with OCD, Bill had significant symptoms of depression. His Beck Depression Inventory—II (BDI–II; Beck, Steer, & Brown, 1996) score at intake was 33, with no suicidal ideation. Although his BDI–II score was high, he fell just short of meeting criteria for any mood disorder. He also did not meet criteria for any other Axis I disorder, and he did not meet criteria for any Axis II disorder. However, he showed elevated levels of schizotypy, with a score of 8 on the Magical Ideation Scale and a score of 52 on the Lucky Beliefs Scale. A summary of the relation these scales have to clinical intervention with OCD clients can be found in McKay and Gruner (2008).

Bill reported an extensive psychological treatment history. Prior to initiating CBT specifically tailored for OCD, he tried general CT, relaxation training, and systematic desensitization in imagery. He had also undergone "general psychotherapy," as well as "Jungian psychoanalysis," whereby the therapist postulated that the causative factor in maintaining his symptoms was job dissatisfaction, a conclusion derived from his report on two occasions of anxiety-based dreams of performance problems at work.

At the start of treatment, Bill was taking several medications, namely sertraline, risperidone, and alprazolam. Prior to this medication regimen, Bill had tried several other SSRIs as well as other antianxiety agents. Although he was prescribed alprazolam for sleep, he frequently took this medication during the day. According to Bill, he did this because he would get increasingly anxious throughout the day as he accumulated blasphemes that would later require washing.

Given all these symptoms, Bill's social and role functioning was seriously impaired. He rarely went out on weekends. Because of his primary symptom of concern over contact with blasphemous information, going out socially, in his view, increased his risk of encountering this kind of material. Because he had to check faucets and the stove, leaving was often a challenge anyway. He could travel, however, as his wife was willing to drive. Prior to initiating CBT, his symptoms had begun to worsen, as he had recently heard the Pope suggest that couples who were remarried try to refrain from sex with their second spouses. Although he was neither Catholic nor remarried, he took this message to potentially apply to him because he had been engaged before meeting his wife. Therefore, because he had been ostensibly committed to another person, he felt that it was possible that God viewed him as effectively married once previously. He had been reluctant to engage in sexual relations with his wife over the preceding six months, although he did not report his concerns to her, instead telling her that he was exhausted from his symptoms. Severity ratings of his obsessive–compulsive symptoms were high, with an obsession score of 16 and a compulsion score of 14 on the Yale–Brown Obsessive–Compulsive Scale (Y-BOCS; Goodman et al., 1989).

Treatment Development

The first session after the intake meeting involved psychoeducation, and treatment was described. Bill was hesitant because he felt that his symptoms were not amenable to direct intervention, particularly the blasphemous symptoms, and because he still lent credibility to the suggestions of his previous therapist who indicated that his problems were a result of job dissatisfaction. After more detailed discussion, Bill noted that work was the one place where, despite the accumulation of blasphemous symptoms, he felt the least depressed and lowest concern with other obsessive–compulsive symptoms. Next, his symptoms were rank ordered from least to most likely amenable to intervention. He indicated that his driving concerns and lucky and unlucky numbers might be easiest to start with, with any symptoms associated with blasphemy rated least likely to respond.

Treatment-Amenable Symptoms

Given the severity and diversity of Bill's symptoms, treatment was initiated twice weekly, for 90 minutes per session. As per the ordered list of symptoms to treat, his fears of hitting pedestrians while driving were targeted first. During the first session, he drove with no anxiety through neighborhoods and parking lots for shopping centers accompanied by the therapist. During these sessions he had "transferred responsibility" to the therapist. Bill readily admitted that he felt there was, to his surprise, little risk of harming anyone so long as he had a passenger in the car. Given that there was growing ill will in his marriage, he was instructed to drive whenever he went out with his wife as a means of demonstrating some immediate treatment gains. Two sessions later, driving exercises were undertaken whereby Bill drove with the therapist following behind in his vehicle. Following this, driving exercises took place with Bill and the therapist driving separate routes to meet at locations away from the office, then ultimately rendezvousing back at the therapist's office. This phase of treatment progressed well, but Bill was still convinced that his concerns over blasphemy would not respond well to treatment.

The next area that was addressed was his concern with lucky and unlucky numbers. Treatment for this symptom also moved swiftly. First, Bill was instructed to write down the unlucky numbers, in ink, in the therapist's office, and then discard them. He then wrote the numbers on paper to keep in his wallet and kept a notebook with 13 pages, all paginated with the number *13* (i.e., page 1 was numbered 13, page 2 numbered 13, etc.), on which he would keep track of other incidental symptoms that might arise each day. Bill reported few difficulties with these activities, even though he initially dreaded these special numbers. To further weaken the association of unlucky numbers to other numbers generally, he later began to intersperse lucky with unlucky numbers on the same page of the notebook (i.e., number 7, a prime number, alongside the numbers 6, *13*, and *22*). He was encouraged to demonstrate to his wife that this symptom was improving, again in the spirit of alleviating the marital distress his OCD symptoms had caused.

Difficult-to-Treat Symptoms

When it came time to address his concerns over blasphemy, Bill had completed eight therapy sessions over a 1-month period. He stated that he was feeling slightly better, although test data suggested he was progressing better than he stated. His BDI–II was now 21, and his obsession score was a 10 and compulsion score an 11 from the Y-BOCS. However, he remained pessimistic that the concerns over blasphemy could respond to therapy. He was also not confident that the problems related to symmetry and ordering would be amenable to treatment.

Because research has suggested that symmetry and ordering symptoms respond well to treatment, that symptom area was targeted next. Two sessions were conducted at Bill's home. Rather than start with an area of high personal relevance, it was decided that if Bill was going to respond to treatment at all, it would be in the kitchen in places that have relatively little order but where he spends some time each day. Bill was instructed to deliberately misplace a fork and spatula by switching the drawers in which these were stored. He reported no anxiety for this intervention because it happened deliberately and therefore conformed to a certain orderliness anyway. Additional areas were therefore targeted to deliberately create asymmetry and make less orderly, such as the bathroom (particularly the medicine chest), bedroom drawers, closet (by intermingling some of his clothes with those of his wife), and his homework space. Throughout this portion of treatment, Bill was gently reminded that he was being "less godly," which produced minor anxiety but not so much that Bill undid any of the interventions during the course of the sessions.

Although it appeared that Bill was not undoing the session work, in the third session in which symmetry and ordering were addressed (Session 11), he reported that he was still concerned with orderliness and was not convinced that he had made any gains in that area. Instead, Bill reported that the possessions that were deliberately put in different spots were in order now, because he could remember where everything was, having not himself misplaced any objects. Bill reasoned that it would be ungodly if he himself misplaced an object. However, he reported that he was now less concerned with symmetry. He arrived at this conclusion, he said, because during an earlier session at the therapist's office, he recalled a poster on the wall of a natural canyon scene that was highly asymmetrical. Because the canyon was a work of God, he reasoned that symmetry was not an essential component of godliness.

At this point, Bill reported that his wife was becoming impatient because he had not yet shaken the thought regarding sexual relations that was prompted by the Pope's comment about second marriages. Shortly after starting treatment, Bill reported the real reason he had for avoiding sexual contact with his wife. Following this, Bill had heard the argument from his wife numerous times that (a) he was never previously married and (b) he was not Catholic. The therapist approached this from the perspective of societal norms and by carefully parsing the Pope's words. On the first count, society, even among remarried Catholics whose first spouse had died, would not expect this level of chastity. Would Bill feel that the vast majority of society was not on God's good side? How could so many people, even Catholics, flaunt the word of the man who is supposed to have a direct line to God? Bill countered that it is really more of a problem in that he particularly remembered that the Pope had these words to say, and that if other people had heard them, or remembered them, then more people would engage in appropriate restraint. Here Bill was demonstrating a problem of overimportance of thought as well as overimportance of memory, as he was taking the comment beyond just that of the Pope (who suggested refraining from sex) to ultimately mean that he should not engage in sex. This involved then parsing the Pope's words further. Bill was slightly more persuaded by this, because it was not recommended that remarried couples never engage in sex. Although Bill was hesitant, a behavioral experiment was set up for him to engage in intimate contact with his wife, without intercourse, and that if God really did not want him to do this, there should be some indicator later, such as loss of a client at work or some other minor negative event. Because of concerns over undetermined time following the activity, Bill and the therapist suggested that the sign would likely come within 24 hours of the sexual act. Bill was able to complete this exercise, and although he felt highly anxious for the following 24 hours, no aversive events occurred. He reported feeling better but still was not convinced that he now had license to have sex with his wife. Furthermore, because he felt so nervous about this activity, he was reluctant to pursue it further.

Given Bill's reluctance in addressing his sexual difficulties, attention was turned to his hand washing associated with exposure to blasphemous ideas. At this point (Session 13), Bill reported that he did not like the hand washing but was not convinced that the blasphemy could be alleviated by any other means. Another home session was scheduled, this time to observe Bill's method of hand washing as a consequence of exposure to blasphemous thoughts. Rather than aggregate a day's worth of blasphemes, the therapist provided a small set of identified blasphemes (i.e., "Nostradamus was a moron," "Gandhi was a show-off by appearing so virtuous," and various foul words) and reading aloud material he deemed blasphemous, such as articles from the satirical newspaper *The Onion*. At the beginning, instead of eliminating his hand washing, the aim was to find ways to reduce the intensity or frequency. His form of hand washing for blasphemes was very brief, by observation. Therefore, it was suggested to Bill that because he was already thinking of blasphemes he was exposed to during the day, perhaps he could organize them into categories and just wash for each category. He liked this idea, and his hand washing quickly reduced from as much as 200 in an evening to less than 10.

When Bill got his hand washing into the single digits each day, he reported that he did not see how he could wash less frequently. He practiced over several sessions, even under more intense exposure whereby the therapist exposed him to other blasphemes, all variations on the same themes. Additional exposure included driving past houses of worship while playing music with blasphemous themes (a dual purpose exposure because Bill would be driving, with music, although this symptom was significantly improved). Nonetheless, he could not eliminate the need to wash, however briefly, for the sake of eliminating his concerns over blasphemous thought content.

After 20 sessions, Bill reported that he did not feel he could improve further. He felt that he had done quite well in therapy, better than any prior treatment experience. He had been attending 90-minute sessions twice weekly for 11 weeks (he missed a session one week). Given the long-standing nature of his symptoms, it was suggested that he continue therapy on a weekly basis at the very least. He agreed to these terms. Bill continued to struggle with the residual concern that he needed to wash away blasphemous ideas that accrued during the day. After 11 more weekly sessions, Bill had made the following symptom-related gains: restored sexual relations with his wife; rarely checked to see if he hit pedestrians while driving, and could drive with music playing; no longer had difficulties with lucky and unlucky numbers; and only checked the faucets and stove before going to bed. Residual symptoms were his concerns over godliness from ordering, although symmetry was no longer a problem, and his remaining concerns over blasphemy. He stated that he did not feel he could benefit further from therapy and ended treatment. Follow-up contact was made after 6 months, whereupon it was found that Bill had decreased his medication substantially but still felt the need to wash for blasphemous ideas. He stated that he typically washed only five to eight times each night. At the end of treatment, his depression was substantially lower than at the start, with his BDI–II at 11. His obsessive-compulsive symptoms were likewise substantially lower, with an obsessions score of 8 and a compulsions score of 5 on the Y-BOCS. At 6-month follow-up, his BDI–II score was 7, Y-BOCS obsessions was 6, and Y-BOCS compulsion was 4.

Bill's symptoms are not unusual for someone with severe OCD. He had significant difficulties in a number of important areas related to the disorder, such as contamination fears, checking, and symmetry/orderliness. Several symptoms responded very readily to treatment, such as his concerns over driving and lucky and unlucky numbers. However, several symptoms were slow to respond to treatment. Contamination fear was particularly difficult to treat and remained a residual problem after treatment ended. This is noteworthy because, as reported earlier, contamination fear is often among the symptoms that respond readily to ERP (Abramowitz et al., 2003). However, contamination fear is typically functionally based on disease-based concerns, whereas Bill's contamination fear was related to an idea or value. Further, the values that were functionally tied to his contamination fear were associated with basic teachings that are typically established early on and held scrupulously. As noted earlier, attitudes of this kind often pose substantial difficulty for clinicians because these are at the intersection of dysfunctional behaviors and societal moral codes. Clinicians therefore face important ethical decisions when embarking on exposure for clients who hold strong scrupulous beliefs. In fact, the treatment decisions in these cases are akin to the decisions necessary in conducting exposure for some religious beliefs (i.e., exposure to places associated with pork products for different religious groups). In the case of Bill, his residual concerns over blasphemy were not completely overcome, and although he was satisfied with his course of treatment, the potential is there for future difficulties because he was unable to eliminate the need for washing following exposure to blasphemous information.

CONCLUSIONS AND FUTURE DIRECTIONS

OCD is a complex, heterogeneous, and typically chronic disorder. Empirically supported treatments have been developed, with among the most effective involving ERP. A careful assessment and case formulation can help the clinician identify and overcome treatment barriers. The clinician's odds of success are enhanced if he or she is conversant with the current state of knowledge concerning OCD etiology and treatment, as well as knowledgeable about the various barriers to treatment success. Creativity on the part of the clinician is also important for tailoring interventions to a given client's problems.

Unfortunately, even the most skilled, creative clinicians have their fair share of treatment failures, and there is a good deal of room for improving both psychosocial and pharmacological treatments for OCD. Many studies have looked at the most obvious ways of improving treatment efficacy, that is, by combining the most promising treatments such as by combining ERP with either cognitive restructuring or serotonergic medications. The results so far have been disappointing and highlight the old maxim that more is not necessarily better (Pull, 2007).

There are at least two important approaches for future research for improving treatment outcomes in OCD; the first is likely to pay dividends in the long term, whereas the second may provide short-term (although incomplete) benefits. The first approach is to develop better biopsychosocial models of OCD; with a better understanding of the disorder, it should be possible to develop interventions that target critical mechanisms, with interventions tailored to a specific OCD subtype or to a specific OCD client. This research approach is part of what Thomas Insel, Director of the National Institutes of Mental Health, has called *cure therapeutics*, defined by the goal of searching for treatments that provide complete and permanent remission (Insel & Scolnick, 2006). This goal is likely to take some time to attain.

The second approach to improving treatment outcome is to persist with the empirically driven "more is better" program of clinical research, with the hope that there exist some combinations of interventions that might outperform the best monotherapies available thus far. At the present time, the research suggests that three kinds of interventions might be profitably combined with ERP-based interventions to augment treatment outcome. ERP could be combined with one or more of the following to improve treatment adherence and to reduce attrition: (a) motivational interviewing methods, which could be used to increase client motivation to engage in ERP (Tolin & Skeketee, 2007); (b) medications that may improve insight in OCD, such as antipsychotic medications like quetiapine (Skapinakis, Papatheodorou, & Mavreas, 2007); and (c) medications that could facilitate distress reduction during ERP, such as the drug D-cycloserine, which has been shown to facilitate exposure therapy for other anxiety disorders (Hofmann, 2007). These approaches to augmenting ERP are promising but require further evaluation. However, the cure-therapeutics approach may eventually prove to be the best way to maximize the effectiveness of the heterogeneous constellation of symptoms that currently fall under the rubric of OCD.

REFERENCES

Abramowitz, J. S. (1996). Variants of exposure with response prevention in the treatment of obsessive–compulsive disorder: A meta-analysis. *Behavior Therapy, 27,* 583–600.

Abramowitz, J. S. (1997). Effectiveness of psychological and pharmacological treatments for obsessive–compulsive disorder: A quantitative review. *Journal of Consulting and Clinical Psychology, 65,* 44–52.

Abramowitz, J. S., Franklin, M. E., Schwartz, S. A., & Furr, J. M. (2003). Symptom presentation and outcome of cognitive–behavioral therapy for obsessive–compulsive disorder. *Journal of Consulting and Clinical Psychology, 71*, 1049–1057.

Abramowitz, J. S., Franklin, M. E., Street, G. P., Kozak, M. J., & Foa, E. B. (2000). Effects of comorbid depression on treatment for obsessive-compulsive disorder. *Behavior Therapy, 31*, 517–528.

Abramowitz, J. S., McKay, D., & Taylor, S. (2005). Subtypes in obsessive–compulsive disorder. *Behavior Therapy, 36*, 367–369.

Abramowitz, J. S., McKay, D., & Taylor, S. (Eds.). (2008). *Clinical handbook of obsessive–compulsive disorder and related problems*. Baltimore, MD: Johns Hopkins University Press.

Abramowitz, J. S., Taylor, S., & McKay, D. (2005). Potentials and limitations of cognitive treatments for obsessive–compulsive disorder. *Cognitive Behaviour Therapy, 34*, 140–147.

American Psychiatric Association. (2000). *Diagnostic and statistical manual of mental disorders* (4th ed., text rev.). Washington, DC: Author.

Antony, M. M., Purdon, C., & Summerfeldt, L. J. (Eds.). (2007). *Psychological treatment of obsessive–compulsive disorder: Fundamentals and beyond*. Washington, DC: American Psychological Association.

Beck, A. T., Steer, R. A., & Brown, G. K. (1996). *Beck Depression Inventory—Second edition manual*. San Antonio, TX: Psychological Corporation.

Bennett-Levy, J., Butler, G., Fennell, M., Hackman, A., Mueller, M., & Westbrook, D. (2004). *Oxford guide to behavioural experiments in cognitive therapy*. Oxford, England: Oxford Press.

Bland, R. C., Newman, S. C., & Orn, H. (1988). Period prevalence of psychiatric disorders in Edmonton. *Acta Psychiatrica Scandinavica, 77*(Suppl. 338), 33–42.

Brown, T. A., Campbell, L. A., Lehman, C. L., Grisham, J. R., & Mancill, R. B. (2001). Current and lifetime comorbidity of the *DSM–IV* anxiety and mood disorders in a large clinical sample. *Journal of Abnormal Psychology, 110*, 585–599.

Clark, D. A. (2004). *Cognitive–behavioral therapy for OCD*. New York: Guilford Press.

Denys, D., Tenney, N., van Megan, H. J. G. M., de Gaus, F., & Westenberg, H. G. M. (2004). Axis I and II comorbidity in a large sample of patients with obsessive–compulsive disorder. *Journal of Affective Disorders, 80*, 155–162.

Flament, M. F., & Bisserbe, J. C. (1997). Pharmacologic treatment of obsessive–compulsive disorder: Comparative studies. *Journal of Clinical Psychiatry, 58*(Suppl. 12), 18–22.

Foa, E. B. (1979). Failure in treating obsessive–compulsives. *Behaviour Research and Therapy, 17*, 169–176.

Foa, E. B., & Kozak, M. (1986). Emotional processing of fear: Exposure to corrective information. *Psychological Bulletin, 99*, 20–35.

Freeston, M. H., Ladouceur, R., Gagnon, F., Thibodeau, N., Rheume, J., Letarte, H., & Bujold, A. (1997). Cognitive–behavioral treatment of obsessive thoughts: A controlled trial. *Journal of Consulting and Clinical Psychology, 65*, 405–413.

Freeston, M. H., Ladouceur, R., Thibodeau, N., & Gagnon, F. (1991). Cognitive intrusions in a nonclinical population: I. Response style, subjective experience, and appraisal. *Behaviour Research and Therapy, 29*, 585–597.

Frost, R. O., & Tolin, D. F. (2008). Compulsive hoarding. In J. S. Abramowitz, D. McKay, & S. Taylor (Eds.), *Clinical handbook of obsessive–compulsive disorder and related problems* (pp. 76–94). Baltimore, MD: Johns Hopkins University Press.

Goodman, W. K., Price, L. H., Rasumssen, S. A., Mazure, C., Fleischmann, R. L., Hill, C. L., et al. (1989). The Yale-Brown Obsessive–Compulsive Scale: I. Development, use, and reliability. *Archives of General Psychiatry, 46*, 1006–1011.

Hantouche, E. G., Bouhassira, M., Lancrenon, S., & Ravily, V. (1995). Prévalence des troubles obsessionnels-compulsifs dans une large population française de patients consultant en psychiatrie [Epidemiological survey of obsessive–compulsive disorder and obsessive–compulsive syndromes in a large French outpatient psychiatric population]. *L'Encephale, 21*, 571–580.

Hofmann, S. G. (2007). Enhancing exposure-based therapy from a translational research perspective. *Behaviour Research and Therapy, 45*, 1987–2001.

Insel, T. R., Mueller, E. A., Alterman, I., Linnoila, M., & Murphy, D. L. (1985). Obsessive–compulsive disorder and serotonin: Is there a connection? *Biological Psychiatry, 20*, 1174–1188.

Insel, T. R., & Scolnick, E. M. (2006). Cure therapeutics and strategic prevention: Raising the bar for mental health research. *Molecular Psychiatry, 11*, 11–17.

Jenike, M. A. (1998). Theories of etiology. In M. A. Jenike, L. Baer, & W. E. Minichiello (Eds.), *Obsessive–compulsive disorders: Practical management* (3rd ed., pp. 203–221). St. Louis, MO: Mosby.

Keeley, M. L., Storch, E. A., Merlo, L. J., & Geffken, G. R. (2008). Clinical predictors of response to cognitive–behavioral therapy for obsessive–compulsive disorder. *Clinical Psychology Review, 28*, 118–130.

Kozak, M. J., & Foa, E. B. (1994). Obsessions, overvalued ideation, and delusions in obsessive–compulsive disorder. *Behaviour Research and Therapy, 32*, 343–353.

Mataix-Cols, D., Marks, I. M., Greist, J. H., Kobak, K. A., & Baer, L. (2002). Obsessive–compulsive symptom dimensions as predictors of compliance with and response to behaviour therapy: Results from a controlled trial. *Psychotherapy and Psychosomatics, 71*, 255–262.

McKay, D., Abramowitz, J., Calamari, J., Kyrios, M., Radomsky, A., Sookman, D., et al. (2004). A critical evaluation of obsessive–compulsive disorder subtypes: Symptoms versus mechanisms. *Clinical Psychology Review, 24*, 283–313.

McKay, D., & Gruner, P. (2008). Obsessive–compulsive disorder and schizotypy. In J. S. Abramowitz, D. McKay, & S. Taylor (Eds.), *Clinical handbook of obsessive–compulsive disorder and related problems* (pp. 126–138). Baltimore, MD: Johns Hopkins University Press.

Minichiello, W. E., Baer, L., & Jenike, M. A. (1987). Schizotypal personality disorder: A poor prognostic indicator for behavior therapy in the treatment of obsessive–compulsive disorder. *Journal of Anxiety Disorders, 1*, 273–276.

Moritz, S., Fricke, S., Jacobson, D., Kloss, M., Wien, C., Rufer, M., et al. (2004). Positive schizotypal symptoms predict treatment outcome in obsessive–compulsive disorder. *Behaviour Research and Therapy, 42*, 217–227.

Neziroglu, F., Stevens, K., Yaryura-Tobias, J. A., & McKay, D. (2001). Predictive validity of the overvalued ideas scale: Outcome in obsessive–compulsive and body dysmorphic disorders. *Behaviour Research and Therapy, 39*, 745–756.

Pato, M. T., & Zohar, J. (Eds.). (2001). *Current treatments of obsessive–compulsive disorder* (2nd ed.). Washington, DC: American Psychiatric Association.

Pull, C. B. (2007). Combined pharmacotherapy and cognitive–behavioural therapy for anxiety disorders. *Current Opinion in Psychiatry, 20*, 30–35.

Rachman, S., & Hodgson, R. J. (1980). *Obsessions and compulsions*. Englewood Cliffs, NJ: Prentice-Hall.

Rauch, S. L., & Savage, C. R. (2000). Investigating cortico-striatal pathophysiology in obsessive–compulsive disorders: Procedural learning and imaging probes. In W. K. Goodman, M. V. Rudorfer, & J. D. Maser (Eds.), *Obsessive–compulsive disorder: Contemporary issues in treatment* (pp. 133–154). Mahwah, NJ: Erlbaum.

Richard, D. C. S., & Gloster, A. T. (2007). Exposure therapy has a public relations problem: A dearth of litigation amid a wealth of concern. In D. C. S. Richard & D. L. Lauterbach (Eds.), *Handbook of exposure therapies* (pp. 409–425). Amsterdam: Academic Press.

Salkovskis, P. M. (1985). Obsessional-compulsive problems: A cognitive–behavioural analysis. *Behaviour Research and Therapy, 25*, 571–583.

Skapinakis, P., Papatheodorou, T., & Mavreas, V. (2007). Antipsychotic augmentation of serotonergic antidepressants in treatment-resistant obsessive–compulsive disorder: A meta-analysis of the randomized controlled trials. *European Neuropsychopharmacology, 17*, 79–93.

Stanley, M. A., Turner, S. M., & Borden, J. W. (1990). Schizotypal features in obsessive–compulsive disorder. *Comprehensive Psychiatry, 31*, 511–518.

Taylor, S., Abramowitz, J. S., & McKay, D. (2007). Cognitive–behavioral models of obsessive–compulsive disorder. In M. M. Antony, C. Purdon, & L. J. Summerfeldt (Eds.), *Psychological theories of obsessive–compulsive disorder: Fundamentals and beyond* (pp. 9–29). Washington, DC: American Psychological Association.

Taylor, S., McKay, D., & Abramowitz, J. (2005). Is obsessive–compulsive disorder a disturbance of security motivation? Comment on Szechtman & Woody (2004). *Psychological Review, 112*, 650–656.

Tolin, D. F., & Steketee, G. (2007). General issues in psychological treatment for obsessive–compulsive disorder. In M. M. Antony, C. Purdon, & L. J. Summerfeldt (Eds.), *Psychological treatment of obsessive–compulsive disorder: Fundamentals and beyond* (pp. 31–59). Washington, DC: American Psychological Association.

Torres, A. R., Prince, M. J., Bebbington, P. E., Bhugra, D., Brugha, T. S., Farrell, M., et al. (2006). Obsessive–compulsive disorder: Prevalence, comorbidity, impact, and help-seeking in the British National Comorbidity Survey of 2000. *The American Journal of Psychiatry, 163*, 1978–1985.

6

GENERALIZED ANXIETY DISORDER

MICHAEL R. RITTER, MICHELLE A. BLACKMORE,
AND RICHARD G. HEIMBERG

Generalized anxiety disorder (GAD) is a chronic and disabling disorder, with a lifetime prevalence of 6.1% (Kessler, Berglund, et al., 2005). GAD is frequently comorbid with depression, other anxiety disorders, and substance abuse (e.g., Kessler, Chiu, Demler, Merikangas, & Walters, 2005; Stein, 2002), and it is associated with significant impairment in occupational and social functioning (Kessler, Dupont, Berglund, & Wittchen, 1999). Unfortunately, rates of response to psychological treatments of GAD are poorer than those for other anxiety disorders (Borkovec & Ruscio, 2001; Fisher & Durham, 1999), in part because of our limited understanding of GAD relative to other anxiety disorders.

Major shifts in the diagnostic criteria for GAD from the third to the fourth editions of the *Diagnostic and Statistical Manual of Mental Disorders* (*DSM–III, DSM–IV*; American Psychiatric Association, 1980, 1994) reflect our improving understanding of GAD. One of the more important changes in the *DSM–IV* is recognition of excessive and pervasive worry as a central feature of GAD and the difficulty persons with GAD have in controlling their worry. Additionally, the specific content of worries was no longer considered in the diagnostic criteria, and it was recognized that worry could occur regardless of the number of events or activities in one's life that were affected (e.g., minor matters, work, health, interpersonal relationships). Unlike most other anxiety disorders, GAD is not characterized by excessive autonomic arousal, as previously thought, but rather by central nervous system activation and suppression of autonomic reactivity (Brown, Chorpita, & Barlow 1998; Thayer, Friedman, & Borkovec, 1996). Thus, the current conceptualization of GAD in the *DSM–IV* excludes a number of the autonomic symptoms (e.g., heart palpitations, sweating) that were a part of previous criteria sets. In *DSM–IV*, the essential feature of GAD is excessive worry occurring more days than not for at least 6 months (but note that both the excessiveness and duration criteria have been questioned; Kessler, Brandenburg, et al., 2005; Ruscio et al., 2005). The worry content may concern a number of different domains or activities (e.g., finances, health, social relationships, minor matters) and must be difficult to control. In addition, the worry or anxiety must be associated with at least three (one for children) of the following six symptoms: (a) restlessness, (b) fatigue, (c) impaired concentration, (d) irritability, (e) muscle tension, and (f) sleep disturbance. The worry must lead to significant distress or impairment and must not be due to another Axis I disorder, general medical condition, or a substance use disorder, and it may not occur solely during the course of a mood disorder (American Psychiatric Association, 1994).

EFFECTIVE TREATMENTS FOR GENERALIZED ANXIETY DISORDER

More accurate diagnosis and improved understanding of the central role of worry in GAD have improved our conceptualizations of the disorder and advanced the development of psychological treatment approaches. Although cognitive–behavioral therapies (CBTs) have been subjected to the most thorough evaluation in the empirical literature to date and has received the greatest empirical support (Nathan & Gorman, 2007), earlier CBT approaches were more generic and nonspecific. Increased knowledge of the disorder has encouraged the development of theory-driven, disorder-specific treatments (e.g., Barlow, Rapee, & Brown, 1992; Borkovec & Newman, 1999; Dugas & Robichaud, 2006; Roemer & Orsillo, 2005; Wells & Carter, 1999). Because of space limitations, we briefly discuss the treatments for GAD on the basis of the theoretical models developed by Borkovec, Alcaine, and Behar (2004); Dugas, Gagnon, Ladouceur, and Freeston (1998); and Wells and Carter (1999).

Borkovec's Avoidance Theory of Worry and Treatment

Combined self-control desensitization and cognitive therapy (SCD/CT; Borkovec & Newman, 1999) is among the most thoroughly studied treatments for GAD. It is based on the avoidance theory of worry, one of the most comprehensive models for the role of worry in GAD (Borkovec et al., 2004). Worry is described as an anticipatory cognitive process, consisting primarily of ruminative, verbal linguistic content (Borkovec, Ray, & Stöber, 1998). Borkovec et al. (2004) proposed that worry acts as a form of avoidance, given that the verbal linguistic nature of worry leads to a more abstract and disengaged experience of emotional topics than would be produced by more elaborated cognitive processing (i.e., images). Thus, worry is negatively reinforced because it temporarily spares the individual from more threatening content and reduces autonomic and emotional responding. However, this kind of short-term suppression of physiological and emotional responding is maladaptive in the long run as it does not allow for the full processing of threatening information necessary for anxiety reduction (Borkovec et al., 2004; Foa & Kozak, 1986). This avoidant cycle may prevent the individual from attending to and integrating evidence from the environment that would disconfirm his or her anxiety-related beliefs. Worry-related beliefs are less likely to be challenged and, therefore, more likely to be maintained.

The SCD/CT treatment has most typically been administered in 16 weekly sessions. Initial sessions focus on psychoeducation regarding the physiological, cognitive, and behavioral aspects of anxiety and a description of the treatment components and rationale. The first component of treatment involves teaching clients to self-monitor so that they can identify internal and external triggers that contribute to their anxiety (e.g., situations, thoughts, interpretations) and their idiosyncratic patterns of responding. In addition to helping clients better understand their anxiety, self-monitoring also begins to teach them to be more present-focused and aware of their present-moment experience (Borkovec, 2002).

Given the important role of psychophysiological characteristics in GAD, clients are then trained in a variety of relaxation skills (Bernstein, Borkovec, & Hazlett-Stevens, 2000), beginning with instruction in diaphragmatic breathing in the first session and progressive muscle relaxation in the second. Clients are taught how to breathe more slowly and deeply from the abdomen rather than the chest. Clients are initially taught to use these skills at times when they do not feel anxious.

The third component of treatment involves training in applied relaxation (Bernstein et al., 2000; Öst, 1987), applying abbreviated versions of learned relaxation skills in the context of increasingly anxiety- or worry-provoking situations. After being introduced to and practicing the various relaxation procedures, clients are encouraged to choose which techniques work best for them in a given situation and to utilize those techniques throughout the remainder of treatment and in their daily lives. A hierarchy consisting of a graduated list of situations, thoughts, worries, feelings, and physical sensations that contribute to the client's anxiety is developed.

SCD techniques (Goldfried, 1971) are taught early in treatment and involve training clients to vividly imagine anxiety-provoking situations and the thoughts, worries, images, and physical responses that are produced. Clients are then instructed to use their relaxation skills during these imaginal exposures in an effort to teach them how to bring about and terminate their anxiety. They are asked to progressively confront anxiety-provoking situations on their hierarchy, beginning with situations that elicit low to moderate anxiety. As clients learn to utilize coping skills to manage their anxiety in these situations, they then turn to the more anxiety-provoking situations on their hierarchy.

The fourth component of treatment involves CT. In addition to relaxation skills, clients are taught alternative ways to cope with their anxiety and worry utilizing cognitive restructuring techniques (e.g., identifying and challenging cognitive distortions, developing alternative interpretations, testing interpretations through behavioral experiments). The CT component also encourages the client to engage in expectancy-free living (i.e., to give up expectations or attempts to predict outcomes). This component allows clients to further practice present-moment living as they are taught to enter situations and experience each situation for what it is, without expectations. A *worry outcome diary* is often used to encourage clients to test their worry predictions. That is, clients are asked to write down each worry they have throughout the day and the associated feared outcome. At the end of the day, they rate whether the outcome and their ability to cope turned out better or worse than expected.

All four treatment components are introduced in the initial therapy sessions and built upon throughout the remainder of treatment, with an emphasis on living in the present moment. Once clients have gained some level of mastery over their anxiety and worry and are able to be more present-focused, they are taught to identify their life values, develop value-oriented perspectives, and engage in value-guided behavior (Borkovec & Sharpless, 2004).

Dugas's Intolerance of Uncertainty Model and Treatment

Dugas et al. (1998) highlighted the important role of worry and intolerance of uncertainty in the maintenance of GAD. *Intolerance of uncertainty* is the predisposition to react with strong, negative affect to ambiguous or uncertain situations and try to control these typically uncontrollable events to reduce anxiety. Dugas's model also proposes that poor problem solving, inaccurate positive beliefs about the value of worry, and cognitive avoidance also play primary roles in the etiology and maintenance of GAD.

Dugas and colleagues designed a CBT package on the basis of this model, which consists of 12 to 16 weekly sessions administered in either individual or group format (see Dugas et al., 2003; Dugas & Robichaud, 2006). During initial treatment sessions, clients receive psychoeducation regarding GAD and the role of worry and a description of the treatment components and rationale. The cycle of excessive worry is then targeted through training in worry awareness, in which clients are asked to monitor daily worries and distinguish between worries related to current problems and worries related to hypothetical situations (i.e., worries about situations that might or might not occur in some imagined future). The concept of intolerance of uncertainty is then introduced, and its role in the worry cycle is reviewed. Ways to increase tolerance of uncertainty are explored, and behavioral experiments (e.g., completing paperwork and turning it in before proofreading) that allow clients to practice progressively tolerating and accepting anxiety-provoking situations with uncertain outcomes are incorporated throughout the rest of treatment. Sessions then begin to incorporate education regarding positive worry beliefs (e.g., "Worry helps prevent bad things from happening") and how such beliefs perpetuate worry. These beliefs are then challenged and their usefulness reevaluated. Negative problem orientation and dysfunctional beliefs about problem solving (e.g., "I'm not a good problem solver") are then confronted, and more adaptive beliefs are targeted in session. Additionally, clients undergo problem-solving training that includes instruction in defining the problem, implementing solutions, and evaluating the effectiveness of implemented solutions. In later treatment sessions, core fears, often involving hypothetical situations, are confronted through imaginal exposure. In the final therapy sessions, skills learned in treatment are reviewed and a relapse prevention plan is developed.

Wells's Metacognitive Model and Treatment

The *metacognitive model* of GAD (Wells, 1995) also emphasizes the central role of worry in GAD and differentiates worry about specific events or situations (Type 1 worry) from metaworry (Type 2 worry) or negative appraisals of worry as itself dangerous and uncontrollable. Type 1 worry is hypothesized to be associated with positive beliefs about worry as a coping strategy. That is, the client is likely to believe that worry is beneficial because potential negative outcomes are generated and anxiety is reduced as responses are planned. Type 1 worry can, therefore, become problematic if worry is used in place of more adaptive coping strategies (e.g., emotional processing of feared situations) or elicits illusions of control. However, during Type 1 worry, a person may begin to engage in *metaworry*, or worrying about worrying (e.g., "I will go crazy because I can't stop worrying"), which increases his or her sense of threat and physiological arousal and, in turn, elicits more metaworry. The metacognitive model suggests that worry persists and becomes problematic because of the conflicting positive beliefs about worry and the negative beliefs that worry is dangerous and cannot be controlled. Further, to prevent worry, individuals may attempt to suppress thoughts that trigger worry. Paradoxically, attempts to suppress thoughts often lead to an increase in the frequency of those thoughts (Purdon, 1999; Wegner, Schneider, Carter, & White, 1987).

Positive and negative metacognitive beliefs and associated factors that maintain worry are the primary targets in metacognitive therapy. The treatment is typically conducted in 6 to 12 weekly sessions and incorporates a number of cognitive and behavioral experiments. Treatment begins by developing an individual case formulation using the metacognitive model to conceptualize a recent worry episode experienced by the client. The case formulation is then presented to the client to help him or her understand the role of metacognitive beliefs about worry and maladaptive coping strategies, as well as to explain the rationale behind metacognitive therapy. Treatment then focuses on challenging negative metacognitive beliefs about the uncontrollability of worry through worry-postponement experiments or mindfulness exercises (e.g., "watching" worry as a passive observer rather than trying to suppress thoughts). Ineffective strategies for the control of worry and the role of positive beliefs about worry in perpetuating it are discussed. Next, sessions focus on challenging and modifying beliefs about the danger of worry through cognitive restructuring and idiographically designed behavioral experiments (e.g., purposeful worrying to test if the client will "go crazy"). Sessions then focus on challenging and modifying positive beliefs about worry. This is done through behavioral experiments such as the mismatch strategy (Wells, 1997), in which the client is asked to list his or her worried outcomes and compare them with the actual outcomes that occurred in a situation that evoked worry. Another behavioral experiment, termed *worry modulation*, asks clients to worry more on certain occasions and less in others to determine if worry is associated with more positive outcomes. In the final sessions of treatment, a copy of the case formulation is given to the client, residual metacognitive beliefs are addressed, treatment techniques and skills learned are reviewed, and relapse prevention strategies are discussed.

EFFICACY OF COGNITIVE–BEHAVIORAL THERAPY FOR GENERALIZED ANXIETY DISORDER

Randomized controlled trials have evaluated relaxation training, cognitive restructuring, and multiple-component cognitive–behavioral approaches in the treatment of GAD. Whereas a full review of the efficacy of treatments for GAD is beyond the scope of this chapter, the following provides a brief account of the efficacy of different cognitive and behavioral treatments. Two recent studies compared the impact of applied relaxation and CT for the treatment of GAD. Öst and Breitholtz (2000) found that both applied relaxation and CT yielded clinically significant improvements. The proportions of clients who demonstrated clinically significant improvement were 53% and 62% at posttreatment and 67% and 56% at follow-up for applied relaxation and CT, respectively. Arntz (2003) also found both treatments to have similar effects at 6-month follow-up, with 55% of clients receiving cognitive and 53% of those receiving applied relaxation showing clinically significant improvement. Siev and Chambless (2007) came to a similar conclusion in a recent meta-analytic comparison of CT and relaxation therapy for GAD.

Several studies have investigated the impact of multiple-component treatments on GAD. Although some of these studies found differences between treatment groups, others failed to show such differences. For example, Borkovec et al. (1987) compared the efficacy of (a) progressive muscle relaxation training plus CT with (b) progressive muscle relaxation training plus nondirective therapy. The combination of progressive muscle relaxation training plus CT produced significantly greater improvement at posttreatment than did progressive muscle relaxation training plus nondirective therapy. However, a later study (Barlow et al., 1992) found that the efficacy of progressive muscle relaxation training plus CT was no different from progressive muscle relaxation training alone or CT alone in treating GAD. In addition, Borkovec and Costello (1993) compared the impact of (a) multicomponent CBT, (b) applied relaxation alone, and (c) nondirective therapy on GAD. Multicomponent CBT and applied relaxation were significantly more effective than nondirective therapy. However, applied relaxation was as effective as multicomponent CBT at posttreatment.

Borkovec and Ruscio (2001) reviewed the methodological characteristics and outcomes of 13 controlled trials of CBT for GAD. Their meta-analysis demonstrated that multicomponent treatments, as compared with wait-list or nonspecific control conditions, consistently produced the largest effect sizes at posttest and at follow-up. In contrast, the results of the meta-analysis were less clear when multicomponent CBT was compared with CT, applied relaxation, or SCD alone. That is, some studies showed that multicomponent CBT was superior to single component treatments, whereas other studies showed no difference. Later, Borkovec, Newman, Pincus, and Lytle (2002) provided GAD clients with (a) applied relaxation and SCD, (b) CT, or (c) the three components combined. All treatment groups showed significant improvements in anxiety at posttest and follow-up assessments. However, again, no single treatment group showed superior results. Borkovec et al. (2002) concluded that it was time to begin looking elsewhere (i.e., beyond traditional CBT) in order to find ways to improve treatment outcomes for GAD.

Consistent with Borkovec et al.'s (2002) conclusions, researchers have looked beyond traditional approaches to develop new and innovative psychological treatments for GAD. For example, Ladouceur et al. (2000) developed a treatment focusing on a GAD client's characteristic intolerance of uncertainty. Posttreatment data from a randomized controlled trial showed that 77% of clients no longer met criteria for GAD. These treatment gains were largely maintained at 6- and 12-month follow-up. In a second randomized controlled trial, Dugas et al. (2003) tested the same treatment for GAD in a group format. Sixty percent of participants were responders (i.e., they showed a change of 20% or more from pretest to posttest), and 65% met criteria for high end-state functioning (i.e., they demonstrated a posttreatment score within one standard deviation of the mean of normative samples on at least five of seven measures).

Wells (1997) also developed a novel approach to treating GAD, focusing on metacognitive beliefs about worry, described earlier. Results from a recent open trial (Wells & King, 2006) showed promising recovery rates (87.5% at posttreatment and 75% at 6- and 12-month follow-ups). However, these results should be considered cautiously, given the limited sample size ($N = 10$) and the absence of a control group. Finally, Roemer and Orsillo (2007) developed an innovative treatment for GAD, integrating mindfulness and acceptance-based approaches with more traditional CBT. Data from their open trial ($N = 16$) showed significant changes in clinician-rated severity of GAD and significant improvements in quality of life at posttest and follow-up. These new approaches continue to show promise but much more research is needed to further help individuals with GAD. Although CBT has been shown to be efficacious for GAD (Borkovec & Ruscio, 2001), GAD is generally regarded as the least CBT-responsive anxiety disorder (Campbell & Brown, 2002).

FACTORS THAT LEAD TO POOR TREATMENT RESPONSE

Future treatments may benefit by identifying specific predictors of poor treatment response. However, few studies of the treatment of GAD have made strong efforts to identify factors that predict positive or negative treatment response. Durham (2006) reviewed the available literature and identified variables that may predict treatment outcome, and these are reviewed next.

Demographic Variables

Research has shown that demographic variables can be predictive of treatment outcome in GAD. For example, individuals of low socioeconomic status (SES), who are single (or widowed), or who are 65 years of age or older (Wetherell et al., 2005) are less likely to respond to treatment and have a significantly lower likelihood of maintaining treatment gains (Durham, Allan, & Hackett, 1997). These persons have fewer resources to cope with daily stressors than their married/cohabitating, younger, higher SES counterparts. Although the specific reasons that these variables predict poorer treatment response are unknown, one might speculate that any variable that is associated with higher numbers of uncontrollable daily stressors, lower social position, and/or fewer coping resources may increase vulnerability to difficult cognitions and emotions.

Interpersonal Difficulties

Relationship difficulties have also been shown to predict poor treatment response in GAD. Borkovec et al. (2002) found that pretherapy interpersonal problems (i.e., tendencies toward being domineering, vindictive, or overly nurturing) are associated with poor end-state functioning both after therapy and at 6-month follow-up. Similarly, Durham et al. (1997) found that married and cohabitating clients with GAD had a greater probability of improvement and a decreased probability of relapse. However, this finding was dependent on the general quality of the relationship. That is, the amount of disharmony or tension in those relationships was a powerful predictor of relapse. As noted previously, the mechanism by which these interpersonal difficulties influence treatment outcomes is not known. However, one might speculate that reoccurring interpersonal difficulties and an increased propensity to worry about social concerns (Roemer, Molina, & Borkovec, 1997) might act to increase real or perceived environmental threats and result in an increase in worry and anxiety. Furthermore, increased interpersonal difficulties may act to diminish social support that might otherwise be available to help keep worries in perspective.

Symptom Severity and Comorbidity

Evidence suggests that the severity of GAD symptoms has a negative impact on treatment outcome (Butler, 1993; Durham et al., 2004; Wetherell et al., 2005). That is, the frequency and intensity of anxiety and worry at the initiation of therapy is likely to affect clients' response to treatment. This finding is widely consistent with research regarding predictors of psychotherapy treatment outcome in general (e.g., Clarkin & Levy, 2004). Symptom severity is often exacerbated by other comorbid disorders, and, in the case of GAD, comorbidity is a common occurrence. In fact, GAD has been found to be one of the most frequent additional diagnoses in clients who have another anxiety or mood disorder (Brown, Campbell, Lehman, Grisham, & Mancill, 2001). Existing GAD outcome research has suggested that the presence of an additional Axis I disorder is strongly related to decreased posttreatment outcomes and to subsequent relapse at follow-up (Durham et al., 1997). For example, one study showed that GAD with comorbid depression was associated with poorer treatment outcomes than was GAD alone (Barlow et al., 1992). Although research has not examined the impact of Axis II disorders on the outcome of treatment for GAD, it seems reasonable to think that such comorbidity would decrease the likelihood of a positive prognosis after treatment and at follow-up (Clarkin & Levy, 2004).

Client Motivation

Research has also identified client motivation as another predictor of outcome (Dugas et al., 2003; Léger, Dugas, Langlois, & Ladouceur, 1998). Client motivation can negatively affect treatment outcomes in a variety of ways. Compared with other psychological treatment approaches, CBT requires more client-initiated effort between treatment sessions. For example, a person receiving CBT for GAD may have multiple homework assignments to complete before the next session (e.g., daily self-monitoring, daily practice of diaphragmatic breathing or relaxation skills, and conduct of various behavioral experiments). In CBT, homework assignments are considered essential for transferring skills learned in session into the client's real life and for accelerating treatment gains. However, motivating clients to comply with such assignments can be extremely challenging.

CASE EXAMPLE

Mary was a 27-year-old single woman who presented to treatment for chronic worry and depression. Mary had a 2-year-old daughter and was employed as a fifth-grade teacher in an inner city public school. Mary reported that she was fortunate to grow up in a home with two loving parents. She noted, however, that both of her parents have struggled with worry and anxiety. She reported being a worrier for as long as she could remember and noted an increase in her anxiety and worry as she began taking on more adult responsibilities (e.g., teaching, motherhood). When Mary presented for treatment (toward the end of the fall semester), she was experiencing excessive and uncontrollable worry concerning a number life domains, including areas that seemed relatively minor (e.g., getting to work and other appointments on time, mechanical problems with her car, computer viruses). She reported having trouble making decisions and completing her day-to-day tasks and responsibilities. She endorsed having difficulty concentrating; being easily fatigued; having muscle tension in her face, neck and shoulders; and experiencing increased irritability.

Mary reported that her anxiety and worry became increasingly excessive and uncontrollable with the introduction of a new principal at the beginning of the school year. The new principal made it clear that her employment status each year would now be largely dependent upon her students' annual standardized test scores. In addition, the new principal required teachers to submit weekly teaching plans for his review and would regularly stop by classrooms to observe the teachers without prior warning. For Mary, this increased pressure was like pouring salt on an open wound. Mary had worried about losing her job since she started teaching 5 years ago. Although her performance as a teacher had never been questioned, she did not believe she measured up to other teachers in her school. She explained that the other teachers seemed to garner much more love and respect from the children than she did. She reasoned that if she were a better teacher, then her kids would have better grades and fewer behavioral problems in her classroom. The added pressure and scrutiny from the new principal led her to believe that her job was seriously at risk. Mary noted that she had been spending an excessive amount of time preparing her teaching plan for the principal each week. She believed that if she spent extra time on the plan that the principal would be less likely to discover her incompetence. She noted, however, that the extra time spent preparing her teaching plans had caused her to fall behind in other aspects of her job (e.g., grading student homework and quizzes). This led her to further question her competence as a teacher and gave her additional reasons to worry.

Mary also worried about her current and future finances. She was ashamed to admit that she was dependent on her parents to meet her basic financial needs. Although Mary was grateful to her parents for providing child care for her daughter, she believed that she would feel better about herself if she were able to take care of her own needs. She worried about having enough money for retirement. She was concerned that she would never be able to save money on a teacher's salary. She often found herself thinking about other careers she could pursue that would provide greater financial security. However, her beliefs about her own incompetence as a teacher caused her to seriously doubt whether she would be any more successful in another career.

Mary also worried excessively about contracting diabetes. Although she had a positive family history for Type 2 diabetes, her annual medical examinations revealed no cause for concern at the current time. Nevertheless, she worried that her high level of stress would increase her probability of developing diabetes. Self-monitoring during the initial sessions of treatment showed that she sometimes misinterpreted her psychological symptoms (e.g., fatigue, irritability, difficulty concentrating) as early signs of diabetes. These misinterpretations were typically associated with immediate increases in her anxiety and worry. Mary also worried about the health of her parents, their getting older and eventually dying, and how she would cope without them.

Mary completed an assessment interview using the Anxiety Disorders Interview Schedule for DSM–IV (Brown, DiNardo, & Barlow 1994) that showed her principal diagnosis was GAD and that she met criteria for an additional diagnosis of major depressive disorder, single episode, mild. The interview confirmed that Mary's depression was brought about by excessive negative thoughts about her future (i.e., worry). Although Mary may not be considered a refractory case by some standards, as will be demonstrated, her treatment needs were multifaceted. As is typical with many GAD clients, Mary's treatment proved to be a complex undertaking.

Treatment

Mary's treatment plan was based primarily on the model of CBT developed by Borkovec (Borkovec et al., 2002; Borkovec & Sharpless, 2004). The primary treatment components consisted of psychoeducation, early cue detection through self-monitoring, relaxation training, mindfulness, CT, response prevention, applied relaxation, and SCD.

Psychoeducation and Self-Monitoring

As part of psychoeducation, Mary was instructed that anxiety is related to her thoughts, physiological responses, and behaviors. The therapist was interested in helping Mary become familiar with the typical ways that she thinks, feels, and behaves in response to interactions with her internal and external world. It was also hypothesized that self-monitoring would help her to become more focused on the present moment. Like most individuals with GAD, Mary spent too much time "in her head," wrapped up in her own thoughts, and too little time interacting with present-moment reality. It was also important that she use the self-monitoring form as soon as she recognized an increase in anxiety so that she could learn to catch the earliest shifts towards anxiety. Developing this awareness would help her to implement more adaptive coping responses. Mary was also asked to monitor any moments when she felt pleasant emotions. GAD is characterized by increased attention to threat in the environment. In an effort to counter this attentional bias, Mary was asked to keep a diary of events or situations in which she experienced emotions ranging from neutral to pleasant. She was also asked to list five things each day for which she could express a sense of gratitude.

It is common for clients to have problems complying with self-monitoring, and there are several ways to improve compliance. First, therapists should inquire whether clients understand the rationale behind self-monitoring (e.g., "How will you benefit by daily self-monitoring?" or "Why would an investment in self-monitoring be beneficial?"). Such questions can assess the client's level of understanding and provide an opportunity for further dialogue as needed. Second, the therapist can help clients identify any obstacles that might prevent them from fully complying with immediate self-monitoring. For example, Mary noted that it would be difficult to record when she was teaching but agreed to record afterward as soon as she could. Mary also decided that having easy access to her self-monitoring form would be helpful (e.g., in her pocket or purse, on her nightstand or desk).

Mindful Diaphragmatic Breathing

The therapist introduced Mary to the concept of mindfulness. She was given a handout that defined *mindfulness* as "paying attention in a particular way: on purpose, in the present moment, and nonjudgmentally" (Kabat-Zinn, 1994, p. 4). After further discussing mindfulness and its application to GAD

(Borkovec & Sharpless, 2004), the therapist introduced Mary to the practice of mindful diaphragmatic breathing. A common way to practice mindfulness is to attend to one's breathing while nonjudgmentally experiencing any thoughts or difficult sensations that might be present while doing so. After practicing in session, Mary agreed to practice at least twice a day for 10 minutes. Initially, the therapist did not discuss how diaphragmatic breathing could be utilized to decrease tension, but this was discussed in a later session. The goal was for Mary to gain experience with mindfulness before employing breathing techniques for anxiety reduction. In a later session, the therapist completed a mindful raisin exercise (Segal, Williams, & Teasdale, 2002) as a way to give Mary an experiential "taste" of the present moment. The exercise uses a raisin as the object of mindful attention, during which the participant was asked to focus her awareness on different aspects of the raisin and to experience the raisin as if she were a child who had never seen or tasted one before (i.e., beginner's mind; Segal et al., 2002).

Relaxation Skills

We taught Mary a variety of relaxation techniques as a way to help her cope with anxiety: progressive muscle relaxation, relaxation by recall, cue-controlled relaxation, and imagery relaxation (Bernstein et al., 2000). First, the therapist explained the rationale for using relaxation exercises in general and progressive muscle relaxation more specifically. Mary responded well to her first experience with progressive muscle relaxation in session. She was amazed at how well a relatively short exercise could reduce her anxiety and tension. However, twice daily practice proved to be a significant barrier to her progress in treatment. Mary felt that she could not find the time in her busy schedule to practice relaxation skills. Also, once she arrived home from work, she did not feel comfortable asking her parents to watch her daughter while she spent time relaxing.

Like Mary, many clients have great difficulty practicing relaxation twice a day. Yet, there are a number of strategies that therapists can use to help motivate this practice. The therapist asked Mary to close her eyes and imagine how her life might be different a year from now if she were able to deploy the same relaxation response that she experienced in session without the aid of a therapist. Although Mary believed that relaxation was an important skill to learn, she could not commit to practicing twice a day. As a compromise, Mary agreed to practice once in the evenings before bedtime.

It is important for therapists to consistently emphasize the importance of relaxation practice as clients will struggle with various barriers to compliance. In this case, the therapist helped Mary to identify and implement solutions that increased the probability of regular practice. Clients may also struggle with relaxation practice because of misunderstandings or problems that inhibit a full and satisfying relaxation response in session. As needed, the therapist should help the client make adjustments to in-session practice until deep relaxation is achieved (see Bernstein et al., 2000). Clients typically feel more motivated to practice relaxation between sessions when they have experienced a satisfying relaxation response in session with the therapist. Another strategy is to use analogies (e.g., learning to ride a bike) to further illustrate how relaxation is learned by consistent and regular practice. Rygh and Sanderson (2004) offered the following analogy to increase the perceived value of progressive muscle relaxation:

> Relaxation is like rain. Relaxation replenishes the body and mind's reservoir of energy. When people allow their bodies and minds to relax, they actually have more energy and become more efficient and productive in the long run. When they deprive themselves of relaxation, their bodies and minds are quickly drained of energy and become less efficient overall. (p. 131)

Some clients, despite the therapist's patience, validation, persistence, and motivation, will have difficulty completing relaxation exercises. Although progressive muscle relaxation can be an important part of a client's treatment, it is most important for clients to feel that they can be open and honest about their adherence to between-session homework assignments. First, as the outcome literature has suggested, progressive muscle relaxation is not an essential component of treatment success (e.g., Ladouceur et al., 2000). In Mary's case, however, one of her primary worry triggers was her chronic neck and facial tension. Thus, we believed that progressive muscle relaxation would benefit her greatly. Second, allowing clients room to openly discuss homework noncompliance without shame or guilt may be beneficial to the therapeutic relationship and to the client's ultimate treatment success.

During another session, the therapist introduced Mary to imagery relaxation. Mary identified a pleasant beach scene and was asked to describe the scene in detail (e.g., colors, sights, sounds, smells, tactile sensations). Mary selected "Let go, and get away" as the phrase she would use to quickly cue the relaxing image in response to incipient anxiety. She practiced turning the image on after stating "Let go, and get away" and keeping the image clearly in mind (i.e., picturing herself as if she was actually there) until the therapist told her to stop visualizing the scene. The practice continued until Mary could effectively turn the image on, keep it vividly in her mind, and turn it off on command. Mary was instructed to practice visualizing the scene (as previously described) during the relaxation enjoyment period of her home relaxation practice. Over time, she advanced through seven-muscle group and four-muscle group relaxation exercises and learned to effectively use relaxation by recall and cue-controlled relaxation (Bernstein et al., 2000).

As Mary became more confident with progressive muscle relaxation and relaxation by recall, she was introduced to applied relaxation. In applied relaxation, Mary was instructed to use a relaxation response between sessions at the earliest detection of anxiety (i.e., a shift away from a relaxed state). To encourage the use of applied relaxation between sessions, the therapist coached her to use her relaxation skills in session anytime she experienced a slight increase in anxiety.

Cognitive Therapy

We first introduced Mary to CT when she was taught the relationship among thoughts, somatic sensations, and behaviors. We helped her to assess the accuracy of her thoughts and beliefs by providing a list of common thinking errors to facilitate this process. Throughout therapy, we used a number of cognitive techniques, including logical analysis, examination of evidence, and considering the probability of feared outcomes. After generating alternative beliefs or thoughts, she was guided to test these new perceptions in the real world through collaboratively designed behavioral experiments. Given the inflexible and rigid nature of many persons with GAD, it is important to build flexibility into the typical way they perceive and think about worrisome situations or events (Borkovec & Sharpless, 2004). To initiate this process with Mary, the therapist proposed that they practice generating novel and multiple perspectives by playing a game called What Can You Do With That? In this game, the therapist and client take turns selecting an object in the therapy room, generating an alternative nonsensical way to use the object, and demonstrating how to use the object in the suggested way. For example, after explaining the rules of the game, the therapist showed Mary a pencil and then impersonated a baseball player using the pencil as a baseball bat. The therapist handed the pencil to Mary, who needed a little encouragement but eventually stood up and used the pencil as if it were a key to unlock the door. This process continued back and forth between Mary and the therapist with various objects until it was apparent that Mary understood the exercise. Mary was then asked to continue this exercise as homework with various objects she encountered during the week. The playful and humorous nature of the task facilitates a more flexible and novel interpretation of objects in the client's present-moment environment (for review, see Borkovec & Sharpless, 2004).

As Mary became more comfortable with generating novel perspectives with ordinary objects, she was encouraged to begin working with increasingly anxiety- and worry-related themes. Mary recalled that she had received an e-mail from the principal asking her to meet with him the following week. The request made her extremely nervous; she had generated a number of catastrophic reasons for the meeting and the worst possible outcomes (e.g., poor performance, increased scrutiny, job loss). Once her worries were identified, Mary began generating alternative reasons for meeting with the principal using What Can You Do With That? Mary was able to generate a number of alternative thoughts, some of them humorous and some with more utility (e.g., "The principal wants to ask me on a date"; "The principal has never talked with me individually, so he may be interested in building rapport"; "Perhaps one of my students is having trouble at home, and the principal wants to talk with me about it"). After listing several different possibilities, Mary was encouraged to narrow the list down by assessing several factors (e.g., likelihood of occurrence, impact on her anxiety). After a few minutes, she reduced the list to three alternative possibilities that were written on paper and given to her. In this case, Mary's actual meeting with the principal served as a behavioral experiment. As it turned out, the principal met with Mary about a topic that she had not considered but that was also not catastrophic. Over the course of treatment, Mary developed a more flexible relationship with her thoughts and her perceptions of "reality." She learned to quickly identify less adaptive thoughts and to take multiple perspectives in reaction to any single event or situation.

Modifying Core Beliefs. Individuals with GAD have a number of core beliefs that contribute to their difficulty with anxiety. Core beliefs are so fundamental to clients' experience that they are often unable to articulate them. Nevertheless, these ideas are regarded by the person as absolute truths (i.e., "just the way things are"; Beck, 1995). Research has identified a few core beliefs associated with GAD (e.g., positive or negative beliefs about worry, intolerance of uncertainty); however, many problematic core beliefs are likely be more idiographic in nature. The therapist used the downward arrow technique as a way to identify Mary's core beliefs. In this technique, the therapist first identifies a key thought that is suspected to stem from a dysfunctional belief. Next, the therapist asks the client to articulate the meaning of that thought. The client's response is typically another thought, which the therapist questions in similar fashion. The therapist continues questioning each successively revealed thought until he or she has uncovered one or more important beliefs. Beck (1995, p. 145) noted that asking "what a thought means about the patient" typically reveals a core belief. Using the downward arrow technique, we discovered that Mary's concern about incompetence was, in reality, part of a deeper rooted fear of failure (e.g., in her career, as a mother, with her finances), which is a common core theme among individuals with GAD.

Consistent with a mindfulness perspective, we wanted Mary to begin placing more value on the process of living in the present moment and less value on specific outcomes. Individuals with GAD tend to place excessive value on future goal attainment while heavily discounting their present-moment experience. To help her to place more value on the present moment, we utilized the downhill skiing metaphor (Hayes, Strosahl, & Wilson, 1999). The metaphor juxtaposes the goal or outcome of skiing with the process of skiing. More specifically, Mary was asked to imagine a beautiful ski slope covered with fluffy white new snow. She arrives at the top of the ski lift only to see a man walk up to her and ask where she is going. Mary points down and says, "I am going down to the bottom toward the ski lodge." At this point, the man throws her back on the ski lift heading down the hill, which drops her off at the lodge. This process continues repeatedly until she says, "Hey, I am not here to ride the ski lift, I am here to ski." This story initiated a conversation regarding the value of the present moment, the value of living to achieve future outcomes, and how to strike a healthy balance. We were also interested in reframing her negative beliefs about failure. One way that we did this was to discuss a number of famous American icons who built their success on top of numerous failures (e.g., Abraham Lincoln, Thomas Edison). Second, we discussed American culture's obsession with success and its lack of emphasis on virtues like persistence, resilience, and humility. Third, we presented her with a handout that listed alternative ways to view failure (e.g., "I can learn from my failure"; "Everyone fails eventually"; "Behaviors fail, not people"; viewing difficulty/failure as a challenge; see Leahy, 2005). We talked about each alternative viewpoint and discussed relevant examples with her. Finally, as a way to solidify her new beliefs about failure, Mary was asked to develop her own Bill of Rights for someone who is "good enough." This was an assignment in which she was to declare that she had the right to be less than perfect, to have a learning curve, and to grow through experiences like all other human beings (Leahy, 2005).

Positive Beliefs About Worry. We were interested in identifying any positive beliefs that Mary had about her worry habits. It is common for individuals to have one or more positive beliefs about worry, including the following: (a) "Worry motivates me," (b) "Worry facilitates problem solving," (c) "Worry can magically prevent threatening outcomes," (d) "Worry shows care and concern," and (e) "Worry can prepare me for the worst possible outcome" (Borkovec & Roemer, 1995). Failure to help clients identify and challenge these beliefs allows them to remain in a "love–hate" relationship with their worry habit. That is, individuals with GAD may be reluctant to fully jettison their worry because of the perceived benefits it provides. The Why Worry II Questionnaire (Holowka, Dugas, Francis, & Laugesen, 2000) is a reliable and efficient device for the assessment of these beliefs. The therapist reviewed Mary's responses to this questionnaire with her in session. This quick assessment showed that Mary held several positive beliefs about worry. For example, Mary believed that worrying about her competence as a teacher would motivate her to improve her teaching skills and would also prepare her for the worst possible outcome. Mary also endorsed the belief that worrying about other people (e.g., parents, children in her classroom) showed that she was a kind, caring, and thoughtful person.

On the basis of this assessment, the therapist helped Mary reevaluate whether her worry habit was as beneficial as she might believe. The major aim was to help Mary develop greater flexibility regarding these beliefs by viewing them as interpretations rather than as facts. After a brief discussion, Mary had little difficulty abandoning her belief that worry aided in motivation. For example, she acknowledged that her worries regarding her perceived incompetence only hindered her efforts to become a better teacher. She also acknowledged that the benefits of preparing for the worst possible outcome were completely outweighed by the costs. However, Mary did believe that worrying about other people was an important way to show her concern and love. In an effort to challenge this belief, we asked Mary to engage in the lawyer–prosecutor role-play (see Dugas & Robichaud, 2006). In this exercise, Mary first played the role of a lawyer whose goal was to convince the jury how worry can help you to be a more compassionate and caring person. After playing the role of the lawyer, Mary played the role of the prosecutor who tried to convince the jury how worry was detrimental to being a compassionate and carrying person. The role-play allowed Mary to become more aware of the costs of worrying about others and to acknowledge other things she could do to show her concern for people that would cause less emotional distress on her part.

Safety Behaviors

Many individuals with GAD engage in safety behaviors. Salkovskis (1991) defined *safety behaviors* as behaviors performed specifically to prevent or minimize feared consequences. Research has shown that the removal of client safety behaviors significantly improves treatment outcomes (Salkovskis, Clark, Hackmann, Wells, & Gelder, 1999). Although cognitive reframing will help clients reconsider the need to worry, clients will continue to experience strong urges to engage in a number of habitual safety behaviors. Clients with GAD may be able to acknowledge and identify some of their safety behaviors but be unaware of other habitual ways of responding to their anxiety. Years of negative reinforcement may have conditioned them to reduce negative affect by performing a number of excessive and/or unnecessary coping behaviors. Individuals with GAD may be motivated to perform these behaviors from a strong fear of their own anxious responding (Mennin, Heimberg, Turk, & Fresco, 2002). Thus, the therapist's task is to help clients understand how safety behaviors maintain worry and anxiety and to provide them with strategies to help reduce the need to engage in safety behaviors. The therapist explains that safety behaviors may temporarily reduce anxious arousal, but they also interfere with clients' ability to learn whether their threat perceptions are accurate. The therapist further explains how repeated exposure and response prevention will help clients learn that the feared consequences are unlikely to occur and that they can successfully cope without engaging in safety behaviors.

For example, Mary noted that she spent an unreasonable amount of time completing her weekly teaching plans for the principal. Mary was spending approximately 6 to 7 hours editing her existing teaching plans each week whereas other teachers were spending approximately 1 to 2 hours. Mary agreed that the extra time and effort spent was aimed at preventing negative events from occurring. The therapist explained that overpreparing prevented her from learning that it was her own effort and skill as a teacher that kept her "out of trouble" with the principal. Mary agreed with the therapist's intuition but was hesitant to reduce the amount of time she spent creating teaching plans. The therapist suggested a behavioral experiment in which Mary would incrementally reduce the amount of time she spent on teaching plans each week and see if any of her predicted negative consequences occurred. The therapist also stressed the importance and need for healthy levels of risk taking and for tolerating uncertainty (Dugas et al., 1998). That is, the therapist wanted Mary to recognize that a certain degree of risk taking can be a normal and healthy coping response and by spending less time on her teaching plan she was obviously increasing her risk. After a brief period of Socratic questioning, Mary agreed that spending less time on many of her tasks would be a risk worth taking to be a more effective teacher. She agreed to reduce the amount of time she spent on her teaching plan by 1 hour each week until she was spending an average of 2 to 3 hours per week. It took Mary 6 weeks before she was able to successfully complete her teaching plan within the specified time frame. Over the course of treatment, she learned that she did not need to invest as much time in her teaching plans as she had in the past.

Later, the therapist discovered that Mary was engaging in other safety behaviors. For example, Mary was actively avoiding places in which she might come into contact with the principal. Mary reasoned that the principal would be less likely to scrutinize her if she remained out of his presence (i.e., "out of sight, out of mind"). The therapist explained that her continued avoidance of the principal reinforced her belief that she was inadequate, incompetent, or under constant scrutiny. The therapist helped Mary to develop a list of places that she avoided for this reason. Mary was able to work through this minihierarchy within a few weeks, and the therapist added "amount of principal avoidance" to her weekly self-monitoring form as a way to remind Mary to continue her approach behavior.

Self-Control Desensitization

The purpose of SCD (Goldfried, 1971) was to increase Mary's control over worry. Like applied relaxation, SCD provides a way of interrupting the client's spiral of worry and anxiety by catching increases in anxiety early and applying a relaxation response. From a theoretical perspective, the repeated pairing of anxiety-evoking stimuli with a relaxation response works to strengthen the associations between the fearful stimuli and the incompatible response. SCD is completed in session by first constructing a hierarchy of worry triggers and worry responses (e.g., cognitions, physiological arousal, behaviors). The therapist worked closely with Mary to construct a hierarchy of items that represented her various worry episodes/themes (e.g., contracting diabetes, finances) and different intensity levels of anxiety. The therapist and client arranged the worry themes from the least to the most anxiety provoking. The therapist and Mary worked collaboratively to build a hierarchy that touched on many of her major worry themes.

Once the therapist explained the procedure to Mary, they began SCD by first bringing Mary into a relaxed state. Any relaxation techniques that have been effective for the client in the past can be used (e.g., progressive muscle relaxation, relaxation imagery, relaxation by recall). After Mary was deeply relaxed, external and internal anxiety cues descriptive of the particular hierarchy item were verbally presented by the therapist until Mary signaled (raised her finger) a slight increase in anxiety. For example, one of the items (worry triggers) on Mary's hierarchy represented her fear of contracting diabetes. A common trigger for this worry theme occurred whenever she overheard her parents talking about current or impending diabetes-related health problems. She would become anxious and begin to worry and wonder if she would ever have a better quality of life. She was also concerned whether she would be able to take care of her daughter or her future grandchildren if she had diabetes. Thus, the therapist began by presenting a verbal description of Mary's feared future and her anxious thoughts about this situation. Mary was asked to imagine in her "mind's eye" the different images being described to her.

Next, the therapist continued to provide a combination of anxiety cues and relaxation instructions (i.e., "let go" and "relax"). While listening to the therapist's monologue (as just described), Mary deployed her relaxation response. Once Mary returned to a relaxed state, she lowered her finger and continued to imagine herself in the situation for an additional 20 seconds while the therapist simultaneously encouraged her to relax even more deeply without presenting additional anxiety cues. The final sequence of SCD was to allow Mary to focus exclusively on the relaxation she had just generated for 20 seconds. The therapist repeated each item on the hierarchy until Mary was able to reduce her anxiety within 7 seconds of its occurrence or she was able to remain relaxed after a 1-minute presentation of an anxiety cue on three occasions. Under the guidance of her therapist, Mary completed the SCD hierarchy for several of her most common worry triggers. She reported that SCD helped her reduce the intensity of her anxious responding and her tendency to begin worrying when confronted with these worry themes.

Assessing the Impact of Treatment

It is important for therapists to review with the client improvements that have occurred since entering treatment. When treatment has failed to produce desired results, the therapist and client should work to identify barriers to progress and discuss different treatment options. However, even when treatment has been "successful," it is common for clients to minimize or fail to notice the changes that have occurred. One way to review client improvement is to review their pretreatment scores on self-report questionnaires (e.g., Penn State Worry Questionnaire [PSWQ]; Meyer, Miller, Metzger, & Borkovec, 1990) and or derived from a semistructured interview (e.g., Anxiety Disorders Interview Schedule for *DSM–IV*; Brown et al., 1994) and compare them with more recent scores and verbal symptom reports. The therapist and Mary reviewed her scores on the PSWQ and made mention of the individual items that showed dramatic improvement. At posttreatment assessment, Mary's PSWQ scores had dropped from 66 to 41. The therapist explained to Mary that her PSWQ scores were inidicative of individuals who would not typically seek treatment for worry (Behar, Alcaine, Zuellig, & Borkovec, 2003). In addition, they reviewed the diagnostic criteria for GAD and depression (American Psychiatric Association, 1994) and noted that she no longer met criteria for either disorder. We believe that Mary's improvement was due to a number of different treatment strategies, such as (a) identifying barriers to practicing relaxation, (b) focusing on the value of present-moment experience, (c) increasing her cognitive flexibility, (d) identifying and challenging her positive beliefs about worry, (e) identifying and eliminating safety behaviors, and (f) SCD.

Relapse Prevention

Once the therapist and Mary agreed to conclude treatment, two additional sessions were scheduled 2 weeks apart to discuss relapse prevention. For Mary to maintain her treatment gains, we informed her that she would need to continue practicing the skills learned in treatment on a regular basis. The therapist explained that she should continue practicing these skills until they become fully internalized habitual responses. It is very common for clients to stop using skills learned in treatment when they begin to feel better. The therapist helped Mary to determine how she might maintain the use of these skills in the absence of weekly treatment sessions. It is also important for therapists to prepare clients for the possibility of relapse. A return of painful symptoms is often perceived in negative terms by clients (e.g., "I am a failure"). Therapists can help clients to see that relapses are simply an opportunity to learn additional ways of coping with anxiety. In addition, therapists should encourage clients to return for booster sessions whenever their own efforts prove to be ineffective.

CONCLUSIONS AND FUTURE DIRECTIONS

At this point in time, CBT provides the best psychological approach to treating GAD. However, only 50% of individuals receiving CBT for GAD obtain clinically significant change (Fisher, 2006). We reviewed factors that negatively affect initial and long-term outcomes of CBT for GAD. Research has shown that client motivation (Leger et al., 1998), demographic variables (e.g., SES, single/widowed; Durham, 2006), relationship difficulties (Borkovec et al., 2002), symptom severity, and diagnostic comorbidity (Durham et al., 2004) are all predictive of poor treatment outcomes.

GAD is generally regarded as the anxiety disorder least responsive to CBT (Campbell & Brown, 2002). Although GAD continues to be considerably less studied than most of the other anxiety disorders (Dugas, 2000), new innovative treatments have recently been developed, and promising results have been reported (e.g., Dugas et al., 2003; Mennin, 2006; Roemer & Orsillo, 2007; Wells & King, 2006). Treatments that emphasize acceptance and regulation of emotional experience, focus on the present moment, and making decisions according to one's values rather than one's anxiety and worry may be especially worthy of future research attention. It is clear that additional research is needed to improve the treatment outcomes for individuals who suffer with GAD. Given the substantial amount of heterogeneity among individuals who receive the diagnosis, Antony (2002) suggested that perhaps the challenge presented to GAD researchers will be to identify which clients are likely to benefit from different interventions. Following this line of thinking, it would be interesting to determine whether subtypes of the disorder can be reliably identified (e.g., those who are highly inhibited in their behavioral choices vs. those who respond to distress by chaotically moving from one worry to another; those with more pronounced somatic symptoms vs. those with a predominantly cognitive presentation). The identification of such subtypes may offer considerable treatment utility.

REFERENCES

American Psychiatric Association. (1980). *Diagnostic and statistical manual of mental disorders* (3rd ed.). Washington, DC: Author.

American Psychiatric Association. (1994). *Diagnostic and statistical manual of mental disorders* (4th ed.). Washington, DC: Author.

Antony, M. M. (2002). Enhancing current treatments for anxiety disorders. *Clinical Psychology: Science and Practice, 9*, 91–97.

Arntz, A. (2003). Cognitive therapy versus applied relaxation as treatment of generalized anxiety disorder. *Behaviour Research and Therapy, 41*, 633–646.

Barlow, D. H., Rapee, R. M., & Brown, T. A. (1992). Behavioral treatment of generalized anxiety disorder. *Behavior Therapy, 23*, 551–570.

Beck, J. S. (1995). *Cognitive therapy: Basics and beyond.* New York: Guilford Press.

Behar, E., Alcaine, O., Zuellig, A. R., & Borkovec, T. D. (2003). Screening for generalized anxiety disorder using the Penn State Worry Questionnaire: A receiver operating characteristics analysis. *Journal of Behavior Therapy and Experimental Psychiatry, 34*, 25–43.

Bernstein D. A., Borkovec T. D., & Hazlett-Stevens H. (2000). *New directions in progressive relaxation training: A guidebook for helping professionals*. Westport, CT: Praeger.

Borkovec, T. D. (2002). Life in the future, versus life in the present. *Clinical Psychology: Science and Practice, 9*, 76–80.

Borkovec, T. D., Alcaine, O., & Behar, E. (2004). Avoidance theory of worry and generalized anxiety disorder. In R. G. Heimberg, C. L. Turk, & D. S. Mennin (Eds.), *Generalized anxiety disorder: Advances in research and practice* (77–108). New York: Guilford Press.

Borkovec, T. D., & Costello, E. (1993). Efficacy of applied relaxation and cognitive–behavioral therapy in the treatment of generalized anxiety disorder. *Journal of Consulting and Clinical Psychology, 61*, 611–619.

Borkovec, T. D., Mathews, A. M., Chambers, A., Ebrahimi, S., Lytle, R., & Nelson, R. (1987). The effects of relaxation training with cognitive or nondirective therapy and the role of relaxation-induced anxiety in the treatment of generalized anxiety. *Journal of Consulting and Clinical Psychology, 55*, 883–888.

Borkovec, T. D., & Newman, M. G. (1999). Worry and generalized anxiety disorder. In A. S. Bellack & M. Hersen (Series Eds.) & P. Salkovskis (Vol. Ed.), *Comprehensive clinical psychology: Vol. 4. Adults: Clinical formulation and treatment* (pp. 439–459). Oxford, England: Elsevier Science.

Borkovec, T. D., Newman, M. G., Pincus, A., & Lytle, R. (2002). A component analysis of cognitive behavioral therapy for generalized anxiety disorder and the role of interpersonal problems. *Journal of Consulting and Clinical Psychology, 70*, 288–298.

Borkovec, T. D., Ray, W. J., & Stöber, J. (1998). Worry: A cognitive phenomenon intimately linked to affective, physiological, and interpersonal behavioral processes. *Cognitive Therapy and Research, 22*, 561–576.

Borkovec, T. D., & Roemer, L. (1995). Perceived function of worry among generalized anxiety disorder subjects: Distraction from more emotionally distressing topics. *Journal of Behavior Therapy and Experimental Psychiatry, 26*, 25–30.

Borkovec, T. D., & Ruscio, A. M. (2001). Psychotherapy for generalized anxiety disorder. *Journal of Clinical Psychiatry, 62*, 37–42.

Borkovec, T. D., & Sharpless, B. (2004). Generalized anxiety disorder: Bringing cognitive behavioral therapy into the valued present. In S. Hayes, V. Follette, & M. Linehan (Eds.), *New directions in behavior therapy* (pp. 209–242). New York: Guilford Press.

Brown, T. A., Campbell, L. A., Lehman, C. L., Grisham, J. R., & Mancill, R. B. (2001). Current and lifetime comorbidity of the *DSM–IV* anxiety and mood disorders in a large clinical sample. *Journal of Abnormal Psychology, 110*, 585–599.

Brown, T. A., Chorpita, B., & Barlow, D. H. (1998). Structural relationships among dimensions of the *DSM–IV* anxiety and mood disorders and dimensions of negative affect, positive affect, and autonomic arousal. *Journal of Abnormal Psychology, 107*, 179–192.

Brown, T. A., DiNardo, P. A., & Barlow, D. H. (1994). *Anxiety Disorders Interview Schedule for* DSM–IV *(ADIS-IV)*. New York: Oxford University Press.

Butler, G. (1993). Predicting outcomes after treatment for generalised anxiety disorder. *Behaviour Research and Therapy, 31*, 211–213.

Campbell, L. A., & Brown, T. A. (2002). Generalized anxiety disorder. In M. M. Antony & D. H. Barlow (Eds.), *Handbook of assessment and treatment planning for psychological disorder* (pp. 147–181). New York: Guilford Press.

Clarkin, J., & Levy, K. (2004). The influence of client variables on psychotherapy. In M. Lambert (Ed.), *Bergin and Garfield's handbook of psychotherapy and behaviour change* (5th ed., pp. 194–226). New York: Wiley.

Dugas, M. J. (2000). Generalized anxiety disorder publications: So where do we stand? *Journal of Anxiety Disorders, 14*, 31–40.

Dugas, M. J., Gagnon, F., Ladouceur, R., & Freeston, M. H. (1998). Generalized anxiety disorder: A preliminary test of a conceptual model. *Behaviour Research and Therapy, 36*, 215–226.

Dugas, M. J., Ladouceur, R., Léger, E., Freeston, M. H., Langlois, F., Provencher, M. D., & Boisvert, J.-M. (2003). Group cognitive–behavioral therapy for generalized anxiety disorder: Treatment outcome and long-term follow-up. *Journal of Consulting and Clinical Psychology, 71*, 821–825.

Dugas M. J., & Robichaud, M. (2006). *Cognitive–behavioral treatment for generalized anxiety disorder: From science to practice*. New York: Routledge.

Durham, R. C. (2006). Predictors of treatment outcome. In G. C. L. Davey & A. Wells (Eds.), *Worry and its psychological disorders: Theory, assessment and treatment* (pp. 379–398). Hoboken, NJ: Wiley.

Durham, R. C., Allan, T., & Hackett, C. (1997). On predicting improvement and relapse in generalized anxiety disorder following psychotherapy. *British Journal of Clinical Psychology, 36*, 101–119.

Durham, R., Fisher, P., Dow, M., Sharp, D., Power, K., Swan, J., & Morton, R. (2004). Cognitive behaviour therapy for good and poor prognosis generalized anxiety disorder: A clinical effectiveness study. *Clinical Psychology and Psychotherapy, 11*, 145–157.

Fisher, P. L. (2006). The efficacy of psychological treatments for generalized anxiety disorder? Predictors of treatment outcome. In G. C. L. Davey & A. Wells (Eds.), *Worry and its psychological disorders: Theory, assessment and treatment* (pp. 359–377). Hoboken, NJ: Wiley.

Fisher, P. L., & Durham, R. C. (1999). Recovery rates in generalised anxiety disorder following psychological therapy: An analysis of clinically significant change in STAI-T across outcome studies since 1990. *Psychological Medicine, 29*, 1425–1434.

Foa, E. B., & Kozak, M. J. (1986). Emotional processing of fear: Exposure to corrective information. *Psychological Bulletin, 99*, 20–35.

Goldfried, M. R. (1971). Systematic densensitization as training in self-control. *Journal of Consulting and Clinical Psychology, 37*, 228–234.

Hayes, S. C., Strosahl, K. D., & Wilson, K. G. (1999). *Acceptance and commitment therapy: An experiential approach to behavior change*. New York: Guilford Press.

Holowka, D. W., Dugas, M. J., Francis, K., & Laugesen, N. (2000, November). *Measuring beliefs about worry: A psychometric evaluation of the Why Worry-II Questionnaire*. Presented at the annual meeting of the Association for Advancement of Behavior Therapy, New Orleans, LA.

Kabat-Zinn, J. (1994). *Wherever you go, there you are: Mindfulness meditation in everyday life*. New York: Hyperion.

Kessler, R. C., Berglund, P. D., Demler, O., Olga, J. R., Merikangas, K. R., & Walters, E. E. (2005). Lifetime prevalence and age-of-onset distributions of *DSM–IV* disorders in the National Comorbidity Survey Replication. *Archives of General Psychiatry, 62*, 593–602.

Kessler, R. C., Brandenburg, N., Lane, M., Roy-Byrne, P., Stang, P. D., Stein, D.J., & Wittchen, H. U. (2005). Rethinking the duration requirement for generalized anxiety disorder: Evidence from the National Comorbidity Survey Replication. *Psychological Medicine, 35*, 1073–1082.

Kessler, R. C., Chiu, W. T., Demler, O., Merikangas K., & Walters E. (2005). Prevalence, severity, and comorbidity of 12-month *DSM–IV* disorders in the National Comorbidity Survey Replication. *Archives of General Psychiatry, 62*, 617–627.

Kessler, R. C., Dupont, R. L., Berglund, P., & Wittchen, H. U. (1999). Impairments in pure and comorbid generalized anxiety disorder and major depression at 12 months in two national surveys. *The American Journal of Psychiatry, 156*, 1915–1923.

Ladouceur, R., Dugas, M. J., Freeston, M. H., Léger, E., Gagnon, F., & Thibodeau, N. (2000). Efficacy of a cognitive behavioral treatment for generalized anxiety disorder: Evaluation in a controlled clinical trial. *Journal of Consulting and Clinical Psychology, 68*, 957–964.

Leahy, R. L. (2005). *The worry cure: Seven steps to stop worry from stopping you*. New York: Harmony Books.

Léger, E., Dugas, M. J., Langlois, F., & Ladouceur, R. (1998, November). *Motivation, expectations and therapeutic relationship as predictors of outcome in the treatment of GAD*. Presented at the annual meeting of the Association for Advancement of Behavior Therapy, Washington, DC.

Mennin, D. S. (2006). Emotion regulation therapy: An integrative approach to treatment-resistant anxiety disorders. *Journal of Contemporary Psychotherapy, 36*, 95–105.

Mennin, D. S., Heimberg, R. G., Turk, C. L., & Fresco, D. M. (2002). Applying an emotion regulation framework to integrative approaches to generalized anxiety disorder. *Clinical Psychology: Science and Practice, 9*, 85–90.

Meyer, T. J., Miller, M. L., Metzger, R. L., & Borkovec, T. D. (1990). Development and validation of the Penn State Worry Questionnaire. *Behaviour Research and Therapy, 28*, 487–495.

Nathan, P. E., & Gorman, J. M. (2007). *A guide to treatments that work*. New York: Oxford University Press.

Öst, L. G. (1987). Applied relaxation: Description of a coping technique and review of controlled studies. *Behaviour Research and Therapy, 25*, 397–409.

Öst, L. G., & Breitholtz, E. (2000). Applied relaxation vs. cognitive therapy in the treatment of generalized anxiety disorder. *Behaviour Research and Therapy, 38*, 777–790.

Purdon, C. (1999). Thought suppression and psychopathology. *Behaviour Research and Therapy, 37*, 1029–1054.

Roemer, L., Molina, S., & Borkovec, T. D. (1997). An investigation of worry content among generally anxious individuals. *The Journal of Nervous and Mental Disease, 185*, 314–319.

Roemer, L., & Orsillo, S. M. (2005). An acceptance-based behavior therapy for generalized anxiety disorder. In S. M. Orsillo & L. Roemer (Eds.), *Acceptance and mindfulness-based approaches to anxiety: Conceptualization and treatment* (pp. 213–240). New York: Springer.

Roemer, L., & Orsillo, S. M. (2007). An open trial of an acceptance-based behavior therapy for GAD. *Behavior Therapy, 38*, 72–85.

Ruscio, A. M., Lane, M., Roy-Byrne, P., Stang, P. E., Stein, D. J., Wittchen, H. U., & Kessler, R. C. (2005). Should excessive worry be required for a diagnosis of generalized anxiety disorder? Results from the U.S. National Comorbidity Survey Replication. *Psychological Medicine 35*, 1761 1772.

Rygh, J. L., & Sanderson, W. C. (2004). *Treating generalized anxiety disorder: Evidence-based strategies, tools and techniques*. New York: Guilford Press.

Salkovskis, P. M. (1991). The importance of behaviour in the maintenance of anxiety and panic: A cognitive account. *Behavioural Psychotherapy, 19*, 6–19.

Salkovskis, P. M., Clark, D. N., Hackmann, A., Wells, A., & Gelder, M. G. (1999). An experimental investigation of the role of safety seeking behaviours in the maintenance of panic disorder with agoraphobia. *Behaviour Research and Therapy, 37*, 559–574.

Segal, Z. V., Williams, M. G., & Teasdale, J. D. (2002). *Mindfulness-based cognitive therapy for depression: A new approach to preventing relapse*. New York: Guilford Press.

Siev, J., & Chambless, D. L. (2007). Specificity of treatment effects: Cognitive therapy and relaxation for generalized anxiety and panic disorders. *Journal of Consulting and Clinical Psychology, 75*, 513–522.

Stein, D. J. (2002). Comorbidity in generalized anxiety disorder: Impact and implications. *Journal of Clinical Psychiatry, 62*, 29–34.

Thayer, J. F., Friedman, B. H., & Borkovec, T. D. (1996). Autonomic characteristics of generalized anxiety disorder and worry. *Biological Psychiatry, 39*, 255–266.

Wegner, D. M., Schneider, D. J., Carter, S., & White, T. (1987). Paradoxical effects of thought suppression. *Journal of Personality and Social Psychology, 53*, 5–13.

Wells, A. (1995). Metacognition and worry: A cognitive model of generalized anxiety disorder. *Behavioural and Cognitive Psychotherapy, 23*, 301–320.

Wells, A. (1997). *Cognitive therapy of anxiety disorders: A practice manual and conceptual guide*. Chichester, England: Wiley.

Wells, A., & Carter, C. (1999). Preliminary tests of a cognitive model of generalised anxiety disorder. *Behaviour Research and Therapy, 37*, 585–594.

Wells, A., & King, P. (2006). Metacognitive therapy for generalized anxiety disorder: An open trial. *Journal of Behavior Therapy and Experimental Psychiatry, 37*, 206–212.

Wetherell, J., Hopko, D., Diefenbach, G., Averill, P., Beck, G., Craske, M., et al. (2005). Cognitive–behavioral therapy for late life generalized anxiety disorder: Who gets better? *Behavior Therapy, 36*, 147–156.

7

POSTTRAUMATIC STRESS DISORDER

STEVEN TAYLOR

Posttraumatic stress disorder (PTSD), as defined by the *Diagnostic and Statistical Manual of Mental Disorders* (4th ed., text rev.; American Psychiatric Association, 2000), develops in some people after they have been exposed to a traumatic event such as sexual abuse, a serious road traffic collision, a natural disaster, criminal victimization, or military combat. PTSD is characterized by a range of symptoms: vivid reexperiencing of the trauma (e.g., intrusive memories, recurrent nightmares), avoidance of trauma-related stimuli (e.g., effortful attempts to avoid places, people, or recollections of the trauma), emotional numbing (e.g., difficulty experiencing close emotional connections to other people), and hyperarousal (e.g., hypervigilance, irritability, or insomnia). To be diagnosed with PTSD, a sufficient number of these symptoms must be present for at least a month; that is, at least one reexperiencing symptom, at least three avoidance or numbing symptoms, and at least two hyperarousal symptoms.

PTSD has a lifetime prevalence of 7% to 12% in the United States (American Psychiatric Association, 2000; Breslau, 2002). It often follows a chronic course, although the frequency and severity of symptoms typically fluctuate over time depending on a range of factors, including the person's degree of exposure to subsequent stressors—traumatic or otherwise—that can amplify or exacerbate symptoms (Taylor, 2006). Patients meeting diagnostic criteria for PTSD often have other disorders, including other anxiety disorders, mood disorders, personality disorders, or substance use disorders (American Psychiatric Association, 2000).

To diagnose PTSD, it is necessary to rule out malingering (American Psychiatric Association, 2000). *Malingering* is the intentional production of false or grossly exaggerated symptoms, motivated by external incentives. For example, a survivor of a work-related accident might malinger PTSD to obtain a large workers' compensation or insurance settlement, or a military veteran might malinger PTSD to obtain government disability benefits. Little is known about prevalence of PTSD malingering among treatment-seeking populations. According to one review, "This is largely because practitioners are so conditioned to accept client reports as being ingenuous that they fail to scrutinize the accuracy of the report and, consequently, do not formally assess for malingering" (Guriel & Fremouw, 2003, p. 882). Indeed, there have been many reported cases in which therapists have been fooled by patients who were malingering PTSD (Burkett & Whitely, 1998; Hickling, Blanchard, Mundy, & Galovski, 2002; Pankratz, 1998). In one of the few studies to examine the occurrence of malingering among people seeking treatment for PTSD, Freeman, Hart, and Kimbrell (2005) assessed 33 Vietnam veterans presenting for residential treatment at a U.S. Veterans Affairs facility. The majority of veterans (55%) showed clear evidence of symptom exaggeration, as assessed by a structured interview. How many of our cognitive behavioral therapy (CBT) failures were actually malingering? We return to this controversial but important issue later in this chapter.

RISK FACTORS FOR POSTTRAUMATIC STRESS DISORDER

Four types of variables have been found to be significant risk factors or predictors of PTSD: (a) historical (pretrauma) variables such as family psychiatric history, family instability, and personal past history of PTSD or prior trauma exposure; (b) severity of the index trauma; (c) threat-relevant psychological processes during and immediately after the trauma (e.g., perception of threat, dissociative symptoms); and (d) life stressors and low social support after the trauma (Brewin, Andrews, & Valentine, 2000; Ozer, Best, Lipsey, & Weiss, 2003). Factors closer in time to the traumatic event (e.g., peritraumatic dissociation and the perception of threat at the time of the event) tend to be stronger than historical factors (e.g., personality traits) in predicting PTSD (Ozer et al., 2003).

ETIOLOGIC FACTORS

A vast amount of research has been conducted on the etiology of PTSD, and many theories have attempted to synthesize and account for the salient findings. The highlights are summarized here, but they are reviewed in more detail elsewhere (e.g., Taylor, 2006).

Approximately 80% of the U.S. population has experienced a traumatic event at some point in their lives, yet no more than 12% of the population develops PTSD (American Psychiatric Association, 2000; Breslau, 2002). This suggests that vulnerability factors may be important, and research has indeed indicated that the risk of developing PTSD symptoms is influenced by genetic and other vulnerability factors (Stein, Jang, Taylor, Vernon, & Livesley, 2002). A diathesis-stress conceptualization is a promising framework for understanding the disorder, whereby the risk of developing PTSD depends on the interaction between vulnerability factors and the severity or "dose" of the traumatic stressor. Vulnerability factors could include genetic risk factors—for example, those factors influencing the person's propensity for acquiring conditioned fears, or genetic factors associated with the dysregulation of neurohormonal and neurotransmitter systems implicated in PTSD, such as serotonergic and noradrenergic systems. Particular sorts of pretrauma learning experiences could contribute to cognitive diatheses for the disorder. These include experiences that lead the person to believe that the world is very dangerous and that the self is vulnerable. Such beliefs could lead the person to react with especially strong fear to traumatic events.

There is no single, comprehensive model of PTSD. Much work needs to be done to integrate biological, cognitive, and behavioral findings into such a model. Nevertheless, for the cognitive–behavioral practitioner, one of the most powerful and parsimonious accounts is the emotional processing model (Foa & Rothbaum, 1998; Foa, Steketee, & Rothbaum, 1989). This model proposes that PTSD arises from a "fear structure" stored in long-term memory. The structure contains representations of feared stimuli (e.g., being alone at night), response information (e.g., palpitations, trembling, fear, safety-seeking behaviors), and meaning information (e.g., the concept of danger). In the network, the three types of information—stimuli, responses, and meaning elements—are interlinked. For example, conditioned links among stimuli (e.g., links between "adult men" and "weapons"), links between stimuli and meaning elements (e.g., "sleeping with the lights off" and "danger"), as well as other types of links (e.g., stimulus–response, response–meaning). Links can be innate or acquired by processes such as conditioning. In PTSD, many of these links represent erroneous associations (e.g., "men with red hair" linked with "danger"). Fear structures are activated by incoming information that matches information stored in the network (i.e., matches a stimulus, response, or meaning element). Activation of the network evokes fear and motivates avoidance or escape behavior.

The model holds that traumatic events are so intense that they cause fear conditioning to a wide range of stimuli (e.g., sights, sounds, odors, and bodily sensations associated with the trauma). Thus, a plethora of stimuli and responses are represented in the fear structure. Trauma-related stimuli serve as reminders of the trauma, activating the fear structure and thereby producing hyperarousal and intrusive recollections of the trauma.

Avoidance and emotional numbing are said to arise from mechanisms for deactivating the fear structure in the short term (e.g., via conditioned analgesia; Foa, Zinbarg, & Rothbaum, 1992). They prevent the structure from being modified and thereby contribute to the persistence of PTSD in the longer term. Avoidance also prevents dysfunctional beliefs (meaning elements) from being corrected.

The model also includes the concept of *schemata*, which refers to the person's store of abstracted knowledge and beliefs about a given topic, such as the self. The model, in its current form, consists of *memory records* (i.e., fear structures) that interact with (e.g., influence) schemata. Chronic PTSD is said to be associated with strong negative schemata involving beliefs that one is totally incompetent and that the world is highly dangerous. Such beliefs are said to produce chronic hyperarousal, extreme fear, and widespread avoidance.

The model suggests that the effective treatment of PTSD requires exposure to corrective information. This includes interventions such as (a) imaginal exposure to the trauma until emotional extinction occurs, thereby breaking, weakening, or inhibiting the link between trauma-related stimuli and conditioned emotional arousal; (b) situational exposure to distressing but harmless stimuli, which teaches the person that the stimuli are not dangerous (i.e., incorporates safety information into the fear structure); and (c) cognitive restructuring to help the person make sense out of the traumatic event and to modify maladaptive beliefs. These are the elements involved in the various forms of contemporary CBT.

EFFECTIVE TREATMENTS

Early Interventions

Interventions in the early aftermath of trauma are typically used to prevent symptoms from persisting for longer than a month, which is required to diagnose full-blown PTSD. Among the most widely used early interventions are the various forms of psychological debriefing, such as critical incident stress debriefing (Mitchell & Everly, 2000). Debriefing is implemented in a single session, 24 to 48 hours posttrauma, either individually or in groups. The trauma survivor is presented with information about common reactions to trauma (e.g., PTSD symptoms) and asked to provide the debriefer with a detailed review of the trauma. The debriefer encourages emotional expression and encourages the person to discuss the trauma with others. Avoidance of trauma-related stimuli is discouraged, and the person is encouraged to seek further help if symptoms persist. Despite the widespread use of psychological debriefing, little information about its effects was available until recently. Research has indicated that debriefing, compared with no intervention, is either ineffective or possibly harmful in that it seems to perpetuate PTSD symptoms (Bisson, 2003; Feldner, Monson, & Friedman, 2007; van Emmerik, Kamphuis, Hulsbosch, & Emmelkamp, 2002). A more promising approach is to implement a four- to five-session CBT program 2 to 4 weeks posttrauma. This is similar to CBT for chronic PTSD; both typically involve some combination of imaginal and in vivo exposure to distressing but harmless stimuli, cognitive restructuring of maladaptive beliefs, and training in emotional coping skills such as diaphragmatic breathing or relaxation exercises. Research has indicated that early intervention with CBT can reduce symptoms in the short term and, in the longer term, reduces the risk that the person will develop chronic PTSD (Taylor, 2006).

Treatments for Full-Blown Posttraumatic Stress Disorder

Many randomized controlled trials have shown that CBT is effective in treating PTSD, with gains generally maintained at follow-ups of a year or more (Ballenger et al., 2000; National Institute for Clinical Excellence, 2005). CBT protocols that combine imaginal and in vivo exposure tend to be more effective than imaginal exposure alone (Devilly & Foa, 2001). Adding cognitive restructuring to these forms of exposure generally does not improve treatment outcome, except in cases of severe trauma-related anger or guilt, in which cognitive restructuring is useful (Taylor, 2006).

Randomized controlled studies have shown that CBT is more effective than supportive counseling. There have been comparatively fewer other direct comparisons of CBT with other treatments. Meta-analytic research, which pools outcome studies to compare treatment effects, has indicated that CBT tends to be more effective than hypnotherapy and short-term psychodynamic therapy, and that CBT and eye movement desensitization and reprocessing (EMDR) have comparable efficacy and dropout rates (Bisson et al., 2007; Hembree et al., 2003; van Etten & Taylor, 1998). However, CBT tends to be more acceptable and credible than EMDR to potential consumers of these therapies (Tarrier, Liversidge, & Gregg, 2006).

Meta-analytic studies have indicated that CBT tends to be associated with fewer treatment dropouts than pharmacotherapies and that CBT is equally effective in the short term as the most well-established and efficacious of the PTSD pharmacotherapies—the selective serotonin reuptake inhibitors (SSRIs; e.g., fluvoxamine; see van Etten & Taylor, 1998). It is currently unclear whether CBT is as effective as another, more recently used class of medications, the serotonergic and noradrenergic reuptake inhibitors (SNRIs; e.g., venlafaxine). Preliminary research has suggested that SNRIs may be at least as effective as SSRIs (Davidson et al., 2006), which suggests that CBT and SNRIs may also have equivalent short-term efficacy. It remains to be seen whether CBT and pharmacotherapies differ in their long-term efficacy. Patients tend to maintain their gains after they have completed a course of CBT (e.g., 8–12 weeks of treatment). It remains to be seen whether pharmacotherapy patients maintain their gains over the long term, even if the medication is administered on an ongoing basis.

Although there are a number of empirically supported treatments for PTSD, no treatment is universally efficacious. Even for CBT, there is a good deal of room for improving treatment efficacy. It remains to be seen whether treatment outcome is improved when CBT is combined with SSRIs or SNRIs. Results for other anxiety disorders suggest that there is, at best, a limited and short-lived advantage of such combined treatments, compared with CBT alone (Davis, Barad, Otto, & Southwick, 2006).

FACTORS ASSOCIATED WITH POOR RESPONSE TO COGNITIVE–BEHAVIORAL THERAPY

A major problem in the search for predictors of poor response is that most treatment studies have limited statistical power to conduct such analyses, and so only the most robust predictors can be reliably identified. It is not surprising that there are very few reliable findings in the field. With regard to treatment dropout, pretreatment variables, such as PTSD severity, trauma characteristics, dysfunctional beliefs, and demographic features, are unreliable predictors; that is, they are significant in some studies but not in others (e.g., Bryant et al., 2007; Tarrier, Pilgrim, et al., 1999; Taylor, 2004; Taylor et al., 2001). Treatment credibility is also an inconsistent predictor of treatment dropout (Tarrier, Pilgrim, et al., 1999; Taylor, 2004; van Minnen, Arntz, & Keijsers, 2002).

Concerning treatment outcome, the following are unreliable predictors: demographic features, type of trauma, pretreatment clinical features (e.g., PTSD symptom severity, dysfunctional beliefs, duration of trauma, duration since trauma, comorbid depression, dissociative symptoms, guilt, shame, substance abuse history, comorbid Axis I disorders), and personality variables (e.g., Basoglu, Livanou, Salcioglu, & Kalender, 2003; Forbes, Creamer, Hawthorne, Allen, & McHugh, 2003; Livanou et al., 2002; Taylor, 2004).

Preliminary research has suggested that the patient's interpersonal environment may have important implications for PTSD treatment. Tarrier, Sommerfield, and Pilgrim (1999) found that outcome of CBT tended to be poor when PTSD patients lived with angry or critical significant others. There is some evidence that comorbid chronic pain may predict poor outcome for PTSD treatment (Taylor et al., 2001), even when pain management techniques are included as part of treatment (Wald, Taylor, & Fedoroff, 2004).

PTSD-related compensation-seeking or litigation generally does not predict treatment dropout or outcome (e.g., Brooks & McKinlay, 1992; Grace,

Green, Lindy, & Leonard, 1993; Taylor et al., 2001). However, there are exceptions. Some patients malinger PTSD symptoms and fail to adhere to treatment in the hope of receiving a large financial settlement, as previously noted (Simon, 2003; Taylor, Frueh, & Asmundson, 2007).

In summary, to date there are few variables that reliably predict treatment outcome for cases in which PTSD is the primary presenting problem. Patients who are most likely to benefit from treatment tend to show treatment-related gains within the first few sessions (van Minnen & Hagenaars, 2002).

The following case example illustrates many of the complexities and challenges encountered in the treatment of PTSD.

CASE EXAMPLE

George, a 52-year-old White corporate executive, was assessed by a regional Workers' Compensation Board (WCB) because of complaints of psychological problems and chronic pain after being involved in a multiple-car freeway collision in which another driver was killed. At the time of the accident, he experienced intense fear and thought he was going to die. He also described a period of peritraumatic dissociation shortly after the accident in which he recalled standing by the side of the highway "in a daze" as ambulance workers attended to survivors and fire department personnel doused the flaming vehicles. George sustained some soft tissue injuries to his neck and left shoulder and arm but was otherwise physically unharmed. He was able to escape from his vehicle without assistance and stated that he did not lose consciousness during the collision.

In the following weeks, he presented to his primary care physician for analgesic and anxiolytic medication and took sick leave from work. Months went by without George returning to work. He applied to his company and to WBC for disability-related wage loss compensation. As part of this process, he was asked to undergo a medical and psychological evaluation by the WBC. No physical injuries were identified, although George reported persistent pain in his neck and left shoulder and arm. The WCB psychologist administered the Clinician Administered PTSD Scale (CAPS; Blake et al., 1997) and concluded that George suffered from severe PTSD, in addition to chronic pain. On the basis of George's self-report, the psychologist concluded that he was 100% disabled as a result of his pain and PTSD.

A WCB psychiatrist initiated pharmacotherapy with sertraline. George was also referred to a physiotherapist for physical rehabilitation and to a psychologist for psychosocial treatment. Months went by without any clinical improvement, despite an increase in dose of medication. Progress reports to the WCB from the psychologist eventually revealed that although this clinician claimed to have expertise in PTSD, his treatment consisted largely of supportive counseling, which, as mentioned earlier, is not an empirically supported treatment for this disorder. Accordingly, George was referred to a psychologist with expertise in CBT for PTSD, which was initiated in addition to ongoing pharmacotherapy and physiotherapy.

Prior to initiating treatment, the CBT practitioner reviewed the assessment reports compiled by the WBC and also conducted an intake evaluation consisting of the CAPS, an unstructured interview to assess for other psychiatric disorders, and the following self-report inventories: Trauma Symptom Inventory (Briere, 1995), Posttraumatic Diagnostic Scale (Foa, 1995), Beck Anxiety Inventory (A. T. Beck & Steer, 1990), and Beck Depression Inventory (A. T. Beck & Steer, 1987). The CAPS, Trauma Symptom Inventory, and Posttraumatic Diagnostic Scale suggested that George was suffering from severe PTSD. The findings from validity scales of the Trauma Symptom Inventory were ambiguous with regard to symptom validity. The findings suggested either that he was overendorsing symptoms or that he had severe psychopathology. The clinician decided to give George the benefit of the doubt and interpreted the findings as being consistent with severe PTSD. George also had scores on the Beck inventories suggesting moderate depression and severe general anxiety. There was no evidence of psychotic features or suicide risk.

The CBT clinician treated George for 12 months, mostly on a weekly basis. Treatment consisted of cognitive restructuring of maladaptive beliefs (e.g., "I'm sure to be killed if I get into a car"; "I'll never get better") and a combination of imaginal and in vivo exposure (see Taylor, 2006, for details on these treatment protocols). Pain management methods were also implemented, including cognitive restructuring (e.g., challenging the belief that "hurt equals harm") and relaxation training. Behavioral activation methods were also used (e.g., encouraging George to increase his level of formerly enjoyable activities), which has been found useful in treating both PTSD and depression (Jakupcak et al., 2006). Behavioral activation involves encouraging the patient to increase her or his pursuit of activities that may enhance the patient's sense of mastery or enjoyment. Such activities may also counter the avoidance symptoms associated with PTSD.

In addition, the treating psychiatrist continued treating George with pharmacotherapy. George also continued in physiotherapy and completed a multidisciplinary pain management program, which included, among other things, pharmacotherapy with topiramate, which has shown promise in the treatment of pain and PTSD (Taylor, Wald, & Asmundson, 2004). All treatment was funded by the WCB, and George continued to receive disability-related wage loss compensation. The latter was a considerable sum, given his seniority in the company.

Treatment progress was assessed by means of George's self-reported pain and PTSD symptoms and, more formally, by asking him to periodically complete the Posttraumatic Diagnostic Scale and Beck Inventories. Despite 12 months of intensive, multidisciplinary treatment, George had made little progress and continued to report severe symptoms. His adherence to CBT was poor. Although he dutifully attended sessions, he failed to complete most homework assignments (e.g., relaxation exercises, exposure assignments, cognitive restructuring exercises). He offered various reasons for this, such as difficulty finding time or finding the assignments too difficult.

George continued to report severe and debilitating PTSD and pain. Moreover, he reported the development of new symptoms, such as headache and pains "all over" his body. Repeated medical evaluations, including independent evaluations by a physician specializing in chronic pain and a neurologist, could find no evidence of a neurological or general medical condition that might account for his problems. Both clinicians concurred that George was suffering from severe PTSD.

The CBT practitioner and the WCB psychiatrist made several adjustments to treatment in an attempt to improve outcome. Cognitive–behavioral assignments were altered (e.g., exposure exercises were implemented more gradually, beginning with only mildly distressing exercises), and the frequency of cognitive–behavioral sessions was increased from once to twice a week. The psychiatrist made various adjustments to the patient's medication, including changes in dose and type and using adjunctive medications. None of these modifications had any impact.

After 12 months of treatment, the CBT practitioner left for sabbatical, and George was transferred to another psychologist, who also had expertise in CBT for PTSD. That psychologist concurred with the other mental health practitioners that George suffered from severe PTSD and chronic pain.

Meanwhile, the WCB had, unbeknownst to the health care providers, hired a private investigator to conduct videotape surveillance of George. Although George told the treating clinicians that he was terrified of motor vehicles and of all forms of road travel, the videotape surveillance revealed evidence to clearly refute these claims. Tapes showed George smiling and chatting with friends and then climbing onto his motorcycle and roaring off down a busy city street. He was also filmed standing by the edge of the curb waiting for a taxi. Trucks thundered past, inches from George, and yet he seemed unconcerned and displayed no startle response or other overt reactions. He was filmed casually crossing pedestrian walkways on busy roads, and even jaywalking on such streets, without any behavioral evidence of fear. The WCB screened the video to the second CBT clinician, who conceded that George's behavior was quite inconsistent with how he presented during the treatment sessions. When George was shown the videotapes, he protested that the tapes had simply caught him on "good days." Unconvinced, the WCB discontinued funding for George's treatment because it was ineffective and seemingly unnecessary and rejected his compensation claim. Further information from George's former place of employment suggested that he had never been an outstanding employee and that his performance had deteriorated in recent years when he was promoted (because of seniority) beyond his level of competence. Given his increasingly poor work record and the realistic possibility of being fired, George apparently turned to malingering in an effort to maintain his income and to avoid the humiliating prospect of losing his job.

This vignette illustrates how treatment providers can be easily fooled by people who malinger PTSD and other symptoms in order to receive financial benefits. George apparently fooled the WCB psychologist conducting the initial evaluation, the three psychologist treatment providers, the WCB psychiatrist, and several other health care providers. One of the CBT therapists had screened for symptom exaggeration using the Trauma Symptom Inventory, but unfortunately subsequent research has revealed that this inventory is inadequate for detecting malingering (Elhai et al., 2005). CBT treatment protocols for PTSD are clearly not the best way of addressing malingering. This case example shows how a considerable amount of clinical time and expense can be squandered when clinicians fail to properly screen for malingering in compensation-seeking PTSD patients. It is possible that George did have some genuine symptoms, such as lingering neck and shoulder pain, and that he was simply exaggerating their severity. However, in the absence of a proper assessment of malingering, this possibility could not be properly evaluated. Guidelines for conducting such an assessment in treatment settings are described elsewhere (Taylor et al., 2007).

CONCLUSIONS AND FUTURE DIRECTIONS

The research evidence clearly supports the efficacy of CBT for PTSD, and yet there is ample room for improving treatment efficacy. Little is known about the prognostic indicators of poor treatment response or about the best ways of improving outcome in treatment nonresponders. Cases like the one of George highlight the fact that CBT is unlikely to be effective if treatment is based on a faulty case formulation. In this case, the clinicians involved in George's care based their treatment plans on the erroneous assumption that he actually had PTSD. Most people presenting for treatment of PTSD are probably not malingering. Nevertheless, clinicians should be alert to the fact that some of their putative treatment failures may in fact be malingering.

For those PTSD patients who are not malingering, there are some promising future directions for improving the outcome of CBT. One approach is to add cognitive–behavioral interventions that are used to treat other disorders but are not typically used to treat PTSD. For example, preliminary research has indicated that behavioral activation exercises, as used in CBT for depression, may be beneficial in reducing PTSD symptoms (Jakupcak et al., 2006).

Preliminary research also has suggested that interoceptive exposure, which is an intervention used in CBT for panic disorder, may also be usefully added to CBT for PTSD (Wald & Taylor, 2005, 2007). Interoceptive exposure involves a series of exercises (e.g., voluntary hyperventilation) that help teach the patient that arousal- or anxiety-related sensations (e.g., dizziness, dyspnea) are harmless. The rationale for using this intervention in panic disorder (and in PTSD) is that research has indicated that patients with anxiety disorders tend to be extremely frightened of arousal-related sensations (Taylor, 2000, 2006), which can exacerbate symptoms of PTSD (Wald & Taylor, 2008).

Other sorts of psychosocial interventions also show promise, such as combining CBT with virtual-reality exposure to trauma-related stimuli (J. G. Beck, Palyo, Winer, Schwagler, & Ang, 2007; Rizzo, Rothbaum, & Graap, 2007). For survivors of sexual assault, combining CBT with self-defense training appears promising, not only because such training may reduce the risk for future assault but also because self-defense training entails a form of in vivo exposure for survivors of assault (David, Simpson, & Cotton, 2006; Taylor, 2006). For patients with particular types of comorbidity, such as combined PTSD and substance use disorder, specialized CBT protocols have been developed to concurrently address the combined problems (e.g., Najavits, Gallop, & Weiss, 2006). Preliminary research supports the value of these protocols (Back, Waldrop, Brady, & Hien, 2006). For PTSD with comorbid chronic pain, it sometimes can be useful to combine CBT for PTSD with a multidisciplinary pain management program, although even here it can be difficult to reduce PTSD (Wald et al., 2004).

With regard to adjuvant pharmacotherapy, a promising approach for boosting the efficacy of CBT is to combine it with pharmacologic agents that enhance the exposure component of treatment. One such agent is D-cycloserine. A small but steadily growing body of research has suggested that the therapeutic effects of an exposure session are enhanced if this agent is administered shortly before the exposure session (Davis et al., 2006). D-cycloserine has effects on receptors in the amygdala, which play a role in fear extinction. The benefits of adding D-cycloserine to CBT remain to be fully evaluated in the treatment of PTSD, although research on other anxiety disorders has suggested that this approach holds great promise for PTSD (Davis et al., 2006).

REFERENCES

American Psychiatric Association. (2000). *Diagnostic and statistical manual of mental disorders* (4th ed., text rev.). Washington, DC: Author.

Back, S. E., Waldrop, A. E., Brady, K. T., & Hien, D. (2006). Evidence-based time-limited treatment of co-occurring substance-use disorders and civilian-related posttraumatic stress disorder. *Brief Treatment and Crisis Intervention, 6,* 283–294.

Ballenger, J. C., Davidson, J. R. T., Lecrubier, Y., Nutt, D. J., Foa, E. B., Kessler, R. C., et al. (2000). Consensus statement on posttraumatic stress disorder from the International Consensus Group on Depression and Anxiety. *Journal of Clinical Psychiatry, 61*(Suppl. 5), 60–66.

Basoglu, M., Livanou, M., Salcioglu, E., & Kalender, D. (2003). A brief behavioural treatment of chronic post-traumatic stress disorder in earthquake survivors: Results from an open clinical trial. *Psychological Medicine, 33*, 647–654.

Beck, A. T., & Steer, R. A. (1987). *Manual for the revised Beck Depression Inventory.* San Antonio, TX: Psychological Corporation.

Beck, A. T., & Steer, R. A. (1990). *Manual for the revised Beck Anxiety Inventory.* San Antonio, TX: Psychological Corporation.

Beck, J. G., Palyo, S. A., Winer, E. H., Schwagler, B. E., & Ang, E. J. (2007). Virtual reality exposure therapy for PTSD symptoms after a road accident: An uncontrolled case series. *Behavior Therapy, 38*, 39–48.

Bisson, J. I. (2003). Single-session early psychological interventions following traumatic events. *Clinical Psychology Review, 23*, 481–499.

Bisson, J. I., Ehlers, A., Matthews, R., Pilling, S., Richards, D., & Turner, S. (2007). Psychological treatments for chronic post-traumatic stress disorder: Systematic review and meta-analysis. *The British Journal of Psychiatry, 190*, 97–104.

Blake, D., Weathers, F. W., Nagy, L. M., Kaloupek, D. G., Charney, D. S., & Keane, T. M. (1997). *Clinician Administered PTSD Scale (revised).* Boston: Boston National Center for Post-Traumatic Stress Disorder.

Breslau, N. (2002). Epidemiologic studies of trauma, posttraumatic stress disorder, and other psychiatric disorders. *Canadian Journal of Psychiatry, 47*, 923–929.

Brewin, C. R., Andrews, B., & Valentine, J. D. (2000). Meta-analysis of risk factors for posttraumatic stress disorder in trauma-exposed adults. *Journal of Consulting and Clinical Psychology, 68*, 748–766.

Briere, J. (1995). *Trauma Symptom Inventory professional manual.* Odessa, FL: Psychological Assessment Resources.

Brooks, N., & McKinlay, W. W. (1992). Mental health consequences of the Lockerbie disaster. *Journal of Traumatic Stress, 5*, 527–543.

Bryant, R. A., Moulds, M. L., Mastrodomenico, J., Hopwood, S., Felmingham, K., & Nixon, R. D. V. (2007). Who drops out of treatment for post-traumatic stress disorder? *Clinical Psychologist, 11*, 13–15.

Burkett, B. G., & Whitley, G. (1998). *Stolen valor: How the Vietnam generation was robbed of its heroes and its history.* Dallas, TX: Verity Press.

David, W. S., Simpson, T. L., & Cotton, A. J. (2006). Taking charge: A pilot curriculum of self-defense and personal safety training for female veterans with PTSD because of military sexual trauma. *Journal of Interpersonal Violence, 21*, 555–565.

Davidson, J. R. T., Rothbaum, B. O., Tucker, P., Asnis, G., Benattia, I., & Musgnung, J. J. (2006). Venlafaxine extended release in posttraumatic stress disorder: A sertraline- and placebo-controlled study. *Journal of Clinical Psychopharmacology, 26*, 259–267.

Davis, M., Barad, M., Otto, M., & Southwick, S. (2006). Combining pharmaco-therapy with cognitive behavioral therapy: Traditional and new approaches. *Journal of Traumatic Stress, 19*, 571–581.

Devilly, G. J., & Foa, E. B. (2001). Comments on Tarrier et al.'s study and the investigation of exposure and cognitive therapy. *Journal of Consulting and Clinical Psychology, 69*, 114–116.

Elhai, J. D., Gray, M. J., Naifeh, J. A., Butcher, J. J., Davis, J. L., Falsetti. S. A., et al. (2005). Utility of the Trauma Symptom Inventory's atypical response scale in detecting malingered posttraumatic stress disorder. *Assessment, 12*, 210–219.

Feldner, M. T., Monson, C. M., & Friedman, M. J. (2007). A critical analysis of approaches to targeted PTSD prevention: Current status and theoretically derived future directions. *Behavior Modification, 31*, 80–116.

Foa, E. B. (1995). *The Posttraumatic Diagnostic Scale (PDS) manual.* Minneapolis, MN: National Computer Systems.

Foa, E. B., & Rothbaum, B. O. (1998). *Treating the trauma of rape.* New York: Guilford Press.

Foa, E. B., Steketee, G., & Rothbaum, B. O. (1989). Behavioral/cognitive conceptualizations of post-traumatic stress disorder. *Behavior Therapy, 20*, 155–176.

Foa, E. B., Zinbarg, R., & Rothbaum, B. O. (1992). Uncontrollability and unpredictability in post-traumatic stress disorder: An animal model. *Psychological Bulletin, 112*, 218–238.

Forbes, D., Creamer, M., Hawthorne, G., Allen, N., & McHugh, T. (2003). Comorbidity as a predictor of symptom change after treatment in combat-related posttraumatic stress disorder. *The Journal of Nervous and Mental Disease, 191*, 93–99.

Freeman, T., Hart, H., & Kimbrell, T. (2005). *Symptom exaggeration in Veterans populations with PTSD: Preliminary findings.* Unpublished manuscript, Department of Psychiatry, University of Arkansas Medical Sciences, Little Rock.

Grace, M. C., Green, B. L., Lindy, J. D., & Leonard, A. C. (1993). The Buffalo Creek disaster: A 14-year follow-up. In J. P. Wilson & B. Raphael (Eds.), *International handbook of traumatic stress syndromes* (pp. 441–449). New York: Plenum Press.

Guriel, J., & Fremouw, W. (2003). Assessing malingered posttraumatic stress disorder: A critical review. *Clinical Psychology Review, 23*, 881–904.

Hembree, E. A., Foa, E. B., Dorfan, N. M., Street, G. P., Tu, X., & Kowalski, J. (2003). Do patients drop out prematurely from exposure therapy for PTSD? *Journal of Traumatic Stress, 16*, 555–562.

Hickling, E. J., Blanchard, E. B., Mundy, E., & Galovski, T. E. (2002). Detection of malingered MVA related posttraumatic stress disorder: An investigation of the ability to detect professional actors by experienced clinicians, psychological tests and psychophysiological assessment. *Journal of Forensic Psychology Practice, 2*, 33–53.

Jakupcak, M., Roberts, L. J., Martell, C., Mulick, P., Michael, S., Reed, R., et al. (2006). A pilot study of behavioral activation for veterans with posttraumatic stress disorder. *Journal of Traumatic Stress, 19*, 387–391.

Livanou, M., Basoglu, M., Marks, I. M., de Silva, P., Noshirvani, H., Lovell, K., et al. (2002). Beliefs, sense of control and treatment outcome in post-traumatic stress disorder. *Psychological Medicine, 32,* 157–165.

Mitchell, J. T., & Everly, G. S. (2000). Critical incident stress management and critical incident stress debriefings: Evolutions, effects and outcomes. In B. Raphael & J. P. Wilson (Eds.), *Psychological debriefing: Theory, practice and evidence* (pp. 71–90). New York: Cambridge University Press.

Najavits, L. M., Gallop, R. J., & Weiss, R. D. (2006). Seeking safety therapy for adolescent girls with PTSD and substance use disorder: A randomized controlled trial. *Journal of Behavioral Health Services and Research, 33,* 453–463.

National Institute for Clinical Excellence. (2005). *Post-traumatic stress disorder: The management of PTSD in adults and children in primary and secondary care.* London: Gaskell and the British Psychological Society.

Ozer, E. J., Best, S. R., Lipsey, T. L., & Weiss, D. S. (2003). Predictors of posttraumatic stress disorder and symptoms in adults: A meta-analysis. *Psychological Bulletin, 129,* 52–73.

Pankratz, L. (1998). *Patients who deceive: Assessment and management of risk in providing health care and financial benefits.* Springfield, IL: Charles C Thomas.

Rizzo, A., Rothbaum, B. O., & Graap, K. (2007). Virtual reality applications for the treatment of combat-related PTSD. In C. R. Figley & W. P. Nash (Eds.), *Combat stress injury: Theory, research, and management* (pp. 183–204). New York: Routledge.

Simon, R. I. (2003). *Posttraumatic stress disorder in litigation: Guidelines for forensic assessment* (2nd ed.). Washington, DC: American Psychiatric Publishing.

Stein, M. B., Jang, K. L., Taylor, S., Vernon, P. A., & Livesley, W. J. (2002). Genetic and environmental influences on trauma exposure and posttraumatic stress disorder symptoms: A general population twin study. *The American Journal of Psychiatry, 159,* 1675–1681.

Tarrier, N., Liversidge, T., & Gregg, L. (2006). The acceptability and preference for the psychological treatment of PTSD. *Behaviour Research and Therapy, 44,* 1643–1656.

Tarrier, N., Pilgrim, H., Sommerfield, C., Faragher, B., Reynolds, M., Graham, E., et al. (1999). A randomized trial of cognitive therapy and imaginal exposure in the treatment of chronic posttraumatic stress disorder. *Journal of Consulting and Clinical Psychology, 67,* 13–18.

Tarrier, N., Sommerfield, C., & Pilgrim, H. (1999). Relatives' expressed emotion (EE) and PTSD treatment outcome. *Psychological Medicine, 29,* 801–811.

Taylor, S. (2000). *Understanding and treating panic disorder.* New York: Wiley.

Taylor, S. (2004). *Advances in the treatment of posttraumatic stress disorder: Cognitive–behavioral perspectives.* New York: Springer.

Taylor, S. (2006). *Clinician's guide to PTSD: A cognitive–behavioral approach.* New York: Guilford Press.

Taylor, S., Fedoroff, I. C., Koch, W. J., Thordarson, D. S., Fecteau, G., & Nicki, R. (2001). Posttraumatic stress disorder arising after road traffic collisions: Patterns of response to cognitive–behavior therapy. *Journal of Consulting and Clinical Psychology, 69,* 541–551.

Taylor, S., Frueh, B. C., & Asmundson, G. J. G. (2007). Detection and management of malingering in people presenting for treatment of posttraumatic stress disorder: Methods, obstacles, and recommendations. *Journal of Anxiety Disorders, 21,* 22–41.

Taylor, S., Wald, J., & Asmundson, G. J. G. (2004). Current status and future directions in the cognitive–behavioral treatment of PTSD. In T. A. Corales (Ed.), *Progress in posttraumatic stress disorder research* (pp. 263–284). Hauppauge, NY: Nova Science.

van Emmerik, A. A. P., Kamphuis, J. H., Hulsbosch, A. M., & Emmelkamp, P. M. G. (2002, September 7). Single session debriefing after psychological trauma: A meta-analysis. *The Lancet, 360,* 766–771.

van Etten, M., & Taylor, S. (1998). Comparative efficacy of treatments for posttraumatic stress disorder: A meta-analysis. *Clinical Psychology and Psychotherapy, 5,* 126–145.

van Minnen, A., Arntz, A., & Keijsers, G. P. J. (2002). Prolonged exposure in patients with chronic PTSD: Predictors of treatment outcome and dropout. *Behaviour Research and Therapy, 40,* 439–457.

van Minnen, A., & Hagenaars, M. (2002). Fear activation and habituation patterns as early process predictors of response to prolonged exposure treatment in PTSD. *Journal of Traumatic Stress, 15,* 359–367.

Wald, J., & Taylor, S. (2005). Interoceptive exposure therapy combined with trauma-related exposure therapy for posttraumatic stress disorder: A case report. *Cognitive Behaviour Therapy, 34,* 34–40.

Wald, J., & Taylor, S. (2007). Efficacy of interoceptive exposure therapy combined with trauma-related exposure therapy for posttraumatic stress disorder: A case series. *Journal of Anxiety Disorders, 21,* 1050–1060.

Wald, J., & Taylor, S. (2008). Responses to interoceptive exposure in people with posttraumatic stress disorder (PTSD): A preliminary analysis of induced anxiety reactions and trauma memories, and their relationship to anxiety sensitivity and PTSD symptoms. *Cognitive Behaviour Therapy, 37,* 90–100.

Wald, J., Taylor, S., & Fedoroff, I. C. (2004). The challenge of treating PTSD in the context of chronic pain. In S. Taylor (Ed.), *Advances in the treatment of posttraumatic stress disorder: Cognitive–behavioral perspectives* (pp. 197–222). New York: Springer.

8

EATING DISORDERS

ATA GHADERI

Eating disorders (EDs) are one of the most common psychiatric disorders in young women (Kendler et al., 1991), and there is evidence that the prevalence of these disorders is rising (Götestam & Agras, 1995). The price for EDs is high, both in terms of the costs for the health care system and human suffering (Striegel-Moore, Leslie, Petrill, Garvin, & Rosenheck, 2000). Among the consequences of EDs are heightened risks of mortality, depression, suicide, and chronic medical complications such as cardiovascular and gastrointestinal problems (Becker, Grinspoon, Klibanski, & Herzog, 1999; Hall et al., 1989). The road to recovery is often long, with the average duration of an ED being 9 to 15 years (Milos, Spindler, Schnyder, & Fairburn, 2005).

Anorexia nervosa (AN), *bulimia nervosa* (BN), and the residual category labeled *eating disorders not otherwise specified* (EDNOS) are the three recognized ED diagnoses in the *Diagnostic and Statistical Manual of Mental Disorders* (4th ed., text rev.; American Psychiatric Association, 2000).

AN is characterized by the following aspects: (a) very low weight (below 85% of expected weight in relation to the individual's age, gender, and height, which is equivalent to a body mass index [BMI] below 17.5 for adults); (b) intense fear of gaining weight or becoming fat, even though the person is underweight; (c) amenorrhea in postmenarche females (i.e., absence of at least three consecutive menstrual cycles); and (d) disturbances in the experience of body shape or weight, which in some cases is expressed as an undue influence of body weight or shape on the individual's self-evaluation or denial of the seriousness of the low weight and its consequences. Evidence has suggested that the core features in the development and maintenance of AN are the potent positive reinforcement of a "feeling of being in control" and "feelings of self-satisfaction" (Slade, 1982, pp. 169, 172) and the overvaluation of shape and weight (Fairburn, Cooper, & Shafran, 2003). Moreover, the extreme low weight in AN influences many physiological processes to the extent that the individual's perceptions, emotions, and cognitions become affected in a way that perpetuates the disorder.

BN is a more recent diagnosis than AN and is characterized by (a) recurrent episodes of *binge eating* (i.e., uncontrollably eating significantly larger amounts of food than what is considered normal in the context it occurs); followed by (b) compensatory behaviors such as self-induced vomiting, abusing laxatives or diuretics (*purging behaviors*), fasting, dieting, or extreme exercising (*nonpurging compensatory behaviors*); and (c) self-evaluation that is unduly influenced by body weight and shape. Although AN is perpetuated by a constant striving to gain as much control as possible and to experience the same feelings that were present during the initial phase of AN (i.e., weight loss; feeling of being in control; experiencing uniqueness and strength, which is partly due to a huge amount of stress hormones and beta-endorphin in the body as a reaction to the ongoing weight loss), those with BN often feel a clear lack of control, as their attempts to diet soon result in binge eating and the need to drastically compensate for their intake.

Although AN and BN are the main categories of EDs, the majority of patients in clinical practice do not meet the full criteria for AN or BN; instead, they fall under the residual category diagnosis of EDNOS (Fairburn & Bohn, 2005). There has been very little research on EDNOS, with the exception of *binge eating disorder* (BED), which is similar to BN in many aspects. BED is characterized by recurrent binge episodes without regular compensatory behavior and by its frequent comorbidity with obesity. Because of the residual category status of EDNOS, the conditions listed under this category (e.g., partial or subthreshold AN or BN, BED, regular vomiting, other compensatory behaviors after eating small amounts of food) have received very little attention, and thus many clinicians erroneously view these conditions as being considerably less severe than AN or BN. Consequently, many patients with such diagnoses do not receive adequate treatment, if any at all, because the cases with the full AN or BN diagnoses are prioritized.

Another problem concerning ED classification is encountered with the definition of the severity of the disorders. Empirical research has shown that the arbitrarily chosen limits that define a full or subthreshold ED diagnosis are highly questionable. As an example, those receiving a full or partial BED diagnosis do not differ significantly on measures of weight and shape concern, restraint, distress, and history of seeking treatment for an eating or weight problem (Striegel-Moore, Dohm, et al., 2000) after adjusting for differences in BMI. Similarly, the results from the study on full versus syndromal EDs by Crow, Stewart Agras, Halmi, Mitchell, and Kraemer (2002) emphasized the similarities between full and partial cases, especially concerning AN and BED.

The most recent advances concerning the classification of ED, which bear on the understanding and treatment of these disorders, suggest a transdiagnostic theory and treatment that focuses on the fundamental similarities between all the diagnoses of ED, as well as ED's distinction as a category of disorders compared with other psychiatric problems (Fairburn et al., 2003).

EFFECTIVE TREATMENTS FOR EATING DISORDERS

Meta-analyses, reviews, guidelines, and authoritative papers (e.g., Fairburn & Harrison, 2003; National Institute for Clinical Excellence, 2004; Wilson, 1996) all have suggested that cognitive–behavioral therapy (CBT) should be considered the first-line treatment of choice for BN. Although interpersonal psychotherapy (IPT) results in similar outcomes as CBT at 1 year after the end of the treatment (Agras, Walsh, Fairburn, Wilson, & Kraemer, 2000), it is not suggested as the treatment of choice because the patients recover significantly faster through CBT, which means faster and more effective reduction of suffering for BN patients.

The effect of psychotropic medication, especially antidepressants (primarily the selective serotonin reuptake inhibitor [SSRI] class), has been investigated in many studies (e.g., Mitchell, Raymond, & Specker, 1993), and some SSRIs (e.g., fluoxetine) have been shown to be effective in the treatment of BN and BED. However, the general rate of remission with these medications is low (e.g., Mitchell, Agras, & Wonderlich, 2007), and the prevalence of relapse is high when the medication is withdrawn (e.g., Mitchell et al., 2007; Walsh, Hadigan, Delvin, Gladis, & Roose, 1991). Furthermore, medication is considered to have limited efficacy and is difficult to dose appropriately among low-weight patients with AN (e.g., Ferguson, La Via, Crossan, & Kaye, 1999). The combination of CBT and medication has also been investigated in several studies. In most cases, there are no significant differences between CBT as the sole treatment and CBT combined with medication (e.g., Goldbloom et al., 1997; Mitchell et al., 1990). It should be remembered, though, that these are group-level data, and in some individual cases the combination might be a better choice (see the Factors Leading to Poor Treatment Response section for strategies for treating those with poor treatment response).

For AN, there is still no effective treatment available. However, for nonchronic patients (i.e., those with symptoms for less than 2 years) who have their debut in their early teens, systemic family-based treatments in line with the model used at the Maudsley Hospital (e.g., Lock, Le Grange, Agras, & Dare, 2001), which is largely identical to the behavioral family systems therapy (Robin, 2003), have been shown to be a viable treatment option with good outcome (e.g., Eisler et al., 2000; Robin et al., 1999).

There are virtually no well-designed treatment outcome studies or specifically targeted treatments for the most frequently encountered diagnostic category of ED (i.e., EDNOS), with the exception of BED. A few high-quality studies have shown that CBT is an effective treatment for those with BED (Grilo, Masheb, & Wilson, 2005) and that IPT is a viable option to group CBT (e.g., Wilfley et al., 1993, 2002).

As CBT has not resulted in higher remission than 40% to 50% among those who complete the treatment (usually 80%), considerable efforts have been made to enhance the treatment during the last 10 years on the basis of empirical research and theoretical refinement of the treatment model. The recently completed Oxford-Leicester trial using the enhanced version of CBT (called CBT-E), which is based on a transdiagnostic view of ED, has resulted in considerably better outcome than trials using previous versions of CBT (e.g., Wilson, Fairburn, & Agras, 1997), despite the fact that *remission* and *recovery* have been defined much more stringently than in previous studies (Fairburn, 2007). CBT-E includes methods such as techniques for improving metacognitive awareness, which have been shown to be more potent than conventional cognitive restructuring in the treatment of patients with EDs. In addition, in CBT-E there is a greater focus on several other maintaining mechanisms, such as body checking. Focusing on several maintaining mechanisms helps to overcome the overvaluation of weight and shape. Finally, CBT-E is designed to be extended for those not showing rapid response to CBT, to address further maintaining mechanisms such as low self-esteem, perfectionism, interpersonal difficulties, and affect intolerance. The large number of CBT studies on EDs, especially on BN, have resulted in a better and more functional understanding of mechanisms that maintain EDs. CBT-E reflects the lessons learned from these studies.

CORE BASIS OF THE TREATMENT OF EATING DISORDERS

In this section, the essential elements of CBT for EDs are briefly described, that is, the core elements of CBT and CBT-E. Although the focus of this chapter, and the volume, is on lessons learned from CBT, a short description of IPT is also provided because it serves certain functions in the further analysis of treatment-refractory cases.

In CBT, the focus is on variables maintaining the disorder (Fairburn, Marcus, & Wilson, 1993). One of the most central of these variables is the overvaluation of shape and weight that results in efforts to control weight and shape through restraint, dieting in various forms, and in some cases, starvation. In some patients (mostly those with BN), these behaviors lead to overeating and binge eating as a consequence of hunger and abstinence violation effects (i.e., to relinquish all efforts to control eating and to refrain from overeating whenever rigid, eating-related rules are broken, such as when a small amount of "forbidden" food is consumed). Hence, a vicious cycle emerges between dieting and binge eating. The latter becomes even more established as the individual uses different compensatory behaviors to get rid of the ingested food and the anxiety that binge eating creates. The compensatory behaviors make the binge eating feel less intolerable than it is. Consequently, vomiting, misusing laxatives, excessive exercise, and other forms of compensatory behaviors maintain the binge eating and are in turn maintained by binge eating. With each episode of binge eating, the individual becomes more determined to lose more weight and diet even harder because of the nature of binge eating that encompasses a strong sense of loss of control. In turn, increased restraint and dieting lead to more frequent binges, while the individual becomes more focused on weight and shape and more worried about the consequences of his or her binges. The treatment targets these maintaining variables starting with psychoeducation and helping the patient to stop compensating and to eat regularly. Psychoeducation consists of (a) information on why compensatory behaviors are ineffective to control weight and shape, (b) an explanation of the vicious cycle between dieting and binge eating by using examples from research such as the Minnesota starvation study (Keys, Brozek, Henschel, & Mickelson, 1950), (c) a discussion of the physical and psychological consequences of EDs, and (d) a review of the impact of regular eating on the regulation of hunger and satiety signals. These strategies (i.e., psychoeducation, cessation of compensatory behaviors, and regular eating) alone help reduce binge eating by 70% on average. Focus then shifts toward addressing restraint, dieting, and body image issues as well as the individual's self-esteem and other maintaining variables.

Those diagnosed with AN fall into vicious cycles between overvaluation of control over eating, shape, and weight on the one hand and dieting as well as psychological and physiological consequences of low weight on the other hand, that lead to more focus on weight and shape and dieting. Another subgroup of patients, when categorized on the basis of maintaining variables, present a mixed picture of the above categories, although some are different variants of the first or second category (often diagnosed with BN or some EDNOS variant of BN, or with full, partial, or subthreshold AN).

In systemic or behavioral family therapy for AN, the focus is on empowering the parents to help their child eat and gain weight while major efforts are made to improve the communication among the family members. The family members, particularly the parents, are mobilized by learning about the seriousness of AN and the need for the family to take charge of the situation in order to help the teenage child gain weight and pursue the normal path of development. As the child starts to eat and his or her weight stabilizes, the focus shifts toward addressing adolescence issues such as identity and independence. Parents receive a lot of guidance and support to help their child eat more and gain weight while efforts are made to help the family communicate independent of AN (Lock et al., 2001).

In IPT, the focus is on four major areas that have significant bearing on interpersonal relations: grief, interpersonal conflicts, transitions, and interpersonal deficits (Wilfley, MacKenzie, Welch, Ayres, & Weissman, 2000). The therapy is often given in a group format in which the group members view their current life situation and difficulties in relation to potential loss and grief, conflicts, interpersonal skills deficits, or positive or negative transitions. IPT is an empirically supported, time-limited psychotherapy that focuses on the here and now, with no psychodynamic interpretations or focus on transference or other issues inherent in psychodynamic psychotherapy (Markowitz, Svartberg, & Swartz, 1998).

FACTORS LEADING TO POOR TREATMENT RESPONSE

A sound knowledge of the nature, phenomenology, risk factors, course, and maintaining mechanisms of EDs, as well as the relevant therapeutic methods and techniques, is crucial for understanding, analyzing, and addressing poor treatment response in EDs. In the sections that follow, a short summary of some of these factors that might have a more general relation to poor treatment response is given, followed by more specific variables that lead to poor treatment response. Finally, ways to enhance and improve the treatment so as to help as many people with EDs as possible are discussed.

The origins of EDs are widely considered to be multifactorial. Different combinations of various risk factors interact with each other in different contexts to increase the risk of an individual developing an ED. Although the multifactorial model has been criticized for its lack of specificity and its complexity, currently it fits the empirical data best. Its implication for the treatment of patients not responding to the best available interventions is that it helps the clinician to avoid confirmation bias (i.e., looking only for the information that confirms the clinician's general understanding of the patient's problem on the basis of previous experience rather than what is unique for the individual patient) and to think of other possible early risk factors that might have been missed in the early and ongoing assessment of the patient. Such factors might have become consolidated over time and become maintaining variables, which make the patient unable to focus and work on the target behaviors (in the broad sense of the term—e.g., acts, emotions, cognitions). As an example, obsessive–compulsive tendencies that might be present before an individual develops an ED often make the work on weight gain, normalization of eating habits, and weight and shape concerns very difficult if obsessive–compulsive tendencies are not specifically addressed. Frequent or strong obsessions often diminish the quality of behavioral experiments, cognitive work, and exposure efforts aimed at addressing the ED. The picture is usually quite complex because many obsessive and compulsive tendencies could be a consequence of starvation among low-weight patients, and these tendencies often decrease or disappear after weight restoration. Remaining open to different factors and avoiding overuse of heuristics (i.e., by determining what should be done on the basis of the clinician's previous experience with other patients without paying enough attention to the phenomenology of the problems that the current patient is presenting), which is one of the most frequent forms of bias among clinicians, are extremely important. Attention to different potential risk factors for each individual patient that might function as a maintaining variable is of utmost importance.

The strong genetic predisposition for ED, especially in the cases of patients who are able to starve themselves (Klump, Miller, Keel, McGue, & Iacono, 2001), is also an important variable to bear in mind and to incorporate in the rationale for the treatment. Such a rationale helps the patient to more easily create some distance between him- or herself and the ED, and to take an active stance in handling his or her vulnerability. It also helps patients understand why the significant and rapid weight loss they experienced during the first phase of the AN was as rewarding as it was (due to massive stress response combined with overproduction of endorphins because of the specific genetic predisposition they have) and that weight loss was not a matter of will or character. Furthermore, it is explained that when they achieve a low weight, their body is no longer capable of producing the same rewarding consequences as when they started to loose weight for the first time. Each new effort to lose weight will be less and less rewarding.

The most effective treatments for EDs (e.g., CBT, behavioral or systemic family therapy) focus more on maintaining variables than on potential initial causes. However, a considerable number of patients do not respond to these treatments. In making an informed decision whether to increase the dose or complexity of the treatment, or to refer the patient to another treatment, a critical review of the assessment process, the variables that have been the target of the treatment, potential other maintaining variables, and the relation between the course of the ED and contextual factors is necessary.

EDs are characterized by fluctuations. What the patient subjectively considers to be a "good" period (i.e., weight loss, more control, less eating) is often related to behaviors that maintain the ED. Periods of starvation, dieting, extreme control, and positive feelings are usually followed by episodes of binge eating, overeating, and abandonment of dieting efforts together with feelings of worthlessness, disappointment, and failure. With the patients who do not respond to empirically supported treatments, the clinician needs to pay more attention to contextual factors that contribute to the ups and downs in the course of their ED. For example, the main reason for poor treatment response resulting from failure to engage in the treatment might be the combination of the patient's overvaluation of the significance of the upcoming beach season (i.e., a usual contextual variable) and the patient's past experiences about the importance of being thin enough to wear a favorite bathing suit. Interpersonal relationships that are periodically abusive or stressful are other examples of periodical contextual factors that might make it difficult for the patient to engage in the treatment. Attention to the patient's context in relation to engagement in and response to the treatment cannot be stressed enough.

Understanding the phenomenology of ED for each individual patient has much more treatment utility than the diagnostic labels. Beyond models of the maintenance of ED and nonnegotiable goals, such as weight gain to the level that the low weight is not life threatening, therapists need to meet patients with genuine openness and carefully listen in order to understand and identify the variables that maintain their ED. Showing genuine interest and a frank desire to understand the phenomenology of ED for the individual patient are among the core strategies that help the patient to see both the short- and long-term pros and cons of ED from another perspective than the one contaminated by ED. A common reason for poor treatment response as a consequence of failure to engage in the treatment is the lack of mutual understanding of the ED (i.e., the patient having his or her explanation, or the view that there are no problems at all, and the therapist holding to his or her own perspective). The patient experiences that the treatment is not a team effort but something that is being done to him or her. Taking the time to build a shared understanding of the ED helps to prevent such a dead-end position.

Finally, instead of focusing on the typography of the problems, a functional approach to understanding the past and current behavior of the patient usually leads to more empowerment of the patient and an enhanced therapeutic relationship. A functional approach helps the patient see his or her behaviors as understandable responses to the environmental events and controlled by the consequences. Such an understanding enhances the therapeutic relationship because it provides validation of why the patient has acted in particular ways in the past.

The issues mentioned here, in addition to many other central variables leading to poor treatment response, are elaborated on in more detail later in this chapter.

Failure to Engage in Treatment

One of the major reasons for poor treatment response is failure to engage in treatment, which often results from a lack of a clear consensus about what the problem is (if the patient admits to any problem at all), how it was developed, how it is maintained, and the best way to address the issues at hand. In such circumstances, many therapists classify the patient as unmotivated. Lack of motivation, especially among patients with AN, is well documented. However, *motivation* is defined and measured in various ways, and a more precise definition and operationalization of the term might help the clinician to more effectively overcome the underlying difficulties that are usually called *lack of motivation*. Motivation to change can be assessed within the frame of the transtheoretical model of change. Treasure et al. (1999) investigated the role of readiness to change in the engagement of patients and outcome of CBT for BN. The results showed that although the transtheoretical model of change might be useful, available measures of readiness to change require adaptation to capture the core processes involved in the motivation to change in BN. It is not surprising that Dunn, Neighbors, and Larimer (2003) showed that assessing readiness to change bulimic symptomatology explains a larger portion of variance in bulimic behavior than a general measure of readiness to change. Useful guides are also available for using motivational interviewing (MI) in the treatment of AN (e.g., Treasure & Ward, 1998). Other researchers have criticized the transtheoretical stages of change model as having conceptual and empirical limitations (e.g., Wilson & Schlam, 2004). They pointed out that although the model is frequently associated with MI, no theory links the two. Whether combining MI with CBT enhances the efficacy of CBT remains an empirical question (Wilson & Schlam, 2004), but careful integration or sequencing of well-defined clinical procedures of MI with CBT might be a useful way of addressing lack of motivation in treatment-refractory cases of ED. Failure to engage in treatment because of various variables such as problem formulation, maintaining mechanisms, or the suggested way to address the problem might be another way of operationalizing lack of motivation. As an example, it is not unusual for patients to view their ED as a form of addiction. Such a belief makes them assume that they are biologically vulnerable to certain foods (typically different kinds of sugar) and, when exposed to such food, they become addicted to them (Wilson, 1993). The way to recovery, seen through the lens of the addiction model, is total and nonnegotiable restraint. Such a view is in complete contrast to the CBT approach in which rigid restraint and dieting are considered to maintain ED. Patients viewing their eating problems from an addiction point of view would experience major difficulties following the CBT model and rationale in which all forms of dieting should be stopped and thoroughly dealt with.

Explaining the CBT rationale is in some cases not enough if the patient embraces another theory or explanation that is not compatible with CBT. Thus, the therapist needs to carefully explore the patient's beliefs and assumptions regarding the causes and the treatment of ED and address the similarities and differences between the patient's assumptions and CBT.

In a similar way, a common reason for poor outcome is potential similarity between earlier unsuccessful experiences from other therapies or the patient's own efforts to overcome ED and the current suggested homework assignments, parts of the CBT rationale, or strategies. As an example, many patients with BN have some kind of previous experience of recording their food intake and usually report some efforts on their own to eat a little more regularly to overcome their episodes of binge eating. Regular eating and daily records of food intake are among the most crucial elements of the CBT treatment. If the therapist does not explain in what ways the recommended daily recording of food intake in CBT differs from what the patient has done previously, and if the function of this demanding task is not mapped out for the patient to see meaningful differences compared with his or her earlier experiences, then there will be a major risk of not doing the daily records, or even more frequently, of doing them just to please the therapist, which does not help the patient to see functional relations between food intake and ED symptoms and problems. A good understanding of what patients have done before they entered CBT, their expectations, and their previous experiences of the different methods and strategies used is paramount for delivering a clear CBT rationale that differentiates it from what has been done earlier.

Finally, it should be mentioned that in some instances the clients are unable to engage in CBT for various reasons. If CBT is offered within the frame of a multidisciplinary team, then it might be constructive to openly discuss engaging in some other forms of therapy (e.g., occupational therapy, medication) for a period and reengaging in CBT at a later date (Waller, Cordery, et al., 2007). It is important to stop the treatment before it becomes too aversive.

Can Less Be More?

As Wilson (1996) suggested, when the first-line manual-based treatment fails, the therapist should use other empirically supported treatments, and if they do not work or are not available, then the therapist should resort to the problem-solving (hypothesis-testing) approach that characterizes CBT. Empirical studies show that when CBT fails, IPT or pharmacotherapy do not result in further significant improvements (e.g., Agras et al., 1995; Mitchell et al., 2002). Mitchell et al. (2002) concluded that offering lengthy sequential treatments when CBT fails appears to have little value, and alternative models for therapy need to be tested. The question is whether less can be more. However, accumulating knowledge from empirical studies has shown that a host of various variables seem to be responsible for poor outcome, and as no treatment has yet been constructed to address all such variables, clinicians usually have to rely on their own experience in tailoring the treatment to address the special needs of the patients not responding to the empirically supported treatments.

Given the known biases (e.g., heuristic, availability) that are common even among the most skilled clinicians when they have to rely on their own experience (for a review, see Wilson, 1996), it is paramount to use a structured, theoretically sound, and empirically grounded approach to analyze variables that maintain ED among those with poor treatment response. Critical use of case formulation and behavioral functional analysis (e.g., Famer & Latner, 2007; Ghaderi, 2007; Levander & Schmidt, 2006; Needleman, 1999; Persons & Davidson, 2001) seems to be the best available approaches. The importance of acquiring and enhancing skills in doing such analyses cannot be stressed enough.

Starting Well: The Implications of Depression and Other Obstacles to Treatment

In the new transdiagnostic formulations of CBT, Fairburn (2005) stressed the importance of setting the scene to achieve the best possible start to the therapy. This means identifying obstacles for completing treatment, addressing problems such as crises or major transitions (e.g., starting a new job, change in marital status) before the therapy starts, and using pharmacotherapy for patients with clinical depression. Recent research on the treatment of depression shows, however, that behavioral activation (Dimidjian et al., 2006; Jacobson et al., 1996) might be an alternative treatment for depression that is just as potent as, if not better than, pharmacotherapy. In addition, with younger people (i.e., the majority of patients with ED), it is usually easier to come to an agreement about testing a behavioral treatment for depression rather than using pharmacotherapy. This is, however, based on clinical observations, and empirical studies are needed. Furthermore, agreement with the patient on what treatment should be used among the empirically supported ones (pharmacotherapy or psychotherapy) cannot be stressed enough.

Predictors of Treatment Outcome

A large body of research has been devoted to identifying predictors of treatment outcome. The picture is often one of null results or considerable variation in the outcome of these studies because of methodological shortcomings such as less rigorous methods of assessment and small samples. Consequently, reliable predictors of outcome for CBT, or in fact any other form of psychotherapy, have not been identified. Early response to CBT is an exception, though, and has been one of the best predictors of favorable outcome (Grilo, Masheb, & Wilson, 2006; Wilson et al., 1999). Hence, it is crucial to assess the progress of the patient, retake and broaden the assessment, and revise the treatment if no clinically meaningful sign of improvement can be seen after the first few weeks of treatment (e.g., by Week 4 of the treatment of BN or BED). More research is needed on other proposed predictors of outcome, such as obesity and low weight, as the findings from different studies are contradictory.

Although addressing the core psychopathology of ED helps a substantial portion of the patients to recover from ED, about half of the patients do not benefit enough from CBT (Wilson, 1996). Increased individualization of the treatment on the basis of functional analysis has shown more favorable outcome with BN patients (Ghaderi, 2006) than standard CBT. Parallel to this line of research, the transdiagnostic treatment (CBT-E), which also makes room for further individualization, has shown increased efficacy (Fairburn, 2007) compared with earlier trials of standard CBT. The transdiagnostic trial also showed that patients with more complicated ED benefited more from the broad version of the treatment (working with one or several additional maintaining factors than those related to the core psychopathology of ED), whereas for those with less complicated ED, there were no differences between the broad or focused CBT-E (Fairburn, 2007). A very important lesson learned is to adapt treatment to meet the needs of the patient. Instead of increasing the dose of the treatment for those not responding to the standard intervention, therapists should look for additional maintaining variables besides those that are almost always present among cases with ED.

The additional variables that needed to be addressed in the individualized trial on BN (Ghaderi, 2006) on the basis of ideographic analysis (Ghaderi, 2007) were very similar to areas suggested in the transdiagnostic CBT for ED by Fairburn et al. (2003). The authors suggested that core low self-esteem, clinical perfectionism, interpersonal difficulties, and mood intolerance might be important additional maintaining variables that need to be addressed for a subsample of patients with ED.

The additional variables that usually maintain EDs among patients with poor treatment response must be addressed in the course of the therapy to achieve clinically significant and durable results. As an example, patients with significant interpersonal difficulties (e.g., recurrent role conflicts and disputes) might find it difficult to focus on treatment because their eating-related problems are usually highly affected by negative emotions that they experience because of the specific difficulties in their close relationships. Difficulties in being assertive, expressing primary affects (e.g., feelings of longing or sadness because a spouse spends too much time at work), or effectively discussing and handling conflicts might result in constant invalidation, expression of secondary feelings (e.g., subsequent frustration and anger at the absent spouse), dysfunctional judgments, and maladaptive coping (Fruzzetti, 1996). The negative emotions in relationships are common antecedents of binge eating or dieting. Low self-esteem, and in some cases core low self-esteem (the latter being unconditional and pervasive), is also a common feature among those with ED, which in many ways is intertwined with difficulties in being assertive and expressing one's own needs. In his seminal invited essay, Wilson (1996) mentioned that the Oxford group consistently found that low self-esteem predicts a more negative treatment outcome. Patients with core low self-esteem usually report that they do not feel worthy of the treatment efforts or the engagement of the treatment providers; furthermore, they feel unworthy of living a good and valued life. Consequently, they see no point in engaging in the treatment, and hence, no rapid changes can be achieved that might reinforce increased engagement and hope for working harder to overcome the ED.

Interaction of Complicating Variables: Low Self-Esteem, Low Weight, and Rigidity

The situation is also in some cases complicated by the presence of severe low weight; the increased rigidity (i.e., the demand to follow rules and rituals to even higher degree than before) that is partly a consequence of starvation; and the association of self-worth only with control over eating, weight, and shape (i.e., ED becoming part of the individual's identity). Weight restoration is crucial in these cases, but the discrepancy between the patient's and the treatment providers' agenda usually results in lack of engagement in the treatment, and a pattern of power struggle is unfortunately not uncommon. The patient perceives the treatment as something that is being imposed on him or her, rather than a joint effort to overcome the difficulties. The medical issues of safety, usually the consequences of low weight such as *hypokalemia* (i.e., low blood levels of potassium) or other complicating issues, put a tremendous pressure on the treatment providers to be persuasive and even forceful if needed. The seriousness of the situation makes it, in some cases, very difficult to agree on an agenda and help the patient to create enough distance to be willing to test alternative strategies. Using a functional analytic approach to assessment and treatment of ED, the therapist should frame the weight gain in the treatment rationale as a series of behavioral experiments in which the patient can be helped to test his or her assumption in the face of efforts to gain weight. The patient needs to feel in charge.

It is worth mentioning that some new developments in the field of CBT and behavior analysis, in terms of relational frame theory (RFT; Hayes, Barnes-Holmes, & Roche, 2001) and acceptance and commitment therapy (ACT; Hayes, Strosahl, & Wilson, 1999), would suggest a more radical stance in which the therapist helps the patient to see the impossibility of exerting control over internal states. The function of losing weight is primarily to achieve some internal consequences (e.g., feeling unique, worthy, in control, special) and, initially, some positive social reinforcement before emaciation becomes a fact. The radical approach in ACT is to help the patient to experience the futility of efforts to control internal events in the long run through experiential exercises, analogies, metaphors, and a host of other methods. This is done to help the patient be willing to test other alternatives and be open to new and direct experiences. Although ACT is approaching the status of an empirically supported treatment for some psychological disorders, there is a marked paucity of data on ACT and its efficacy for ED. Hence, although ACT seems to be a promising approach, its use for ED should only be considered in light of rigorous continuous clinical assessment and should be limited to treatment-refractory cases in which other empirically supported treatments have failed.

To increase the patient's willingness to gain weight, it is often very helpful to address issues related to low self-esteem. Recent advances in CBT for addressing low self-esteem (Fennell, 2006) provide a good framework and useful tools for helping ED patients create a more adequate and functional sense of self, their value as humans, and what they value in life, which together with a focus on the core psychopathology of ED and other maintaining factors might increase the probability of favorable treatment response. Fennell (2004) suggested that metacognitive awareness, operationalized in terms of acceptance of the idea that thoughts and beliefs are cognitive events and processes rather than reflections of objective truth, may be an important precursor for many patients to become actively engaged in the therapy. This is in line with findings from RFT research, which show that some forms of verbal behavior (e.g., thinking, assuming) may lead to lack of contact with actual contingencies around us, which in turn might result in increased inflexibility and lack of action in valued directions. The suggested strategies based on the behavioral analysis of cognitions (e.g., distancing, deliteralization, cognitive defusion; Hayes et al., 1999) are in line with the other new methods and strategies (e.g., metacognitive awareness; Teasdale, Moore, Haylurst, Pope, & Williams, 2002; Wells & King, 2006) used in the CBT treatment manuals from recent years. The central process in all of these strategies is to help patients view their thoughts and emotions as nothing more than thoughts and emotions, and not as ultimate truths. Detaching from thoughts and emotions helps the patient to take the steps necessary to experience the world as it is, by exposure, and not as his or her thoughts say it is. Although more studies are needed, available outcome studies of ED using such newer strategies show promising results (Fairburn, 2007; Ghaderi, 2006).

Interpersonal Relations and Difficulties

The importance of interpersonal relations for recovery from ED became more evident when randomized controlled studies of CBT for BN and BED showed that IPT could produce as good long-term outcome as CBT (Agras et al., 2000; Fairburn et al., 1991; Fairburn, Jones, Peveler, Hope, & O'Connor, 1993; Wilfley et al., 1993). However, IPT has not shown any evidence of efficacy in the treatment of AN (McIntosh et al., 2005). Nevertheless, taken together, the lessons learned from ideographic CBT approaches integrated with evidence-based treatment (Ghaderi, 2006) and accumulated knowledge from a large number of empirical studies (for a review, see Fairburn et al., 2003) indicate that interpersonal processes contribute in a variety of ways to the perpetuation of ED. It is interesting that the role of interpersonal difficulties has also been a focal point in other difficult-to-treat psychiatric disorders, such as generalized anxiety disorder (Borkovec, Newman, Pincus, & Lytle, 2002). Because IPT is an empirically supported treatment, methods and strategies from IPT can be integrated into CBT treatment of ED to address interpersonal difficulties. Another alternative is to use more cognitive–behavioral congruent approaches, such as assertiveness training (e.g., Alberti & Emmons, 2001).

Affect Intolerance

Another complicating variable, *affect intolerance*, is defined as an inability to cope with certain emotions, sensitivity to intense mood states, and engagement in dysfunctional mood regulatory behaviors such as self-injury or taking psychoactive substances. Some ED patients have major difficulties regulating their emotions. Studies investigating the predictors of outcome have often focused on the complicating role of personality disorders. Borderline personality disorder is one the common Axis II disorders (American Psychiatric Association, 2000) among patients with ED. Dialectical behavior therapy (DBT; Linehan, 1993) has been developed for helping patients with borderline personality disorder and has shown good evidence of efficacy in several trials (Linehan et al., 1999, 2006). DBT is composed of many modules, one of which is to help patients to pay attention to (i.e., be mindful of) and tolerate their emotions. Using chain analysis, which is a simplified version of functional analysis, patients learn to identify the triggering variables and the consequences of the way they handle their strong emotions, as well as to learn new ways of handling their emotions. All these behaviorally based strategies are easy to incorporate in CBT for ED, which also helps the patient to overcome many difficulties in interpersonal contexts and to build a more adequate sense of self. In a similar way, Waller, Corstorphine, and Mountford (2007b) refer to *emotional invalidation*, which occurs when the expression of emotions leads to negative and undesirable reactions (i.e., punishing reactions from others) or lack of any responses from the environment. Invalidations might result in poor distress tolerance and emotional inhibition. Waller et al. outlined CBT approaches for work on the acceptability of emotions and the core beliefs that underpin the emotional difficulties.

Perfectionism

Severe perfectionism might also be one of the major maintaining variables that needs to be addressed when it is profound and appears to make it difficult for the patient to fully engage in the treatment. *Clinical perfectionism* from a CBT perspective has been defined as the overdependence of self-evaluation on the determined pursuit of personally demanding, self-imposed standards in at least one highly salient domain, despite adverse consequences (Shafran, Coooper, & Fairburn, 2003).

Once again, many potent CBT strategies and methods are available for the treatment of perfectionism (e.g., Antony & Swinson, 1998), and initial trials focusing on ED patients with severe perfectionism show promising results (Riley, Lee, Cooper, Fairburn, & Shafran, 2007).

Body Checking

One of the important maintaining variables that has not received enough attention in earlier trials and CBT treatment manuals is body checking. It can be seen as a variant of safety behaviors observed in anxiety disorders and plays an important role for the maintenance of ED. Although frequent weighing and use of mirrors—or complete avoidance of weighing or mirrors—have been fairly well addressed in early CBT treatment manuals, other forms of body checking, such as constant pinching of parts of the body to check for fat or comparisons with other women, need further attention. The belief that checking the body allows one to judge one's own body and weight has been shown to be related more to bingeing and vomiting than to ED diagnoses (Mountford, Haase, & Waller, 2007). Hence, special attention should be paid to body checking issues among those with such symptoms. Work on other areas such as regular eating and cessation of all forms of dieting is usually affected negatively if the patient is highly engaged in body checking. The effect of exposure and stimulus control will be in part neutralized in the patient's mind through body checking. As an example, the patient might believe that her weight is not increasing dramatically, although she is eating more regularly, because she keeps checking her body. Body checking, as a safety behavior, does not let the patient get in touch with the actual consequences of her regular eating because they will be wrongly attributed to body checking. For example, the typical bulimic patient fails to see that regular eating, despite abstinence from compensatory behaviors, actually does not result in weight gain. She believes that her weight is stable thanks to her constant body checking. For more guidance on how to expand the work on body image issues and body checking, see Waller, Cordery, et al. (2007) and Fairburn, Cooper, Shafran, and Wilson (2008).

Cognitive Deficits

A substantial number of studies have focused on the role of cognitive deficits for the development and maintenance of ED (Lena, Fiocco, & Leyenaar, 2004). Deficits in executive functioning, visual-spatial ability, sustained attention, verbal ability, learning, and memory have been observed.

Although some of the cognitive deficits observed among ED patients might be attributed to starvation and low weight, some studies have shown that certain cognitive deficits do not improve after refeeding and weight gain (e.g., Lena et al., 2004). Furthermore, a subsample of the patients (mostly those diagnosed with AN) suffer from autism spectrum disorders such as Asperger's syndrome, have specific difficulties in perspective taking, and show a test profile characterized by difficulties concerning comprehension (Gillberg, Gillberg, Rastam, & Johansson, 1996). These patients become easily obsessed about details and display significant problems in abstract thinking and comprehending the overall picture in the context. Treating ED patients with comorbid autistic-like disorders is a challenge to even the most skilled clinician. As many features of ED in such cases might be secondary to primary difficulties in perspective taking, excessive rigidity, and cognitive deficits due to the autism spectrum disorders, a thorough functional analysis is invaluable in ascertaining what behaviors and deficits to focus on in order to address the ED-related symptoms.

Finally, a recurrent finding that might be of clinical interest is that patients with BN show a more impulsive cognitive style (Kaye, Bastiani, & Moss, 1995) that is similar to that of patients with attention-deficit/hyperactivity disorder. Such difficulties can in some cases explain the failure to engage in the treatment, and thus attention to possible cognitive deficits among treatment-refractory cases is crucial in reassessing such patients.

Excessive Dominance of Rule-Governed Behavior

Detailed analysis of patients not responding to CBT (Ghaderi, 2006) showed that they were characterized by extreme dominance of rule-governed behaviors and lack of contact with actual contingencies of their behaviors. When a person's behavior is extremely rule-governed, he or she will be insensitive to the actual consequences of the behavior and will continue with the behavior despite adverse effects, because what matters to the person is to follow the rule. Vicious cycles maintaining ED (Fairburn et al., 2003) comprise both contingency-based reinforcements (often negative reinforcement) and rule-governed behavior. As an example, purging increases the probability of future binge eating, as it drastically decreases the anxiety produced by binge eating (negative reinforcement). Purging can also serve another function. It makes the individual feel relaxed through vagal stimulation (positive reinforcement). Furthermore, purging can be rule-governed in that it might make the individual feel "clean," which is not the same as having an empty stomach. It is a rule about the importance of being clean, which is achievable through repeated vomiting (i.e., not only throwing up ingested food but also drinking water and vomiting repeatedly to ensure that no food is left until the thought of being clean, which is perceived as a feeling, is present). In fact, the sensation comes from the vagal stimulation due to vomiting and is mislabeled as being clean. Metacognitive awareness (Teasdale et al., 2002; Wells, 2000) and cognitive defusion (Hayes et al., 1999) are potent strategies to address excessive verbal behavior. The former is included in the new transdiagnostic treatment of ED. For a more detailed description of excessive rule-governed behavior and intervention strategies, see Ghaderi (2007).

Other Factors That Lead to Poor Treatment Response

A large number of other factors might lead to poor treatment response. Although there are clear exceptions, substantial comorbid states, high frequency of impulsive behaviors, a history of trauma, and secondary gains from ED are usually seen among those who fail to benefit from CBT (Waller, Cordery, et al., 2007). For patients with poor treatment response and evidence of comorbidity, additional treatment strategies to address the comorbid state should be considered if the comorbidity is primary, and not secondary, to ED. The core processes in the comorbid state might be issues such as affect intolerance and emotional instability (e.g., for those with ED and borderline personality disorder). A thorough functional assessment (e.g., Ghaderi, 2007) of the client's behavior or cognitive case formulation and reassessment (Needleman, 1999; Persons & Davidson, 2001) might help the clinician to decide what processes to focus on, what behaviors to prioritize, what cognitions and emotions to address, and how to assess progress in therapy in order to be vigilant and ready to revise the treatment. Some of the core processes in some comorbid states might be best classified as therapy-interfering behaviors. DBT provides very helpful guidelines and suggestions for how to best handle such behaviors (Linehan, 1993). Presence of past or present trauma calls for special attention to issues related to patient safety and emotional processing of the trauma. CBT approaches to the treatment of trauma are very successful (Foa, 2006; Paunovic, 2003; Taylor, 2006) and can easily be integrated in the treatment of patients with ED and trauma.

CASE EXAMPLE

Lisa had a history of restrictive AN since age 13. She managed to gain some weight after years of treatment (at four different specialty units for the treatment of ED and a large number of outpatient treatments). During the course of the last outpatient treatment, before she moved from her parents' home at the age of 20, she started to binge and purge. Since she was 20 years old (she was 27 at the time of contact with us), she had been struggling with severe BN and short but recurrent periods of starvation. Lisa had been through virtually all possible treatments and their combinations and had received CBT from two different therapists. A thorough reassessment of the factors maintaining her ED and Lisa's perception of the earlier treatments showed that most of the usual perpetuating factors were present despite years of treatment—that is, dietary restraint; constant preoccupation with thoughts about weight, shape, and food; overvaluation of shape and weight; profound and early impact of starvation when she was younger (e.g., feeling of being in control and unique); the negative reinforcing effect of vomiting; and her beliefs about the powerful effect of compensatory behaviors despite some psychoeducation during the course of CBT.

During the assessment, she displayed and reported extremely low self-esteem, major difficulties in emotion regulation in terms of bursts of anger (which later analysis showed was a way of setting limits because she had not developed the skills necessary to set limits without showing anger or strong disappointment), and extreme rules that guided many of her behaviors (e.g., "I am okay when I am thin, but never lovable anyway"; "I have to be strong whatever happens"; "Everybody will use you and abuse you if you don't show that you are different"; "I am useless if I can't win the battle with food . . . I decide when to eat"; "I need to be thin and small").

Additional maintaining variables were lack of problem-solving skills, poor interpersonal relations, and constant conflicts (leading to binge episodes), especially with those expressing love and appreciation, low stress tolerance (largely due to low weight and chaotic eating but also due to her assumptions that everybody else has an easier life and to her lack of skills to plan and evaluate her actions), viewing the ED as a major part of who she was (i.e., identity issues), and almost meeting criteria for social phobia. Moreover, she had started to imagine how she would commit suicide by jumping from her student room on the fifth floor when her anxiety and sense of worthlessness felt impossible to handle.

During the three assessment sessions, Lisa indicated in various indirect ways that she had been victimized and abused; however, when questioned, she declined any history of abuse or trauma. Lisa had clear difficulties expressing emotions other than anger and disappointment. She had poor eye contact during the interviews. Although part of her limited repertoire of emotions and interpersonal behaviors could be understood in terms of her skills deficits explaining much of her social phobic problems, in later analysis some other aspects showed to be the result of rigid rules and strong and inappropriate verbal consequential control (e.g., "I might look needy if I behave really friendly"; "People expect me to do whatever they want, if I look them in the eyes and really listen to them").

Given Lisa's feelings of worthlessness and hopelessness, considerable efforts were made to validate her and to put her thoughts, feelings, and behaviors in a context in which what she did made sense. High expectations from her parents and some failures during her early teens had set the scene for low self-esteem and hopelessness. Lisa could gradually view most of her thoughts and actions as a way of compensating for her core negative beliefs about herself. What she did made sense given how she viewed herself, and the vicious cycles resulting from her avoidance and dysfunctional behaviors such as rigid dieting to escape feelings that were rooted in her view of herself. Using Lisa's own examples of antecedents to her binge episodes and starvation, as well as consequences and establishing operations (often feeling hungry, humiliated or agitated), an initial CBT model of the maintenance of her problems was formed, which was further developed by her during the therapy. Lisa had become sensitive to therapists telling her what was wrong with her and what she should do. To establish a good collaboration, helping Lisa create a new identity already from the assessment phase and engaging Lisa in the treatment from the beginning, the therapist explained clearly and repeatedly that certain aspects of her complex situation needed to be further analyzed and that she was the only person who could work it out and create a good understanding of her situation that might help her build up a new sense of self and live a valued life. As the therapist was uncertain about the quality of former CBT treatments, he tested the effectiveness of some of the standard techniques in an experimental way before he decided to switch to more advanced methods; for example, cognitive restructuring was tested and shown to be inadequate because of excessive rule-governed behavior. Hence, cognitive defusion and acceptance strategies were used to help Lisa create some distance to her cognitions and be able to acquire new, more contingency-based and less rule-governed experiences through exposure and stimulus control. Lisa agreed to eat more regularly within the frame of a behavioral experiment to test her assumptions about the consequences that she thought would come true after no more than 4 weeks. Early in the treatment, Lisa was encouraged to think through what she valued in life as a way of increasing her motivation to engage in the treatment and find incentives to eat regularly and stop all the compensatory behaviors. She also had to make room for all her fears and the acute anxiety that intensified her thoughts about committing suicide. These problems were addressed by encouraging Lisa to view her thoughts and feelings as thoughts and feelings, and not as definite facts (i.e., the cognitive defusion technique), and by focusing on what she could do to live in accordance with what she valued while observing her feelings (i.e., acceptance). In the treatment contract, Lisa agreed to take as many steps as necessary (listed as different coping strategies, the last one being contact with the emergency room) to avoid harming herself during the course of the therapy. Fortunately, Lisa had two good friends and a sister whom she trusted and who could be supportive when she needed them. The work on values, especially those related to friendship, family, education, and health, and on strategies to enhance Lisa's self-esteem made the work on the core psychopathology of her ED easier. By the 10th session, Lisa and the therapist agreed to focus on assertiveness training and to increase Lisa's social engagement and activity. A slight deterioration took place during 2 weeks, mostly due to Lisa's imagination of the consequences of exposure to some new social situations. To address the problem, a more stepwise plan for building up and training assertiveness skills was agreed upon that helped Lisa feel in control.

Therapy lasted for 24 sessions. Lisa acquired enough interpersonal skills to continue on her own for developing further skills; became better at identifying and expressing different emotions; learned to set limits by expressing her needs and primary emotions; and created a new pattern of communication with her family without constantly arguing about issues related to ED, food, shape, and weight. It was agreed with Lisa and her family that Lisa, as an adult, should take the responsibility for her health and that she would ask the family to help her whenever she needed.

The three central factors leading to poor outcome in earlier treatments seemed to be her profoundly low self-esteem, lack of many skills necessary to communicate effectively and clearly, and excessive rule-governed behavior. Much of what she did (e.g., short periods of starvation) served as safety behaviors that were meant to prevent various imagined consequences (e.g., "If I keep on eating this way, I will never be able to stop"; "If I gain weight, I will be even more worthless"). Strategies and methods that were used to help Lisa develop metacognitive awareness and create distance to her thoughts helped her to be more flexible, dare to enter new situations, take surveys by asking people around her (to test some of her assumptions), be more present in different everyday situations, and pay attention to her experiences instead of solely relying on her thoughts and assumptions. She also started to be more mindful when she ate, and this helped her to work more effectively with mislabeling of her thoughts and emotions.

Lisa continued to make progress, as shown by the 1-year follow-up assessment. She had a BMI of 20.8 (it was 18.2 before the treatment), had stopped bingeing and purging, felt good about herself, and reported relatively high quality of life compared with before the treatment. She had resumed her studies to become a dentist and had become more aware of some of her perfectionist tendencies that were only slightly addressed during the therapy. She had become more receptive to positive comments from people and reported that she often used to ask herself "what kind of glasses I was wearing" whenever she became very critical of herself. "It's a hard work to put the ED glasses away, but—oh, I mean, *and* I am doing well," she said at the end of the follow-up interview.

CONCLUSIONS AND FUTURE DIRECTIONS

Lessons learned from empirical studies of ED in general and CBT treatment studies of ED in particular have helped us to identify a host of variables that might explain poor treatment response to CBT for ED in some cases. Among the potential complicating variables leading to poor treatment response are interpersonal difficulties such as role conflicts and interpersonal skills deficits, affect intolerance, lack of certain skills such as assertiveness, excessive rule-governed behavior, substantial comorbidity, excessive impulsivity, low self-esteem, high level of perfectionism, identity issues, trauma, and secondary gains from ED. However, the best predictor of poor outcome is lack of early response to CBT. Given the diversity of factors that are associated with less favorable outcome, use of individual case formulation or functional analysis to identify the specific factors that prevent successful treatment for the individual patient cannot be stressed enough. Supervision is often invaluable in this context.

CBT for ED is becoming more and more effective. We are gaining a much better understanding of ED, and we use more potent treatment strategies compared with earlier formulations and treatments. However, for favorable outcomes, therapists will probably always need to understand and identify variables, processes, and interactions of factors specific for individual patients who do not respond to the best available treatments. Future research needs to focus on ways of improving not only the treatment in general but also how we can arrive at valid and reliable analyses for the individual patients who present a more complex picture and who are in need of thoughtful adaptations of our best treatments to overcome ED.

REFERENCES

Agras, W. S., Telch, C. F., Arnow, B., Eldredge, K., Detzer, M. J., Henderson, J., et al. (1995). Does interpersonal therapy help patients with binge eating disorder who fail to respond to cognitive–behavioral therapy? *Journal of Consulting and Clinical Psychology, 63,* 356–360.

Agras, W. S., Walsh, T., Fairburn, C. G., Wilson, G. T., & Kraemer, H. C. (2000). A multicenter comparison of cognitive–behavioral therapy and interpersonal psychotherapy for bulimia nervosa. *Archives of General Psychiatry, 57,* 459–466.

Alberti, R. E., & Emmons, M. (2001). *Your perfect right: Assertiveness and equality in your life and relationships* (8th ed.). New York: Impact.

American Psychiatric Association. (2000). *Diagnostic and statistical manual of mental disorders* (4th ed., text rev.). Washington, DC: Author.

Antony, M. M., & Swinson, R. P. (1998). *When perfect isn't good enough: Strategies for coping with perfectionism.* Oakland, CA: New Harbinger.

Becker, A. E., Grinspoon, S. K., Klibanski, A., & Herzog, D. B. (1999). Eating disorders. *The New England Journal of Medicine, 340,* 1092–1098.

Borkovec, T. D., Newman, M. G., Pincus, A. L., & Lytle, R. (2002). A component analysis of cognitive–behavioral therapy for generalized anxiety disorder and the role of interpersonal problems. *Journal of Consulting and Clinical Psychology, 70,* 288–298.

Crow, S. J., Stewart Agras, W., Halmi, K., Mitchell, J. E., & Kraemer, H. C. (2002). Full syndromal versus subthreshold anorexia nervosa, bulimia nervosa, and binge eating disorder: A multicenter study. *International Journal of Eating Disorders*, *32*, 309–318.

Dimidjian, S., Hollon, S. D., Dobson, K. S., Schmaling, K. B., Kohlenberg, R. J., Addis, M. E., et al. (2006). Randomized trial of behavioral activation, cognitive therapy, and antidepressant medication in the acute treatment of adults with major depression. *Journal of Consulting and Clinical Psychology*, *74*, 658–670.

Dunn, E. C., Neighbors, C., & Larimer, M. (2003). Assessing readiness to change binge eating and compensatory behaviors. *Eating Behaviors*, *4*, 305–314.

Eisler, I., Dare, C., Hodes, M., Russell, G. F., Dodge, E., & Le Grange, D. (2000). Family therapy for adolescent anorexia nervosa: The results of a controlled comparison of two family interventions. *Journal of Child Psychology and Psychiatry and Allied Disciplines*, *41*, 727–736.

Fairburn, C. G. (March, 2005). *Transdiagnostic CBT for eating disorders*. Workshop presented at Uppsala University, Uppsala, Sweden.

Fairburn, C. G. (July, 2007). *Invited address*. Presented at the World Congress of Cognitive and Behavioral Therapies, Barcelona, Spain.

Fairburn, C. G., & Bohn, K. (2005). Eating disorder NOS (EDNOS): An example of the troublesome "not otherwise specified" (NOS) category in *DSM–IV*. *Behaviour Research and Therapy*, *43*, 691–701.

Fairburn, C. G., Cooper, Z., & Shafran, R. (2003). Cognitive behaviour therapy for eating disorders: A "transdiagnostic" theory and treatment. *Behaviour Research and Therapy*, *41*, 509–528.

Fairburn, C. G., Cooper, Z., Shafran, R., & Wilson, G. T. (2008). Eating disorders: A transdiagnostic protocol. In D. H. Barlow (Ed.), *Clinical handbook of psychological disorders: A step-by-step treatment manual* (4th ed., pp. 578–614). New York: Guilford Press.

Fairburn, C. G., & Harrison, P. J. (2003, February 1). Eating disorders. *The Lancet*, *361*, 406–417.

Fairburn, C. G., Jones, R., Peveler, R. C., Carr, S. J., Solomon, R. A., O'Connor, M. E., et al. (1991). Three psychological treatments for bulimia nervosa: A comparative trial. *Archives of General Psychiatry*, *48*, 463–469.

Fairburn, C. G., Jones, R., Peveler, R. C., Hope, R. A., & O'Connor, M. (1993). Psychotherapy and bulimia nervosa: Longer-term effects of interpersonal psychotherapy, behavior therapy, and cognitive behavior therapy. *Archives of General Psychiatry*, *50*, 419–428.

Fairburn, C. G., Marcus, M. D., & Wilson, G. T. (1993). Cognitive behaviour therapy for binge eating and bulimia nervosa: A comprehensive treatment manual. In C. G. Fairburn & G. T. Wilson (Eds.), *Binge eating: Nature, assessment and treatment* (pp. 361–404). New York: Guilford Press.

Famer, R. R., & Latner, J. D. (2007). Eating disorders. In P. Sturmey (Ed.), *Functional analysis in clinical treatment* (pp. 379–402). San Diego, CA: Academic Press.

Fennell, M. J. (2004). Depression, low self-esteem and mindfulness. *Behaviour Research and Therapy, 42*, 1053–1067.

Fennell, M. J. (2006). *Overcoming low self-esteem self-help programme*. London: Constable and Robinson.

Ferguson, C. P., La Via, M. C., Crossan, P. J., & Kaye, W. H. (1999). Are serotonin selective reuptake inhibitors effective in underweight anorexia nervosa? *International Journal of Eating Disorders, 25*, 11–17.

Foa, E. B. (2006). Psychosocial therapy for posttraumatic stress disorder. *Journal of Clinical Psychiatry, 67*(Suppl. 2), 40–45.

Fruzzetti, A. E. (1996). Causes and consequences: Individual distress in the context of couple interactions. *Journal of Consulting and Clinical Psychology, 64*, 1192–1201.

Ghaderi, A. (2006). Does individualization matter? A randomized trial of standardized (focused) versus individualized (broad) cognitive behavior therapy for bulimia nervosa. *Behaviour Research and Therapy, 44*, 273–288.

Ghaderi, A. (2007). Logical functional analysis in the assessment and treatment of eating disorders. *Clinical Psychologist, 11*, 1–12.

Gillberg, I. C., Gillberg, C., Rastam, M., & Johansson, M. (1996). The cognitive profile of anorexia nervosa: A comparative study including a community-based sample. *Comprehensive Psychiatry, 37*, 23–30.

Goldbloom, D. S., Olmsted, M., Davis, R., Clewes, J., Heinmaa, M., Rockert, W., et al. (1997). A randomized controlled trial of fluoxetine and cognitive behavioral therapy for bulimia nervosa: Short-term outcome. *Behaviour Research and Therapy, 35*, 803–811.

Götestam, K. G., & Agras, W. S. (1995). General population-based epidemiological study of eating disorders in Norway. *International Journal of Eating Disorders, 18*, 119–126.

Grilo, C. M., Masheb, R. M., & Wilson, G. T. (2005). Efficacy of cognitive behavioral therapy and fluoxetine for the treatment of binge eating disorder: A randomized double-blind placebo-controlled comparison. *Biological Psychiatry, 57*, 301–309.

Grilo, C. M., Masheb, R. M., & Wilson, G. T. (2006). Rapid response to treatment for binge eating disorder. *Journal of Consulting and Clinical Psychology, 74*, 602–613.

Hall, R. C., Hoffman, R. S., Beresford, T. P., Wooley, B., Hall, A. K., & Kubasak, L. (1989). Physical illness encountered in patients with eating disorders. *Psychosomatics, 30*, 174–191.

Hayes, S. C., Barnes-Holmes, D., & Roche, B. (Eds.). (2001). *Relational frame theory: A post-Skinnerian account of human language and cognition*. New York: Plenum Press.

Hayes, S. C., Strosahl, K. D., & Wilson, K. G. (1999). *Acceptance and commitment therapy: An experiential approach to behavior change*. New York: Guilford Press.

Jacobson, N. S., Dobson, K. S., Truax, P. A., Addis, M. E., Koerner, K., Gollan, J. K., et al. (1996). A component analysis of cognitive–behavioral treatment for depression. *Journal of Consulting and Clinical Psychology, 64*, 295–304.

Kaye, W. H., Bastiani, A. M., & Moss, H. (1995). Cognitive style of patients with anorexia nervosa and bulimia nervosa. *International Journal of Eating Disorders, 18,* 287–290.

Kendler, K. S., MacLean, C., Neale, M., Kessler, R., Heath, A., & Eaves, L. (1991). The genetic epidemiology of bulimia nervosa. *The American Journal of Psychiatry, 148,* 1627–1637.

Keys, A., Brozek, J., Henschel, A., & Mickelson, O. (1950). *The biology of human starvation.* Minneapolis: University of Minnesota Press.

Klump, K. L., Miller, K. B., Keel, P. K., McGue, M., & Iacono, W. G. (2001). Genetic and environmental influences on anorexia nervosa syndromes in a population-based twin sample. *Psychological Medicine, 31,* 737–740.

Lena, S. M., Fiocco, A. J., & Leyenaar, J. K. (2004). The role of cognitive deficits in the development of eating disorders. *Neuropsychological Review, 14,* 99–113.

Levander, A., & Schmidt, U. (2006). Cognitive behavioral case formulation in complex eating disorders. In N. Tarrier (Ed.), *Case formulation in cognitive behaviour therapy: The treatment of challenging and complex cases* (pp. 238–262). New York: Routledge.

Linehan, M. M. (1993). *Cognitive–behavioral treatment of borderline personality disorder.* New York: Guilford Press.

Linehan, M. M., Comtois, K. A., Murray, A. M., Brown, M. Z., Gallop, R. J., Heard, H. L., et al. (2006). Two-year randomized controlled trial and follow-up of dialectical behavior therapy vs therapy by experts for suicidal behaviors and borderline personality disorder. *Archives of General Psychiatry, 63,* 757–766.

Linehan, M. M., Schmidt, H., III, Dimeff, L. A., Craft, J. C., Kanter, J., & Comtois, K. A. (1999). Dialectical behavior therapy for patients with borderline personality disorder and drug-dependence. *American Journal of Addiction, 8,* 279–292.

Lock, J., Le Grange, D., Agras, W. S., & Dare, C. (2001). *Treatment manual for anorexia nervosa: A family-based approach.* New York: Guilford Press.

Markowitz, J. C., Svartberg, M., & Swartz, H. A. (1998). Is IPT time-limited psychodynamic psychotherapy? *Journal of Psychotherapy Practice and Research, 7,* 185–195.

McIntosh, V. V., Jordan, J., Carter, F. A., Luty, S. E., McKenzie, J. M., Bulik, C. M., et al. (2005). Three psychotherapies for anorexia nervosa: A randomized, controlled trial. *The American Journal of Psychiatry, 162,* 741–747.

Milos, G., Spindler, A., Schnyder, U., & Fairburn, C. G. (2005). Instability of eating disorder diagnosis: Prospective study. *The British Journal of Psychiatry, 187,* 573–578.

Mitchell, J. E., Agras, S., & Wonderlich, S. (2007). Treatment of bulimia nervosa: Where are we and where are we going? *International Journal of Eating Disorders, 40,* 95–101.

Mitchell, J. E., Halmi, K., Wilson, G. T., Agras, W. S., Kraemer, H., & Crow, S. (2002). A randomized secondary treatment study of women with bulimia nervosa who fail to respond to CBT. *International Journal of Eating Disorders, 32,* 271–281.

Mitchell, J. E., Pyle, R. L., Eckert, E. D., Hatsukami, D., Pomeroy, C., & Zimmerman, R. (1990). A comparison study of antidepressants and structured intensive group psychotherapy in the treatment of bulimia nervosa. *Archives of General Psychiatry, 47*, 149–157.

Mitchell, J. E., Raymond, N., & Specker, S. (1993). A review of the controlled trials of pharmacotherapy and psychotherapy in the treatment of bulimia nervosa. *International Journal of Eating Disorders, 14*, 229–247.

Mountford, V., Haase, A. M., & Waller, G. (2007). Is body checking in the eating disorders more closely related to diagnosis or to symptom presentation? *Behaviour Research and Therapy, 45*, 2704–2711.

National Institute for Clinical Excellence. (2004). *Eating disorders: Core interventions in the treatment and management of anorexia nervosa, bulimia nervosa and related eating disorders.* London: National Collaborating Centre for Mental Health.

Needleman, L. D. (1999). *Cognitive case conceptualization: A guidebook for practitioners.* Mahwah, NJ: Erlbaum.

Paunovic, N. (2003). Prolonged exposure counterconditioning as a treatment for chronic posttraumatic stress disorder. *Journal of Anxiety Disorders, 17*, 479–499.

Persons, J. B., & Davidson, J. (2001). Cognitive–behavioral case formulation. In K. S. Dobson (Ed.), *Handbook of cognitive behavioral therapies* (2nd ed., pp. 86–110). New York: Guilford Press.

Riley, C., Lee, M., Cooper, Z., Fairburn, C. G., & Shafran, R. (2007). A randomised controlled trial of cognitive–behaviour therapy for clinical perfectionism: A preliminary study. *Behaviour Research and Therapy, 45*, 2221–2231.

Robin, A. L. (2003). Behavioral family systems therapy for adolescents with anorexia nervosa. In A. E. Kazdin (Ed.), *Evidence-based psychotherapies for children and adolescents* (pp. 358–373). New York: Guilford Press.

Robin, A. L., Siegel, P. T., Moye, A. W., Gilroy, M., Dennis, A. B., & Sikand, A. (1999). A controlled comparison of family versus individual therapy for adolescents with anorexia nervosa. *Journal of the American Academy of Child & Adolescent Psychiatry, 38*, 1482–1489.

Shafran, R., Cooper, Z., & Fairburn, C. G. (2003). Clinical perfectionism: A cognitive behavioural analysis. *Behaviour Research and Therapy, 40*, 773–791.

Slade, P. D. (1982). Towards a functional analysis of anorexia nervosa and bulimia nervosa. *British Journal of Clinical Psychology, 21*, 167–179.

Striegel-Moore, R. H., Dohm, F. A., Solomon, E. E., Fairburn, C. G., Pike, K. M., & Wilfley, D. E. (2000). Subthreshold binge eating disorder. *International Journal of Eating Disorders, 27*, 270–278.

Striegel-Moore, R. H., Leslie, D., Petrill, S. A., Garvin, V., & Rosenheck, R. A. (2000). One-year use and cost of inpatient and outpatient services among female and male patients with an eating disorder: Evidence from a national database of health insurance claims. *International Journal of Eating Disorders, 27*, 381–389.

Taylor, S. (2006). *Clinician's guide to PTSD: A cognitive–behavioral approach.* New York: Guilford Press.

Teasdale, J. D., Moore, R. G., Haylurst, H., Pope, M., & Williams, S. (2002). Metacognitive awareness and prevention of relapse in depression: Empirical evidence. *Journal of Consulting and Clinical Psychology, 70,* 275–287.

Treasure, J. L., Katzman, M., Schmidts, U., Troop, N., Todd, G., & de Silva, P. (1999). Engagement and outcome in the treatment of bulimia nervosa: First phase of a sequential design comparing motivation enhancement therapy and cognitive behavioural therapy. *Behaviour Research and Therapy, 37,* 405–418.

Treasure, J. L., & Ward, A. (1998). A practical guide to the use of motivational interviewing in anorexia nervosa. *European Eating Disorders Review, 5,* 102–114.

Waller, G., Cordery, H., Corstorphine, E., Hinrichsen, H., Lawson, R., Mountford, V., et al. (2007). *Cognitive behavioral therapy for eating disorders: A comprehensive treatment guide.* Cambridge, England: Cambridge University Press.

Waller, G., Corstorphine, E., & Mountford, V. (2007). The role of emotional abuse in the eating disorders: Implications for treatment. *Eating Disorders, 15,* 317–331.

Walsh, B. T., Hadigan, C. M., Delvin, M. J., Gladis, M., & Roose, S. P. (1991). Long-term outcome of antidepressant treatment for bulimia nervosa. *The American Journal of Psychiatry, 148,* 1206–1212.

Wells, A. (2000). *Emotional disorders and metacognition: Innovative cognitive therapy.* New York: Wiley.

Wells, A., & King, P. (2006). Metacognitive therapy for generalized anxiety disorder: An open trial. *Journal of Behavior Therapy and Experimental Psychiatry, 37,* 206–212.

Wilfley, D. E., Agras, W. S., Telch, C. F., Rossiter, E. M., Schneider, J. A., Cole, A. G., et al. (1993). Group cognitive–behavioral therapy and group interpersonal psychotherapy for the nonpurging bulimic individual: A controlled comparison. *Journal of Consulting and Clinical Psychology, 61,* 296–305.

Wilfley, D. E., MacKenzie, K. R., Welch, R. R., Ayres, V. E., & Weissman, M. M. (2000). *Interpersonal psychotherapy for groups.* New York: Basic Books.

Wilfley, D. E., Welch, R. R., Stein, R. I., Spurrell, E. B., Cohen, L. R., Saelens, B. E., et al. (2002). A randomized comparison of group cognitive–behavioral therapy and group interpersonal psychotherapy for the treatment of overweight individuals with binge-eating disorder. *Archives of General Psychiatry, 59,* 713–721.

Wilson, G. T. (1993). Binge eating and addictive disorders. In C. G. Fairburn & G. T. Wilson (Eds.), *Binge eating: Nature, assessment and treatment* (pp. 97–120). New York: Guilford Press.

Wilson, G. T. (1996). Treatment of bulimia nervosa: When CBT fails. *Behaviour Research and Therapy, 34,* 197–212.

Wilson, G. T., Fairburn, C. G., & Agras, W. S. (1997). Cognitive behavioral therapy for bulimia nervosa. In D. M. Garner & P. E. Garfinkel (Eds.), *Handbook of treatment for eating disorders* (pp. 67–93). New York: Guilford Press.

Wilson, G. T., Loeb, K. L., Walsh, B. T., Labouvie, E., Petkova, E., Liu, X., et al. (1999). Psychological versus pharmacological treatments of bulimia nervosa:

Predictors and processes of change. *Journal of Consulting and Clinical Psychology*, 67, 451–459.

Wilson, G. T., & Schlam, T. R. (2004). The transtheoretical model and motivational interviewing in the treatment of eating and weight disorders. *Clinical Psychology Review*, 24, 361–378.

9

DEPRESSION

BRUCE A. ARNOW AND LISA I. POST

Evidence has suggested that the median length of a depressive episode is 2 to 5 months (Kessler et al., 2003; Solomon et al., 1997; Spijker et al., 2002). However, a significant subgroup of patients experiences depressive episodes lasting 2 years or more. Findings from the National Institute of Mental Health Collaborative Depression Study revealed that 20% of patients had not recovered within 2 years (Keller & Shapiro, 1982), and 12% remained ill at 5 years (Keller et al., 1992).

The nature of major depressive disorder (MDD) is now understood to be recurrent in most instances and chronic in many others (Fava & Kendler, 2000; Keller, 2003). The *Diagnostic and Statistical Manual of Mental Disorders* (4th ed.; American Psychiatric Association, 1994) includes course modifiers specifying the presence or absence of dysthymia, single versus recurrent episodes, and whether recovery from an episode was full or partial. Figure 9.1 depicts various presentations of dysthymia and major depression (Keller et al., 1995).

Chronic depression presents in several ways. As mentioned previously, some patients experience episodes of major depression lasting 2 years or longer; others, however, experience recurrent episodes without full interepisode recovery. Another subgroup meets criteria for major depression superimposed on antecedent dysthymia. Criteria for dysthymic disorder involve depressed

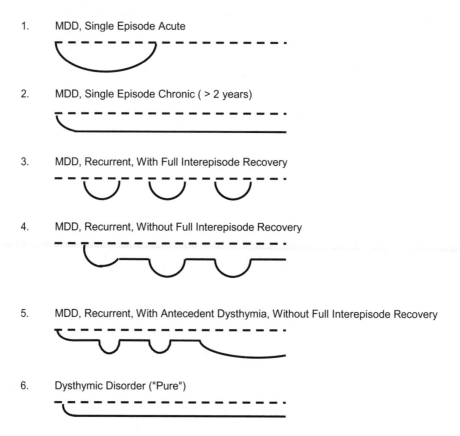

1. MDD, Single Episode Acute

2. MDD, Single Episode Chronic (> 2 years)

3. MDD, Recurrent, With Full Interepisode Recovery

4. MDD, Recurrent, Without Full Interepisode Recovery

5. MDD, Recurrent, With Antecedent Dysthymia, Without Full Interepisode Recovery

6. Dysthymic Disorder ("Pure")

Figure 9.1. Clinical course profiles of major depressive disorder (MDD) and dysthymic disorder.

mood and two additional symptoms persisting for 2 years (i.e., *double depression*). However, the vast majority of patients with dysthymic disorder also experience major depression (Klein, Shankman, & Rose, 2006), and the typical recovery from MDD among these patients is characterized by a return to dysthymia, rather than to a nondepressed baseline (Keller & Lavori, 1984). Overall, 20% to 25% of MDD patients have a chronic course (Mueller & Leon, 1996).

DISABILITY AND COMORBIDITY ASSOCIATED WITH CHRONIC DEPRESSION

Depression is highly disabling (Moussavi et al., 2007). Chronic depression is associated with particularly high work and psychosocial impairment (Friedman, 1995; Hays, Wells, Sherbourne, Rogers, & Spritzer, 1995), as well as medical morbidity (Akiskal, 1982; Gilmer et al., 2005) and high use of health care services (Howland, 1993; Weissman, Leaf, Bruce, & Florio, 1988). Compared with those with acute MDD, chronically depressed individuals show greater functional impairment (Gilmer et al., 2005; Wells, Burnam, Rogers, Hays, & Camp, 1992).

A number of reports have suggested that chronic depression is highly associated with both medical and psychiatric comorbidity. In findings from the Sequenced Treatment Alternatives to Relieve Depression (i.e., STAR-D) project, which evaluated the efficacy of antidepressant treatments, chronic depression was associated with greater medical illness burden than nonchronic depression (Gilmer et al., 2005). Compared with those with acute MDD, individuals with chronic depression have been shown to demonstrate higher rates of Axis I comorbidity (Klein, Taylor, Harding, & Dickstein, 1988). Other findings have suggested higher prevalence of anxiety disorders among those with chronic depression compared with those with acute MDD (Gilmer et al., 2005; Levitt, Jaffe, & MacDonald, 1991), as well as higher prevalence of personality disorders (Klein et al., 1988; Rothschild & Zimmerman, 2002), and higher rates of suicide attempts (Gilmer et al., 2005; Klein et al., 1988).

A number of studies have found chronicity to be associated with psychosocial disadvantage. Two studies reported associations between chronicity and lower levels of education (Gilmer et al., 2005; Swindle, Cronkite, & Moos, 1998). Chronic depression is also associated with unemployment (Gilmer et al., 2005; Sherbourne, Hays, & Wells, 1995) and lower family income (Gilmer et al., 2005; Keller et al., 1984).

EVIDENCE-BASED PSYCHOTHERAPY:
EFFICACY FOR CHRONIC DEPRESSION

Few randomized controlled trials have focused specifically on patients with chronic forms of depression. However, there is some evidence that both cognitive therapy (CT; Beck, Rush, Shaw, & Emery, 1979) and interpersonal therapy (IPT; Klerman, Weissman, Rounsaville, & Chevron, 1984) may be less effective with chronically depressed patients than with nonchronic patients. Additionally, some findings have suggested that these therapies are less effective than medication with chronic patients. In one study, the remission rate for chronically depressed (27%) receiving CT was significantly lower than for acute participants (55%; Thase et al., 1994). In a study with dysthymic patients, Ravindran et al. (1999) reported that the efficacy of medication with or without CT was significantly greater than placebo, whereas CT with placebo was no better than placebo alone. Additionally, combining CT with medication did not add benefit to the latter.

In several randomized clinical trials with chronically depressed patients, IPT has not performed as well as, and/or has not added benefit to, medication. Browne et al. (2002) found that those in IPT improved significantly less than those in sertraline and combined conditions and that IPT did not add to the efficacy of sertraline alone after 6 months of treatment in dysthymic patients. In a randomized controlled trial with participants who met criteria for dysthymia, Markowitz, Kocsis, Bleiberg, Christos, and Sacks (2005) reported that medication was associated with significantly greater efficacy than IPT, and that IPT did not add benefit to medication. Furthermore, in this trial IPT was no more effective than brief supportive therapy, a nonspecific therapy control condition. Finally, de Mello, Myczowisk, and Menezes (2001) reported no advantage for combined medication plus IPT compared with medication alone in a study in Brazil, although this study suffered from a small sample size and had only one therapist carrying out treatment (Arnow & Constantino, 2003). Overall, extant findings have suggested a need to either modify existing evidence-based psychotherapies to address the needs of the chronically depressed or to develop alternative psychotherapy for this subgroup of patients.

COGNITIVE–BEHAVIORAL ANALYSIS SYSTEM OF PSYCHOTHERAPY: EFFICACY

The patient we discuss in this chapter was treated with the *cognitive–behavioral analysis system of psychotherapy* (CBASP; McCullough, 1984, 1991, 2000). CBASP combines elements of both CT and IPT and is the only psychosocial treatment specifically developed for chronic depression (Arnow, 2005). Originally described in uncontrolled case studies, CBASP has been evaluated in a large clinical trial involving nearly 700 patients who met criteria for chronic major depression, major depression superimposed on dysthymia (i.e., double depression), or recurrent major depression with incomplete interepisode recovery and a total duration of illness of 2 years or more (Keller et al., 2000). Patients were randomly assigned to CBASP, nefazodone (MED), or combined CBASP and nefazodone (COMB). The acute phase (12-week) modified intent-to-treat results of that trial revealed response rates of 48% for both MED and CBASP and 73% for COMB. Remission rates also indicated equivalent efficacy between CBASP and MED and a significant advantage for COMB.

The Keller et al. (2000) trial also involved continuation, crossover, and maintenance phases. In the continuation study, those who met responder criteria remained in the cell to which they were randomized. Overall, there were few between-group differences (Kocsis et al., 2003). Relapse rates were extremely low in all three groups: 7% MED, 8% CBASP, and 5% COMB (Kocsis et al., 2003).

In the crossover study, nonresponders to acute phase monotherapy were offered 12 weeks of treatment with the alternative monotherapy. Intention-to-treat results revealed an advantage for those crossed over to CBASP (response rate = 58%) versus MED (42%; Schatzberg et al., 2005). There were no significant differences in the remission rates.

Finally, those who maintained response through the acute and continuation phases of the Keller et al. (2000) trial were offered 1 year of additional maintenance treatment. Those in COMB and MED were randomized to either placebo or maintenance nefazodone. Recurrence rates were 30% MED versus 48% for placebo (Gelenberg et al., 2003); there were no differences in relapse between those who had responded to COMB versus those who had responded to MED only. Responders to CBASP were randomized to either monthly CBASP or assessment only. Klein et al. (2004) found that the recurrence rate in CBASP was only 10% versus 32% in the assessment condition. Thus, evidence to date has suggested that in chronically depressed patients (a) CBASP is equally as effective as single-agent medication; (b) when combined with medication, CBASP is associated with relatively high rates of response and remission; (c) patients who continue to receive CBASP through continuation and maintenance phases have very low rates of relapse; and (d) CBASP is a promising "switch" strategy for patients who do not respond to an initial trial of medication.

COGNITIVE–BEHAVIORAL ANALYSIS SYSTEM OF PSYCHOTHERAPY: ASSUMPTIONS AND PROCEDURES

McCullough (2000, 2003) argued that chronically depressed patients differ from patients presenting with episodic depression in ways that require different therapeutic strategies. A key assumption guiding the CBASP therapy model is that the cognitive style of the chronic patient is consistent with "preoperational" thought as described by Piaget (1926). Such thinking is characterized by (a) impaired understanding of the relationships between thinking, behavior and the outcomes the patient produces; (b) lack of response to intervention relying on logical disputation; (c) egocentricity, with limited ability to integrate the perspective of others; and (d) monologic communication characterized by unresponsiveness to feedback and input from others.

One of the most important goals of treatment is to help the patient to develop an understanding of the consequences of his or her thinking and behavior. A second goal is to counter the tendency toward global construction of one's life situation (e.g., "Nothing I do will improve my life") by teaching patients to focus on problem-solving strategies applied to specific situations. A third goal is to help patients to develop critical behavioral skills that they lack, such as assertiveness.

Situational analysis (SA) is the cornerstone procedure of the CBASP model and is designed to meet the above objectives. Self-monitoring in the

CBASP model is designed to facilitate SA. Each week the patient is asked to fill out a Coping Survey Questionnaire (CSQ; McCullough, 2000), focusing on elements of a problematic interpersonal encounter. The CSQ queries the patient on (a) description of the encounter, (b) thoughts during the event, (c) behavior during the event, (d) actual outcome of the encounter, (e) desired outcome, and (f) whether the desired outcome was achieved.

In the first, or *elicitation*, phase of the SA procedure, the psychotherapist reviews each of these elements with the patient. The key points include making sure that the encounter described is discrete. McCullough (2000, 2003) suggested using the term *slice of time* to convey to patients the necessity of describing a brief vignette with a clear beginning, middle, and end point. In seeking an account of what the patient was thinking during the event, it is often helpful to ask the patient to pinpoint thoughts "as the event was unfolding" in order to ensure that a process-oriented description is captured rather than post-hoc reflections (Arnow, 2005). To carry out the SA procedure effectively, actual and desired outcomes must be stated in behavioral terms. Additionally, therapists sometimes must help patients to focus on one, as opposed to several, desired outcomes.

The second, or *remediation*, phase of SA focuses on analysis of those factors that account for the discrepancy between the actual and desired outcome (typical of the early stages of therapy) or in cases where the desired outcome was achieved, factors accounting for success. This involves engaging the patient in a review of the specific thoughts and behaviors described in the CSQ and how he or she did, or did not, facilitate achieving the desired outcome. Thus, when reviewing a situation in which the desired outcome was not achieved, rather than focusing on the validity of a particular thought, the therapist asks questions that highlight discrepancies between thought and outcomes such as the following: "Given that the outcome you wanted was Y, do you think thought X helped or hurt you?" and "How would thought X have had to change in order to make it more likely for you to be successful in achieving outcome Y?" In reviewing global thoughts (e.g., "I'm incompetent"), the therapist might begin by asking how the thought relates to the specific situation being discussed to underscore for patients how thoughts that are not grounded in the specific experience impede effectiveness.

After arriving at a revised set of thoughts that are both relevant to the situation and likely to facilitate achievement of the desired outcome, the therapist focuses on behavioral changes that are consistent with the outcome the patient wants to accomplish. Using the now-modified thoughts, the therapist begins by asking the patient whether he or she had been thinking the way that we just described (i.e., specifying each thought in turn) and then goes on to ask, "How do think your behavior might have changed to make it more likely that you would have gotten what you wanted from the situation?" Role-plays are often used at this juncture to enhance behavioral skills such as assertiveness and empathic communication.

The third phase of SA is referred to as *generalization*. In most cases, the elements that patients present during the SA procedure are characteristic of patterns that are depression maintaining. The patient who believes that he or she is unlovable and that his or her relationships are doomed to fail, and who copes with such beliefs by avoiding close relationships, will present situations that highlight such beliefs and accompanying behavioral strategies. But to facilitate generalization and transfer of learning, each SA concludes with the therapist asking how what was learned in the current SA applies to other situations in the patient's life and how he or she might apply what was learned to similar situations.

THE THERAPEUTIC RELATIONSHIP IN THE COGNITIVE–BEHAVIORAL ANALYSIS SYSTEM OF PSYCHOTHERAPY

One of the assumptions of the CBASP model is that the patterns maintaining the patient's depression are likely to manifest themselves in the psychotherapy relationship. Session 2 is devoted to a "significant other" history in which the therapist queries the patient about his or her relationships with parents and other significant figures. The therapist poses questions designed to help the patient reflect specifically on how prior critical relationships have influenced current interpersonal relationship patterns (e.g., "Having described your father as harsh and indifferent, how do you think your relationship with him has influenced the way you currently interact with others?"). The data gathered inform the development of *transference hypotheses*, that is, "if . . . then" statements describing beliefs about close relationships with others (e.g., "If I allow myself to rely emotionally on Dr. Post, she will treat me with indifference"). In turn, such hypotheses alert the therapist to interpersonal "hot spots" (McCullough, 2000) in which the patient's constructions regarding the therapist are likely to be enacted in therapeutic encounters.

One procedure for dealing with interpersonal expectancies as they emerge in the therapeutic relationship is the *interpersonal discrimination exercise* (McCullough, 2000). This procedure involves explicitly calling the patient's attention to ways in which interactions with the therapist differ from interactions with significant others in their history. The aim of the exercise is to use the therapeutic relationship to upend the patient's expectancies and provide a corrective emotional experience.

FACTORS ASSOCIATED WITH TREATMENT RESPONSE IN THE COGNITIVE–BEHAVIORAL ANALYSIS SYSTEM OF PSYCHOTHERAPY

Because CBASP is a relatively new treatment, less is known about factors associated with poor treatment response compared with more established therapies such as CT (Beck et al., 1979). Nonetheless, several studies are informative regarding predictors of outcome in CBASP. These are briefly reviewed in this section.

An important question in CBASP is whether success in learning SA is in fact related to outcome. In the Keller et al. (2000) trial, performance and mastery of the SA procedure were rated for all sessions in patients receiving CBASP, with and without medication. Manber et al. (2003) found that patient SA performance at the midpoint of acute treatment predicted depression outcome independent of medication status. Thus, one would expect that patients who do not fill out CSQs, who are resistant to focusing on or learning the SA procedure, or who for other reasons do not make progress in mastering SA, would be likely to have a poorer outcome in CBASP.

In a reanalysis of the Keller et al. (2000) data, Nemeroff et al. (2003) found that those who met criteria for a history of childhood trauma responded significantly better to CBASP than to medication. Additionally, the advantage favoring COMB in the full sample was no longer statistically significant in the subgroup with early childhood trauma. Thus, among chronically depressed patients with a history of trauma and/or loss, psychotherapy appears to confer an advantage relative to medication.

Blalock et al. (2008) reported that changes in escape-avoidant coping and attributional style for negative events met criteria for partial mediation of differences in treatment effect between COMB and MED in the Keller et al. (2000) trial, with escape-avoidant coping accounting for twice as much of the total effect size (51%) as attributional style. In the comparison of COMB versus CBASP, changes in escape-avoidant coping accounted for the 37% of the treatment differential. Thus, patients who present avoidant coping and who do not succeed in making positive changes in that domain are at high risk of a poor response to CBASP treatment.

In an investigation of the relationship between the therapeutic alliance and outcome in the Keller et al. (2000) trial, Klein et al. (2003) found that the early therapeutic alliance significantly predicted subsequent change in depressive symptoms in both the CBASP and COMB conditions after controlling for prior symptom change. Furthermore, Arnow, Blasey, et al. (2007) found that among those receiving CBASP, dropouts had lower early alliance scores than did completers. Thus, compared with those with high-quality therapeutic alliances, patients with lower early alliance scores are likely to have a poorer outcome in CBASP.

Beutler et al. (1991) reported that *high therapeutic reactance*, which has been defined as the tendency toward being "oppositional" (Dowd, Milne, & Wise, 1991), predicted poor outcome to directive treatment, whereas outcomes for those with low reactance were superior in directive compared with nondirective treatment. Although CBASP may be considered a directive treatment, Arnow et al. (2003) found that high reactance predicted better outcome in CBASP alone and did not significantly predict outcome in MED or COMB. One hypothesis to explain the differences in the two studies is that the CBASP model explicitly encourages dealing with therapeutic relationship disruptions, whereas there was no evidence that the therapists in the Beutler et al. (1991) study were given such encouragement or license.

To summarize, there is evidence that mastery of SA is positively associated with outcome in CBASP. Patients with a history of childhood trauma responded better to CBASP than to nefazodone. Changes in avoidant coping and to a lesser extent negative attributional style may be an important mechanism of change in CBASP. High reactant patients did better in CBASP (without medication) than lower reactant patients. And consistent with other findings and other therapy models, a high-quality therapeutic alliance has also been shown to significantly predict outcome in CBASP patients and to be negatively associated with premature treatment termination.

Psychotherapy studies using other therapeutic models may also be instructive in predicting patient factors associated with poor outcome in CBASP. Compliance with homework has been shown to positively predict outcome in CT (Addis & Jacobson, 2000; Burns & Nolen-Hoeksema, 1991; Persons, Burns, & Perloff, 1988). We have observed that patients who do not fill out the CSQs (McCullough, 2000), which are the basis for situational analysis, and who fail to complete other tasks suggested between sessions, are far less likely to respond to treatment than are those who do. Marital status was shown to be associated with better outcome in a study of CT for MDD patients, with married patients demonstrating better response (Jarrett, Eaves, Grannemann, & Rush, 1991). We have found that some of the most difficult patients to work with in CBASP were disconnected in the relationship and work domains, without both romantic partners and steady employment.

CASE EXAMPLE

The patient, John, was enrolled in a clinical trial for chronically depressed patients (Research Evaluating the Value of Augmenting Medication with Psychotherapy; REVAMP). All patients were initially treated with open-label algorithm-guided pharmacotherapy for 12 weeks (Phase 1). Those who did not remit were randomly assigned to receive 12 weeks of treatment (Phase 2) with (a) continued pharmacotherapy options per algorithm only, (b) continued pharmacotherapy options per algorithm plus brief supportive psychotherapy, or (c) continued pharmacotherapy options per algorithm plus CBASP (Arnow, Klein, Manber, Rothbaum, & DeRubeis, 2007).

Patient History

John was a 56-year-old single White male with a history of MDD (recurrent) and dysthymic disorder. At intake, he met criteria for MDD, chronic, with a Hamilton Depression (HAMD-24; Hamilton, 1967) score of 27. He also met criteria for generalized anxiety disorder. His current depressive episode began 3 years ago and was precipitated by a job layoff. He had not been employed since that time. During Phase 1, John completed an unsuccessful 12-week trial of antidepressant medication. John had started on Zoloft, which was titrated to 100 mg/day. At the end of Phase 1, Wellbutrin XL was added, but he experienced adverse effects and discontinued Wellbutrin at Week 10 of Phase 2. His HAMD-24 score remained a 26 at the end of Phase 1, and he was randomized to continued pharmacotherapy plus CBASP. At the end of Phase 2, his HAMD-24 score was 21.

The first psychotherapy interview with John elicited a chronological history of life events. The second session focused on gathering a detailed relationship history with the aim of compiling a list of relevant transference hypotheses. John had never married and had no children. He had two younger siblings. Both parents were deceased. He reported that the onset of depressive symptoms occurred when he was approximately 9 years old. John's childhood was notable for neglect, physical abuse, and domestic violence. He reported that his father was an alcoholic who became physically abusive when intoxicated. His father used corporal punishment with the children and would engage in frightening verbal and physical arguments with his wife. John's parents divorced when he was 14 years old. Subsequently, John's father did not pursue relationships with any of his children.

The impact of his father's violence, his lack of attention, and ultimately his abandonment of the family impacted John's self-esteem, sense of self-efficacy, and behavioral coping style in several ways. First, because his presence in his father's life seemed to have no impact on curbing his father's aggression toward his family and himself, John concluded that "nothing I do will make a difference." He believed he had little or nothing to offer that would elicit or maintain either the interest or commitment of other people and that he was destined to disappoint others. In order to avoid this consequence, John decided that "I don't want to feel like I have to please anyone or owe anyone anything." He stated that if his parents' "relationship didn't work, why should any relationship?" He justified this generalization by stating that he saw himself as a "statistician" who learned by collecting data about interpersonal relationships that "the odds are always against you." When pressed about his wishes for an intimate or sexual partner, John replied, "There is no reason to be romantic." He reported that he did not want to "put myself out there" to be potentially rejected. Furthermore, because he had "lost interest in sex," he reported no motivation to pursue an intimate relationship. Over the course of his adult life he developed three or four important friendships with women. However, he had not had an intimate relationship in nearly 20 years and had last dated in 1989.

Second, as might be expected given his father's violence and neglect, John experienced significant anger toward his father. In the interview, John bluntly stated that his father is "better off dead." Yet, his fear of experiencing and expressing negative emotions was so great that John coped by avoiding memories of his father as much as possible. He reported that after his father moved out he had "no reason to ever think about him." Indeed, he had so distanced himself from these experiences that he could not remember the exact years of his parents' deaths. Additionally, as the eldest son, John felt responsible to care for his younger siblings. He described feeling guilty because he had difficulty controlling his temper and he would "beat up" his siblings. This situation impacted the patient in two ways. First, John identified with his father's violent behavior. At the same time, he was both revolted and frightened by this perceived similarity. Consequently, he was terrified of experiencing anger of any kind. To protect himself and others from potential aggressive behavior, John avoided assertive behavior and never developed effective conflict management skills.

He reported that after his father left, his mother kept the family financially afloat by working several low-paying jobs. Although John acknowledged his mother's ability to persevere in supporting her family, the family continued to experience financial problems. He recalled her as weighed down by her responsibilities and both physically and emotionally absent. In the history he presented, she neither triumphed over adversity nor obtained the rewards that could come from persistence. This led John to develop a belief that most goal-directed efforts would be fruitless. Thus, he avoided formulating desired objectives and gave up prematurely when pursuing academic or career-oriented goals.

The academic, career, and friendship history John presented was similarly bleak. He described himself as a poor student throughout high school, and although he attended college, he did not receive a degree. He characterized himself as a shy person and a loner who did not establish intimate friendships in high school or college. John explained that during his sophomore year of high school, he made a conscious choice to deal with his negative mood through avoidance. He instructed himself to not "get depressed again" and to "shut down" his emotional responses.

After abandoning his education, John worked primarily in the technology industry. His longest period of continuous employment was 6 years. He stated that it was hard for him to "fit in" at established companies because of his "unusual work style." He described himself as "intuitive" but noted that it was difficult for him to function in structured work environments.

As John matured, his lifelong pattern of avoidant coping brought on increasing social marginalization and financial crisis. Shortly after becoming unemployed, he abandoned his job search and ran through his savings. Without the structure of a job, his daily routine became devoid of constructive activity. His sleep cycle was disrupted; he slept in the daytime and was generally awake all night. Except for people with whom he had contact through the Internet, he was socially isolated. Because of his lack of financial resources, he was in danger of becoming homeless. Additionally, he had significant health problems and lacked health insurance. When asked what he hoped to gain from psychotherapy, he replied that he wanted "a silver bullet," a solution to how to be "at peace with the way things are" and how to "sleep through the night."

From the information gathered during the interview process, the therapist developed several transference hypotheses representing John's core interpersonal beliefs:

1. Nothing I do will please Dr. Post or keep her interested in me. If I try to engage her, I will only fail, and she will be disappointed.
2. If I feel negative emotion, I may not be able to control it. If I express it to Dr. Post, she will be overwhelmed.
3. If I put forth effort in therapy, I will only succeed in exposing my inadequacies to Dr. Post, and she will reject me.

The therapist used these hypotheses both to develop a treatment plan targeting the cognitive distortions and problematic behaviors that were negatively impacting John's mood and life and to anticipate possible difficulties in the therapeutic relationship.

Our primary treatment objective was to use SA to help John change these maladaptive beliefs and accompanying avoidant behaviors. We hoped to help him replace his avoidant behavior with more direct, assertive, problem-focused methods of coping with life challenges. We hoped that his mood would improve as he became increasingly able to cope more effectively with the immediate situational crisis by seeking employment, completing the paperwork for state funded health care, and decreasing his social isolation.

Description of Treatment

From the start, John demonstrated reluctance to engage effectively in the therapeutic process. In the initial interviews, he refrained from providing much detail about life events or his relationships. His speech was frequently vague, and he would skip over large periods of time or change the topic. Additionally, when recounting distressing life events, John would sometimes appear emotionally buoyant. When pressed for more information or his emotional reactions, he would reply that he did not remember or that it was inconsequential. He repeatedly referred to himself as a "big-picture thinker" who did not concern himself with "details." This left the therapist with a sense that she had not gotten to know John as well as she would have liked and that he was distancing himself from her.

The therapist addressed this concern in two ways. First, she became more active, repeating questions several times. Second, she commented on the patient's behavior and her reaction to it. For example, "I am really interested in getting to know all about you, and I am having a hard time putting the pieces together. Can you tell me more about how you spend your day?" Despite these interventions, John's tangential and global speech persisted. This behavior continued to be troublesome during SA elicitation when a primary goal was to help John learn to construct a succinct behavioral summary of a situation or a situational outcome. Frequently, the more the therapist pressed the patient for details or behavioral descriptions, the more tangential he would become.

Therapist: How did the event come out for you?

John: It turned out well.

Therapist: Can you be a bit more specific?

John: I strive for harmony between friends in a positive way.

Therapist: How would someone who was watching a videotape of this situation describe its outcome?

John: Whether you are driving with a friend in a car or living life on planet earth, we are together, and we need to work together in more harmony than we do.

John's global pattern of speech was only one part of a pervasive pattern of avoidant behavior that became manifest when he was asked to engage in various aspects of treatment. First, he often did not complete tasks assigned between sessions. Initially, he reported that he did not read the manual on CBASP that was provided, and he habitually failed to bring in his completed CSQs. When questioned as to the obstacles that got in his way, he would quickly attempt to switch topics, noting for instance that he was awake most of the night with "chest pain" or "stomach pain," or he would describe an acute financial predicament. Discussing his apparent avoidance was difficult. The therapist found it hard not to discuss the specific concerns John raised both because of their potential medical severity and because she worried about alienating the patient, with whom the treatment alliance was clearly underdeveloped.

When the therapist would intervene and prompt John to describe a situation that they could analyze in session, he would characteristically challenge the treatment rationale. John questioned the use of SA, stating, "This is not what I was expecting." John reported that he saw therapy as a means to look at "clues to the present that are locked in my memories that I guess you and I are exploring." He voiced concern that the SA would not be helpful, stating, "Anything that you want, odds are against it." Initially, the therapist addressed the patient's motivational reticence by repeatedly redirecting the session toward elicitation of a situation and by reassuring John that they would work together as a team to use the SA procedure to address the acute problems he faced. For a time, the patient began to bring partially completed CSQs to session. Thematically, these CSQs focused on areas relevant to the identified transference hypotheses, reflecting his extreme reluctance to engage in interpersonal situations he feared would be emotionally charged and his belief in his interpersonal incompetence.

Although he began to demonstrate limited willingness to utilize the SA methodology, other aspects of his avoidant style began to interfere with effective use of the SA procedure to effect behavioral change.

Therapist: You say your desired outcome is to tolerate your friend's political views and connect with him. How would you have to be thinking to have that happen? Did the thought, "My friend is trying to get my goat" make it easier or harder for you?

John: I would have to be thinking, "I don't care."

Therapist: "I don't care about . . ."

John: It is a paradox. To tolerate it I would have to not care about anything anybody says. That way, I'm always accepting. I know there is an answer in between caring and not caring, I just . . .

Therapist: What would that be?

John: I don't know, guarded something . . . guarded acceptance . . . guarded nonacceptance. I don't know how when I have strong feelings.

Therapist: Try to stay anchored in the situation. You feel strongly about political issues, and you want to maintain the friendship. How would you have to be thinking?

John: I would actually have to be not thinking. Just cut that part of my brain out. I could just move out of the country. That would solve all of my problems.

Therapist: What about working on smaller goals first, like this situation.

John: That would be too serious.

The therapist tried to elicit an interpretation that would contribute to the patient's ability to obtain his desired outcome. The therapist kept the patient's focus on finding a way of thinking that would resolve an interpersonal dilemma without suggesting a specific alternative cognition herself. She resisted the "pull" to take over the work for the patient in an effort to help him to learn to generate more situation-specific and goal-directed thoughts. Although most of the session addressed this impasse, the patient was unable to revise his thoughts in ways that might have increased the probability that the situation presented could result in a reasonable desirable outcome.

This inability persisted throughout the remainder of treatment, preventing the patient from experiencing the usefulness of the SA. Failing to formulate and link logical thoughts with a desired outcome, he persisted in defaulting to avoidant coping when faced with emotionally painful thoughts or situations. The therapist was unable to prompt him to attempt reasonable proactive behavior outside of the session, such as by seeking employment. As a consequence, he had little evidence that might have prompted him to suspend his belief that his life was hopeless and accept the notion that small changes in his behavior would ultimately be helpful in improving his overall situation.

In the following exchange, the impact on the treatment of John's ambivalence about facing painful events and making necessary behavioral changes is evident.

John: You suggested writing about an event related to my mood or problems, so I wrote about the day I decided not to get up until 8:30 p.m. At about noon I woke up and thought, "I could get up and start my day, I just don't want to." So, I stayed in bed until it was more work to do that than to get up.

Therapist: What were your thoughts while you were in bed?

John: I thought, "This is an escape from reality; I don't want to do anything or think about anything like paying the rent, and I can't stand to stay in bed and pretend I am tired."

Therapist: Okay, and the actual outcome was that you stayed in bed. What was your desired outcome?

John: To escape from reality.

Therapist: Did you get what you wanted?

The therapist attempted to draw John's attention to the futility of using avoidance to deal with the problem of paying the rent.

John: It was hard work staying in bed.

Therapist: I bet. Tell me, what was hard about it?

John: I wanted to sleep and not think.

Therapist: Was this achievable?

John: For a while.

Therapist: Well, let's go back and see if it's a reasonable desired outcome. Is it reasonable to stay in bed all day and try to escape reality given your current life circumstances?

John: Escaping from things for one day is no big deal for me. I needed the rest.

Therapist: But, you introduced this by saying something about it was a problem for you.

The therapist attempted to address the patient's avoidant coping by refocusing him on the problematic nature of this situation.

John: This is an acceptable event. It's like going on vacation.

Therapist: But at the same time, doesn't it represent a larger problem of avoiding? If we look closely at this situation, maybe we can make a dent in improving things. That's the whole point of the SA. What we learn in one small slice of time that can be generalized to other situations.

The therapist tried to help the patient to appreciate that the problems embedded in this situation extended more generally to his life context. John continued to avoid the obvious problems inherent in his choice.

John: The obvious part is the escape from reality, but I don't think it's very important. It's not critical to face all this stuff on any particular day.

For much of the therapy, the therapist chose to persist in using the SA to highlight the patient's depression-maintaining beliefs and behaviors in spite of his continuing resistance to it. In the face of the acute and dire life stresses the patient presented, the therapist attempted to persevere to teach the patient to use SA to address his acute life difficulties. At a certain point, however, the therapist's interventions became more active and confrontational.

Therapist: But this is a troubling story. You know, it's hard for me to accept the answer that it's okay for you to stay in bed and not deal with your life. I think you have an option to do some hard work and face this tendency to avoid and not talk yourself out of it. I don't want to avoid talking about things that keep you depressed.

John: Doesn't escaping help me get my nose back to the grindstone?

Therapist: What do you think? Is that your experience?

John: Maybe I should just go out and get pissed off at somebody. I could write you a story about that.

When the therapist became more directive and confrontational, John experienced an increase in negative emotions with respect to the therapist. Consequently, he began to miss scheduled visits, complaining of serious physical ailments. He became even more reluctant to fill out the CSQ. He began to interpret the therapist's requests for details or clarification as criticisms, and this activated his belief, as identified by the transference hypotheses, that he was failing inside and outside of psychotherapy. Near the end of the 12-week protocol, the therapist began to address the patient's frustration and sense of failure by discussing therapeutic disruptions directly.

John:	I keep leaving here feeling more depressed. I am not sure I have the guts to work on stuff.
Therapist:	That's important. Let's talk about that.
John:	You said that it's hard to get to know me. There must be something wrong with me. What do I have to say to be understood?
Therapist:	Did you feel criticized?
John:	I am nervous. Somehow there is a fear of failure.
Therapist:	Are you worried about failing in here?
John:	I have already failed. When you are such and such an age and you aren't rolling in money and you don't have a family, you are a failure in this society.
Therapist:	Do you think I see you as a failure?
John:	It doesn't feel like that here, but at work in the past this has come up . . .

The therapist was concerned that the patient was deflecting from the issues that may be present in the therapeutic relationship and attempted to bring the discussion back to how this issue may have been manifesting in the moment.

Therapist:	Do you think this has impacted how open you are with me?
John:	When I was in college, I never finished a term paper, and I knew in the back of my mind that as long as you never finish it, no one can judge you on it.
Therapist:	So, if I don't really get to hear about you, I can't judge you?
John:	Yes.
Therapist:	Is that why you missed our last session?
John:	No, but maybe a better route is to never think about this stuff. Drive it down deep.
Therapist:	It sounds like that's how you've been coping with conflict. But that tends to isolate you. We are dealing directly with a tough situation right now. What is it like to talk with me about this right now?

The therapist highlighted the similarity of the patient's current avoidant behavior with his characteristic behavior and once again directed the dialogue back to the interpersonal hot spot.

John:	Okay, but when this happens with other people it really bothers me and sends me to a place where I don't care to be in contact for a while.

Therapist: Well, how about in this case? Are you hanging in there with me?

John: I feel nervous but okay.

This exchange allowed the therapist to help John notice that perhaps he had a greater capacity than he believed to tolerate negative emotions when directly facing interpersonal conflict.

Therapist: That sounds positive. Are you surprised? It sounds like you expected something else to happen.

John: I worry things will blow up.

Therapist: Did they? Did I blow up?

John: No.

Therapist: You don't seem to have blown up either. So, I think this means that sometimes things can turn out differently than you expect. Maybe we can discuss issues between us without harming our relationship. And maybe if we can help you be a little more direct with people like you are being with me right now, things would improve.

John: I don't know how. And we only have a couple meetings left.

John was finally able to tentatively engage in a meaningful discussion of the patterns that maintained his social avoidance when the therapist used data from their interactions to directly address his underlying supposition that she viewed him as a failure. Additionally, the patient was able to participate in the interaction without becoming overwhelmed by negative emotion or conflict. Consequently, the therapist was able to highlight that assertive behavior might be a more effective strategy than avoidance, one that John could use in future situations.

At the time that this interchange occurred, only three additional sessions remained. Although continued attempts were made to address the above issues as they presented in the therapeutic relationship, the therapist acknowledged the patient's observation that little time remained to adequately address the interpersonal problems and significant self-doubt he was experiencing. She validated the progress John had made and expressed her conviction that he was not a failure and could make significant improvements in his life situation if he continued to directly confront his fear of failure and set small reasonable goals in relevant life areas. She praised his willingness to challenge his long-standing belief in his personal inadequacy by directly addressing his worries about treatment and highlighted the importance of his willingness to enter psychotherapy to try to address his difficulties. The therapist and John spent most of the final two sessions formulating a follow-up plan that entailed transferring the patient's care to a qualified community practitioner.

CONCLUSIONS AND FUTURE DIRECTIONS

In examining factors associated with treatment failure in the case of John, we considered several possible contributors: the treatment context and patient and therapist/supervisor factors. Although we organized the discussion under separate headings, these factors are, of course related. In addition to the unique characteristics that the patient and psychotherapist bring separately to the encounter, the two interact with one another. The passive patient can elicit excessive therapist activity. A treatment context in which therapy is limited to a brief time period can compromise the ability of patients who feel hopeless about their prospects for a better life to invest enough effort in psychotherapy to obtain benefit and/or can alter the usual response patterns of psychotherapists.

Treatment Context

As noted previously, John was seen for psychotherapy in a 12-week clinical trial. The treatment context had many positive features, which may have been likely to increase the probability of a successful outcome. John was offered CBASP twice weekly for the first 4 weeks of treatment and weekly for the duration of the trial. In addition to receiving CBASP from Lisa Post, an experienced clinician who met monthly for supervision with Bruce Arnow, an experienced CBASP supervisor, John received concomitant algorithm-driven pharmacotherapy with multiple augmentation and switch strategies from an experienced team. He was seen frequently by a research assistant to complete clinical ratings, and the research assistant (although blind to the treatment condition) provided an extra level of contact and support. Such nonspecific but potentially therapeutic contacts have been discussed as a potential contributor to the high rates of placebo response in clinical trials for depression (Fava, Evins, Dorer, & Schoenfeld, 2003).

On the other hand, certain features of the trial may have reduced the chances of a favorable response. First, it is possible that 12 weeks of treatment is too brief for someone with the combination of long-standing psychopathology and life crises presented by John. We are mindful that more treatment is not necessarily better treatment. The patient who does not demonstrate a response to 12 weeks of CBASP may not respond to 24, 36, or 52 weeks. Nonetheless, some findings have suggested that no more than half of patients would be expected to show clinically significant improvement within the time frame available to us (Lambert, Hansen, & Finch, 2001). Overall, the resources that have been allocated to investigate dose–response relationships in psychotherapy for depression (as well as for other psychological disorders) pale in comparison with those expended to determine these relationships in early phase pharmacotherapy trials. More research is required to establish an empirical basis for the length of clinical trials evaluating the efficacy of psychotherapy for episodic and chronic depression.

Second, clinical trials impose other constraints. Much has been written about the differences between clinical trials and clinical practice, and we do not wish to add to that discussion. We concur that randomized controlled trials are critically important to our field and the best way we have of drawing causal inferences (Hollon, 2006). Nonetheless, no methodology is perfect, and one undeniable difference between clinical practice and the randomized controlled trial is that in the former the primary goal is to help relieve the patient of his symptoms, whereas in the latter the chief aim, apart from ensuring the patient's safety, is to test the efficacy of a treatment or treatments. As our primary responsibility in the REVAMP trial was to test the efficacy of CBASP, we could not use interventions from other models if they were not consistent with CBASP, even if we thought they might be helpful. For instance, motivational interviewing (Miller, 1996) or a more focused behavioral activation approach (Dimidjian et al., 2006) may or may not have been helpful with John, but we did not have the opportunity in this context to find out.

Third, clinical trials differ in the extent to which subsequent contact with the study therapist is permitted. In the REVAMP trial, contact with study psychotherapists was proscribed after the study's conclusion. Although this may confer certain benefits in assessing long-term follow-up, it may also confer costs that compromise acute phase response, particularly with patients with whom the therapist experiences clear ruptures of the therapeutic alliance. Attempts to deal directly with the therapeutic relationship in the context of a brief trial in which the possibility of continuing with the therapist is foreclosed may be particularly difficult for socially isolated patients who have little experience addressing such issues. It is not clear what the optimal solution is to the trade-off between providing the fairest possible test of an acute phase treatment versus assessment of long-term results, but we believe that the disadvantages of prohibiting future therapist contact may fall most heavily on patients such as John, who have a lifelong history of social isolation and impaired attachments to others.

Fourth, we know little about the change beliefs of patients receiving concomitant psychotherapy and pharmacotherapy, and more research in this area is needed. Over the past 2 decades, practice patterns have changed, with more patients being treated with antidepressants and receiving combined treatment than was the case before the advent of selective serotonin reuptake inhibitors (Olfson, Marcus, Druss, Pincus, & Weissman, 2003). This may impact patients in ways that are largely unknown. For example, we have observed that in some patients receiving psychotherapy and concurrent pharmacotherapy, the individual's investment in the former is sometimes compromised as he or she waits for the psychiatrist to try a new drug or for the new drug or increased dose to "kick in." We do not know the extent to which

John's overall emotional investment and willingness to attend psychotherapy sessions or complete homework assignments may have been affected by his simultaneous participation in aggressive pharmacotherapy. Furthermore, differences in the designs of clinical trials are likely to attract different groups of patients with different theories about the nature of, or best treatment for, depression. A trial comparing two different psychotherapies and offering no medication will attract a different slice of the depressed universe than a trial like REVAMP in which all patients had to accept treatment with pharmacotherapy alone before entering the randomized phase.

Patient Factors

In a recent report on extreme nonresponse to CT for depression, the patients most likely not to benefit at all from CT had high baseline symptom severity scores, low Global Assessment of Functioning (GAF) scores, and Axis IV ratings indicating primary psychosocial support and environmental problems (Coffman, Martell, Dimidjian, Gallop, & Hollon, 2007). Although not quite meeting criteria for extreme nonresponse, John had all of these markers. His baseline HAMD-24 score was 27. His GAF was 55. Although he was not specifically rated as having primary support group problems, he lacked a primary support network. He was coded on Axis IV for problems related to the social environment, occupational problems, economic problems, and problems with access to health care services. Patients like John, whose avoidance was sufficiently pervasive to bring about profound disengagement both from the world of employment and from the world of meaningful interpersonal relationships, are among the most difficult to treat under any circumstances.

The question arises, had we been seeing John outside of a clinical trial where we were not constrained by a 12-week limit and his nonresponse persisted, would we have continued to focus on CBASP, and if not, what would we have done? One issue that confronts evidence-based psychotherapies for depression is developing empirically based strategies to guide treatment for those patients who do not respond to an initial psychotherapy trial (of course, John also did not respond to a course of algorithm-driven pharmacotherapy). Theoretically, a shift could be made to another psychotherapy model such as IPT or time-limited dynamic psychotherapy, which has also demonstrated efficacy in clinical trials (Leichsenring, 2001). However, in practice this is difficult. The psychotherapist who is well-trained in and comfortable with CBASP may not be sufficiently well-trained in IPT or time-limited dynamic psychotherapy to make such a switch. This is not the case for pharmacotherapists, who, we believe, experience comparatively less difficulty shifting from one medication to another. An important area of future research is the development of feasible second- and third-step strategies for evidence-based psychotherapies.

Therapist and Supervisor Factors

Reviewing a treatment-refractory case is a humbling experience. We have discussed both treatment context and patient factors that may have contributed to a negative outcome. But there were a great many areas in which, in hindsight, we feel that better execution of the treatment may have produced better results. Space does not permit full discussion of all of these. But one clear error that we were surprised to see in our review was persisting with the SA methodology in the early part of treatment even in the face of the patient's resistance to it. This misjudgment and its consequences were highlighted by Castonguay, Goldfried, Wiser, Raue, and Hayes (1996) in a detailed analysis of CT cases. They found that poor response was associated with therapists dealing with patient resistance to CT procedures and the attendant strains in the therapeutic alliance by continuing to attempt to persuade the patient of the CT rationale or other CT tasks. John questioned the usefulness of the SA methodology, yet we continued to try to engage him in it without a full discussion of his doubts, concerns, and feelings about it. We were aware from the transference hypotheses we developed that the patient had fears of being judged inadequate and that his accustomed strategy was to not engage in tasks that might expose him to scrutiny. Yet when he enacted his avoidant pattern in the sessions, did not bring in CSQs, and did not engage effectively in the SA problem-solving procedure, we persisted for a number of weeks, attempting to apply the specific therapeutic tasks. Later in treatment, we did begin to discuss his avoidant pattern as it arose in the therapeutic relationship, but by then little time remained. It is impossible to know whether earlier attention to John's resistance to SA and the strains in the alliance would have changed the outcome, but we are reasonably certain that persisting with SA in the face of the patient's reluctance was not helpful.

We were surprised to see this misstep, because we consider ourselves reasonably competent at tracking the therapeutic relationship, identifying therapeutic ruptures, and responding effectively to them. In asking ourselves what may have interfered with our ability to respond more effectively to John in a timely fashion, two possibilities stand out. First, the treatment context may have caused us to alter our usual patterns of response. In this 12-week clinical trial with a patient who had entrenched psychopathology and acute life crises, we were somewhat panicked about the prospect of providing help within what we experienced (at least with this patient) to be a narrow window. This may have caused us to spend too much time with the specific problem-solving strategy.

Alternatively, we cannot ignore the possibility that the treatment context was less important a factor than we suggested previously. Of all the tools available to us with John, we believed that the SA method was likely to be most helpful in addressing the life crises he faced. Confronted with a patient who was in danger of becoming homeless and who was not responding adequately to the crisis, we found it difficult to slow down, shift gears, and spend time inquiring about the patient's reservations about the SA procedure or about how it may have been affecting his experience of the therapeutic relationship. Like many psychotherapists, we are believers in the unique elements of the treatment models we apply. Perhaps we make the mistake of applying these techniques in the face of patient opposition more frequently than we think. Yet, in our view, one of the lessons of this case is to remind us of the perils of perseverating on specific techniques in the face of obvious resistance and compromise to the therapeutic alliance.

REFERENCES

Addis, M. E., & Jacobson, N. S. (2000). A closer look at the treatment rationale and homework compliance in cognitive–behavioral therapy for depression. *Cognitive Therapy and Research, 24,* 313–326.

Akiskal, H. S. (1982). Factors associated with incomplete recovery in primary depressive illness. *Journal of Clinical Psychiatry, 43,* 266–271.

American Psychiatric Association. (1994). *Diagnostic and statistical manual of mental disorders* (4th ed.). Washington, DC: Author.

Arnow, B. A. (2005). Cognitive behavioral analysis system of psychotherapy for chronic depression. *Cognitive and Behavioral Practice, 12,* 6–16.

Arnow, B. A., Blasey, C., Manber, R., Constantino, M. J., Markowitz, J. C., Klein, D. N., et al. (2007). Dropouts versus completers among chronically depressed outpatients. *Journal of Affective Disorders, 97,* 197–202.

Arnow, B. A., & Constantino, M. J. (2003). Effectiveness of psychotherapy and combination treatment for chronic depression. *Journal of Clinical Psychology, 59,* 893–905.

Arnow, B. A., Klein, D. N., Manber, R., Rothbaum, B. O., & DeRubeis, R. J. (2007). *Results of the revamp chronic depression trial.* Symposium presented at the 115th Annual Meeting of the American Psychological Association, San Francisco, CA.

Arnow, B. A., Manber, R., Blasey, C., Klein, D. N., Blalock, J. A., Markowitz, J. C., et al. (2003). Therapeutic reactance as a predictor of outcome in the treatment of chronic depression. *Journal of Consulting and Clinical Psychology, 71,* 1025–1035.

Beck, A. T., Rush, A. J., Shaw, B. F., & Emery, G. (1979). *Cognitive therapy of depression.* New York: Guilford Press.

Beutler, L. E., Engle, D., Mohr, D., Daldrup, R. J., Bergan, J., Meredith, K., et al. (1991). Predictors of differential response to cognitive, experiential, and self-directed psychotherapeutic procedures. *Journal of Consulting and Clinical Psychology, 59,* 333–340.

Blalock, J. A., Fouladi, R. T., Cinciripini, P. M., Markowitz, J. C., Arnow, B. A., Manber, R., et al. (2008). Cognitive and behavioral mediators of combined pharmacotherapy and psychotherapy in the treatment of chronic depression. *Cognitive Therapy and Research, 32,* 197–211.

Browne, G., Steiner, M., Roberts, J., Gafni, A., Byrne, C., Dunn, E., et al. (2002). Sertraline and/or interpersonal psychotherapy for patients with dysthymic disorder in primary care: 6-month comparison with longitudinal 2-year follow-up of effectiveness and costs. *Journal of Affective Disorders, 68,* 317–330.

Burns, D. D., & Nolen-Hoeksema, S. (1991). Coping styles, homework compliance, and the effectiveness of cognitive–behavioral therapy. *Journal of Consulting and Clinical Psychology, 59,* 305–311.

Castonguay, L. G., Goldfried, M. R., Wiser, S., Raue, P. J., & Hayes, A. M. (1996). Predicting the effect of cognitive therapy for depression: A study of unique and common factors. *Journal of Consulting and Clinical Psychology, 64,* 497–504.

Coffman, S. J., Martell, C. R., Dimidjian, S., Gallop, R., & Hollon, S. D. (2007). Extreme nonresponse in cognitive therapy: Can behavioral activation succeed where cognitive therapy fails? *Journal of Consulting and Clinical Psychology, 75,* 531–541.

de Mello, M. F., Myczcowisk, L. M., & Menezes, P. R. (2001). A randomized controlled trial comparing moclobemide and moclobemide plus interpersonal psychotherapy in the treatment of dysthymic disorder. *Journal of Psychotherapy Practice and Research, 10,* 117–123.

Dimidjian, S., Hollon, S. D., Dobson, K. S., Schmaling, K. B., Kohlenberg, R. J., Addis, M. E., et al. (2006). Randomized trial of behavioral activation, cognitive therapy, and antidepressant medication in the acute treatment of adults with major depression. *Journal of Consulting and Clinical Psychology, 74,* 658–670.

Dowd, E. T., Milne, C. R., & Wise, S. L. (1991). The Therapeutic Reactance Scale: A measure of psychological reactance. *Journal of Counseling and Development, 69,* 541–545.

Fava, M., Evins, A. E., Dorer, D. J., & Schoenfeld, D. A. (2003). The problem of the placebo response in clinical trials for psychiatric disorders: Culprits, possible remedies, and a novel study design approach. *Psychotherapy and Psychosomatics, 72,* 115–127.

Fava, M., & Kendler, K. S. (2000). Major depressive disorder. *Neuron, 28,* 335–341.

Friedman, R. A. (1995). Social and occupational adjustment in chronic depression. In J. H. Kocsis & D. N. Klein (Eds.), *Diagnosis and treatment of chronic depression* (pp. 89–102). New York: Guilford Press.

Gelenberg, A. J., Trivedi, M. H., Rush, A. J., Thase, M. E., Howland, R., Klein, D. N., et al. (2003). Randomized, placebo-controlled trial of nefazodone maintenance treatment in preventing recurrence in chronic depression. *Biological Psychiatry, 54,* 806–817.

Gilmer, W. S., Trivedi, M. H., Rush, A. J., Wisniewski, S. R., Luther, J., Howland, R. H., et al. (2005). Factors associated with chronic depressive episodes: A preliminary report from the STAR-D project. *Acta Psychiatrica Scandinavica, 112,* 425–433.

Hamilton, M. (1967). Development of a rating scale for primary depressive illness. *British Journal of Social and Clinical Psychology, 6*, 278–296.

Hays, R. D., Wells, K. B., Sherbourne, C. D., Rogers, W., & Spritzer, K. (1995). Functioning and well-being outcomes of patients with depression compared with chronic general medical illnesses. *Archives of General Psychiatry, 52*, 11–19.

Hollon, S. (2006). Randomized clinical trials. In J. C. Norcross, L. E. Beutler, & R. F. Levant (Eds.), *Evidence-based practices in mental health: Debate and dialogue on the fundamental questions* (pp. 96–105). Washington, DC: American Psychological Association.

Howland, R. H. (1993). General health, health care utilization, and medical comorbidity in dysthymia. *International Journal of Psychiatry in Medicine, 23*, 211–238.

Jarrett, R. B., Eaves, G. G., Grannemann, B. D., & Rush, A. J. (1991). Clinical, cognitive, and demographic predictors of response to cognitive therapy for depression: A preliminary report. *Psychiatry Research, 37*, 245–260.

Keller, M. B. (2003). Paroxetine treatment of major depressive disorder. *Psychopharmacological Bulletin, 37*(Suppl. 1), 42–52.

Keller, M. B., Klein, D. N., Hirschfeld, R. M., Kocsis, J. H., McCullough, J. P., Miller, I., et al. (1995). Results of the *DSM–IV* mood disorders field trial. *The American Journal of Psychiatry, 152*, 843–849.

Keller, M. B., Klerman, G. L., Lavori, P. W., Coryell, W., Endicott, J., & Taylor, J. (1984). Long-term outcome of episodes of major depression: Clinical and public health significance. *JAMA, 252*, 788–792.

Keller, M. B., & Lavori, P. W. (1984). Double depression, major depression, and dysthymia: Distinct entities or different phases of a single disorder? *Psychopharmacology Bulletin, 20*, 399–402.

Keller, M. B., Lavori, P. W., Mueller, T. I., Endicott, J., Coryell, W., Hirschfeld, R. M., et al. (1992). Time to recovery, chronicity, and levels of psychopathology in major depression: A 5-year prospective follow-up of 431 subjects. *Archives of General Psychiatry, 49*, 809–816.

Keller, M. B., McCullough, J. P., Klein, D. N., Arnow, B., Dunner, D. L., Gelenberg, A. J., et al. (2000). A comparison of nefazodone, the cognitive behavioral-analysis system of psychotherapy, and their combination for the treatment of chronic depression. *The New England Journal of Medicine, 342*, 1462–1470.

Keller, M. B., & Shapiro, R. W. (1982). "Double depression": Superimposition of acute depressive episodes on chronic depressive disorders. *The Amercian Journal of Psychiatry, 139*, 438–442.

Kessler, R. C., Berglund, P., Demler, O., Jin, R., Koretz, D., Merikangas, K. R., et al. (2003). The epidemiology of major depressive disorder: Results from the national comorbidity survey replication (NCS-R). *JAMA, 289*, 3095–3105.

Klein, D. N., Santiago, N. J., Vivian, D., Blalock, J. A., Kocsis, J. H., Markowitz, J. C., et al. (2004). Cognitive–behavioral analysis system of psychotherapy as a maintenance treatment for chronic depression. *Journal of Consulting and Clinical Psychology, 72*, 681–688.

Klein, D. N., Schwartz, J. E., Santiago, N. J., Vivian, D., Vocisano, C., Castonguay, L. G., et al. (2003). Therapeutic alliance in depression treatment: Controlling for prior change and patient characteristics. *Journal of Consulting and Clinical Psychology, 71,* 997–1006.

Klein, D. N., Shankman, S. A., & Rose, S. (2006). Ten-year prospective follow-up study of the naturalistic course of dysthymic disorder and double depression. *The American Journal of Psychiatry, 163,* 872–880.

Klein, D. N., Taylor, E. B., Harding, K., & Dickstein, S. (1988). Double depression and episodic major depression: Demographic, clinical, familial, personality, and socioenvironmental characteristics and short-term outcome. *The American Journal of Psychiatry, 145,* 1226–1231.

Klerman, G. L., Weissman, M. M., Rounsaville, B. J., & Chevron, E. S. (1984). *Interpersonal psychotherapy for depression.* New York: Basic Books.

Kocsis, J. H., Rush, A. J., Markowitz, J. C., Borian, F. E., Dunner, D. L., Koran, L. M., et al. (2003). Continuation treatment of chronic depression: A comparison of nefazodone, cognitive behavioral analysis system of psychotherapy, and their combination. *Psychopharmacology Bulletin, 37,* 73–87.

Lambert, M. J., Hansen, N. B., & Finch, A. E. (2001). Patient-focused research: Using patient outcome data to enhance treatment effects. *Journal of Consulting and Clinical Psychology, 69,* 159–172.

Leichsenring, F. (2001). Comparative effects of short-term psychodynamic psychotherapy and cognitive–behavioral therapy in depression: A meta-analytic approach. *Clinical Psychology Review, 21,* 401–419.

Levitt, A. J., Joffe, R. T., & MacDonald, C. (1991). Life course of depressive illness and characteristics of current episode in patients with double depression. *The Journal of Nervous and Mental Disease, 179,* 678–682.

Manber, R., Arnow, B., Blasey, C., Vivian, D., McCullough, J. P., Blalock, J. A., et al. (2003). Patient's therapeutic skill acquisition and response to psychotherapy, alone or in combination with medication. *Psychological Medicine, 33,* 693–702.

Markowitz, J. C., Kocsis, J. H., Bleiberg, K. L., Christos, P. J., & Sacks, M. (2005). A comparative trial of psychotherapy and pharmacotherapy for "pure" dysthymic patients. *Journal of Affective Disorders, 89,* 167–175.

McCullough, J. P. (1984). Cognitive–behavioral analysis system of psychotherapy: An interactional treatment approach for dysthymic disorder. *Psychiatry, 47,* 234–250.

McCullough, J. P. (1991). Psychotherapy for dysthymia: A naturalistic study of ten patients. *The Journal of Nervous and Mental Disease, 179,* 734–740.

McCullough, J. P. (2000). *Treatment for chronic depression: Cognitive behavioral analysis system of psychotherapy (CBASP).* New York: Guilford Press.

McCullough, J. P. (2003). Treatment for chronic depression using cognitive behavioral analysis system of psychotherapy (CBASP). *Journal of Clinical Psychology, 59,* 833–846.

Miller, W. R. (1996). Motivational interviewing: Research, practice, and puzzles. *Addictive Behavior, 21,* 835–842.

Moussavi, S., Chatterji, S., Verdes, E., Tandon, A., Patel, V., & Ustun, B. (2007, September 8). Depression, chronic diseases, and decrements in health: Results from the world health surveys. *The Lancet, 370*, 851–858.

Mueller, T. I., & Leon, A. C. (1996). Recovery, chronicity, and levels of psychopathology in major depression. *Psychiatric Clinics of North America, 19*, 85–102.

Nemeroff, C. B., Heim, C. M., Thase, M. E., Klein, D. N., Rush, A. J., Schatzberg, A. F., et al. (2003). Differential responses to psychotherapy versus pharmacotherapy in patients with chronic forms of major depression and childhood trauma. *Proceedings of the National Academy of Sciences, USA, 100*, 14293–14296.

Olfson, M., Marcus, S. C., Druss, B., Pincus, A. H., & Weissman, M. M. (2003). Parental depression, child mental health problems, and health care utilization. *Medical Care, 41*, 716–721.

Persons, J. B., Burns, D. D., & Perloff, J. M. (1988). Predictors of dropout and outcome in cognitive therapy for depression in a private practice setting. *Cognitive Therapy and Research, 12*, 557–575.

Piaget, J. (1926). *The language and thought of the child.* New York: Harcourt Brace.

Ravindran, A. V., Anisman, H., Merali, Z., Charbonneau, Y., Telner, J., Bialik, R. J., et al. (1999). Treatment of primary dysthymia with group cognitive therapy and pharmacotherapy: Clinical symptoms and functional impairments. *The American Journal of Psychiatry, 156*, 1608–1617.

Rothschild, L., & Zimmerman, M. (2002). Personality disorders and the duration of depressive episode: A retrospective study. *Journal of Personal Disorders, 16*, 293–303.

Schatzberg, A. F., Rush, A. J., Arnow, B. A., Banks, P. L., Blalock, J. A., Borian, F. E., et al. (2005). Chronic depression: Medication (nefazodone) or psychotherapy (CBASP) is effective when the other is not. *Archives of General Psychiatry, 62*, 513–520.

Sherbourne, C. D., Hays, R. D., & Wells, K. B. (1995). Personal and psychosocial risk factors for physical and mental health outcomes and course of depression among depressed patients. *Journal of Consulting and Clinical Psychology, 63*, 345–355.

Solomon, D. A., Keller, M. B., Leon, A. C., Mueller, T. I., Shea, M. T., Warshaw, M., et al. (1997). Recovery from major depression: A 10-year prospective follow-up across multiple episodes. *Archives of General Psychiatry, 54*, 1001–1006.

Spijker, J., de Graaf, R., Bijl, R. V., Beekman, A. T., Ormel, J., & Nolen, W. A. (2002). Duration of major depressive episodes in the general population: Results from the Netherlands mental health survey and incidence study (NEMESIS). *The British Journal of Psychiatry, 181*, 208–213.

Swindle, R. W., Jr., Cronkite, R. C., & Moos, R. H. (1998). Risk factors for sustained nonremission of depressive symptoms: A 4-year follow-up. *The Journal of Nervous and Mental Disease, 186*, 462–469.

Thase, M. E., Reynolds, C. F., III, Frank, E., Simons, A. D., Garamoni, G. G., McGeary, J., et al. (1994). Response to cognitive–behavioral therapy in chronic depression. *Journal of Psychotherapy Practice and Research, 3*, 204–214.

Weissman, M. M., Leaf, P. J., Bruce, M. L., & Florio, L. (1988). The epidemiology of dysthymia in five communities: Rates, risks, comorbidity, and treatment. *The American Journal of Psychiatry, 145*, 815–819.

Wells, K. B., Burnam, M. A., Rogers, W., Hays, R., & Camp, P. (1992). The course of depression in adult outpatients: Results from the medical outcomes study. *Archives of General Psychiatry, 49*, 788–794.

10

SUBSTANCE USE DISORDERS

ROISIN M. O'CONNOR AND SHERRY H. STEWART

A national U.S. survey found that 23% of the adult population engage in heavy episodic binge drinking at least once a month, 8% currently use illicit drugs, and 25% identify as smokers (Substance Abuse and Mental Health Services Administration, 2007). Moreover, 9% of the adult population meets the *Diagnostic and Statistical Manual of Mental Disorders* (4th ed.; American Psychiatric Association, 1994) criteria for substance dependence or abuse. Similar prevalence rates have been observed in Canada, where 26% of the adult population engage in heavy episodic drinking at least once a month, 14% use illicit drugs (Adlaf, Begin, & Sawka, 2005), and 19% identify as smokers (Heart and Stroke Foundation, 2007). Together these reports suggest that substance misuse and disorders are a widespread problem.

Cognitive–behavioral therapy (CBT) ranks among the most effective and widely used treatments for alcohol use disorders (e.g., Finney & Monahan, 1996; Oei, Lim, & Young, 1991). There is also growing support for CBT's efficacy for treating illicit substance use disorders (SUD; e.g., cocaine: Carroll et al., 2004; methamphetamine: Rawson, Gonzales, & Brethen, 2002) and as a smoking cessation approach (e.g., Hall, Muñoz, & Reus, 1994). Myriad randomized controlled trials have demonstrated overall support for CBT as comparable to alternative credible psychotherapies, such as 12-step programs and motivational enhancement therapy (e.g., Project MATCH Research

Group, 1997, 1998). As a stand-alone treatment, CBT for SUD is comparable to other manual-guided treatments, but in combination with other treatments, it demonstrates a clear enhancement to overall treatment effectiveness (Epstein, Hawkins, Covi, Umbricht, & Preston, 2003; Krishnan-Sarin et al., 2006). The empirical support, combined with the theoretical underpinnings and client satisfaction with CBT (Donovan, Kadden, DiClemente, & Carroll, 2002), have suggested that it is a valuable treatment for SUD.

CBT is a time-limited psychotherapy that is rooted in social learning theory (Bandura, 1977). Social learning theory posits that expectations about the outcome of a given behavior are proximal predictors of actual behavior and mediate the effects of other intra- and extraindividual level factors (Bandura, 1997). Accordingly, outcome expectancies directly influence the likelihood of using and maintaining use of a substance. Although social learning theory has been primarily applied to understanding alcohol use disorders (Maisto, Carey, & Bradizza, 1999), it can be broadly applied to understanding SUD. Marlatt and Gordon's (1985; see also Marlatt & Donovan, 2005) cognitive–behavioral model, which is rooted in social learning theory, has shown particular utility in understanding SUD, and relapse to substance misuse specifically.

According to social learning theory, vicarious learning and reinforcement are critical to substance use behaviors (Maisto et al., 1999). It is through direct and indirect experience that the positive and negative reinforcing effects of substances are learned. In particular, the euphoric and pleasant sensory effects of substance use are positively reinforcing, whereas the perceived tension reduction, pain relief, and reduced social inhibition effects are negatively reinforcing (e.g., Greeley & Oei, 1999; Pomerleau, Fagerström, Marks, Tate, & Pomerleau, 2003). Marlatt and Gordon's (1985) model posits that these learned expectancies, when combined with low levels of self-efficacy, lead to risk for problematic use. *Self-efficacy* is the belief that one can cope successfully without the use of substances. For example, those who believe they do not have the skills to socialize at a party or relax after a stressful day at work on their own, without the use of substances, are at increased risk of SUD (Bandura, 1997; Marlatt & Gordon, 1985). Specifically, as depicted in Figure 10.1, when individuals are presented with a subjectively high-risk situation for which they lack effective coping responses, there is a subsequent decrease in self-efficacy. This diminished self-efficacy combined with the activation of previously formed positive outcome expectancies (e.g., expecting relaxation or euphoria from substance intake) lead to the increased inclination to engage in substance use. Marlatt and Gordon's cognitive–behavioral model further accounts for continued use (i.e., relapse), as it posits that the beliefs one holds about his or her violation of abstinence (e.g., guilt, catastrophic thinking), combined with the perceived rewarding effects of the substance, lead to continued use.

The lack of adaptive coping skills is pivotal to risk of SUD. Accordingly, coping skills training is the core focus of CBT for SUD. Monti, Kadden,

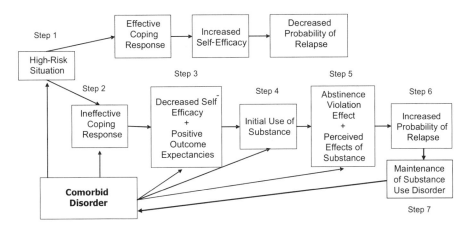

Figure 10.1. Cognitive–behavioral model of substance use disorder for explaining maintenance of substance use and comorbid disorders. From *Relapse Prevention: Maintenance Strategies in the Treatment of Addictive Behaviors* (p. 38), by G. A. Marlatt and J. R. Gordon, 1985, New York: Guilford Press. Copyright 1985 by Guilford Press. Adapted with permission. Also from *Anxiety and Substance Use Disorders: The Vicious Cycle of Comorbidity* (p. 250), by S. H. Stewart and P. J. Conrod, 2008, New York: Springer. Copyright 2008 by Springer. Adapted with permission.

Rohsenow, Cooney, and Abrams's (2002) manualized coping skills treatment for alcohol dependence is widely used and has been adapted for use in treating illicit SUD and tobacco dependence. In brief, the focus of these coping-based CBT approaches is on overcoming skills deficits. Clients are taught specific cognitive and behavioral coping methods that they can implement in their daily lives to deal with interpersonal (e.g., conflicts with others) and intrapersonal (e.g., negative mood) triggers. To increase interpersonal effectiveness, skills such as assertiveness, listening, and drink/drug refusal are taught, whereas such skills as managing urges, increasing pleasant activities, and anger management are taught to increase intrapersonal success (Monti et al., 2002). The goal is to increase the ability to cope with the high-risk situations that typically precede substance use and subsequent relapse. A body of literature supports the positive association between adaptive skills and decreased substance use or abstinence (e.g., Rohsenow, Martin, & Monti, 2005). However, there is still a lack of empirical support for the theorized mediational chain proposed in the CBT model that CBT increases coping skills, which reduces substance use (Stewart & Conrod, 2005).

Cue exposure is another component often included in CBT for SUD. It is rooted in social learning theory and classical and operant conditioning models. According to theory (Abrams & Niaura, 1987), certain cues (e.g., places, internal states) become conditioned with substance use, and exposure to these cues increases the urge to use. Monti et al.'s (2002) CBT treatment incorporates cue exposure. In brief, the treatment involves repeated exposures to individually relevant cues and teaching skills to cope with urges. The goal is to reduce the strength of the internal reactions to the cues and to equip clients with coping skills that can be used in vivo. Empirical evidence has supported the positive association between heightened cue reactivity (e.g., physiological arousal, narrowed attention) and problematic substance use (e.g., Sayette et al., 1994; Waters et al., 2003). There is some evidence to support the efficacy of cue exposure treatment for reducing alcohol abuse (Loeber, Croissant, Heinz, Mann, & Flor, 2006); however, the support is not consistent. Furthermore, there is some evidence suggesting that cue exposure treatments are not effective for smoking cessation and the treatment of other SUDs (Marissen, Franken, & Blanken, 2007; Niaura et al., 1999). Because of the limited research in this area, no definitive conclusions can be made regarding the effectiveness of cue exposure therapy for SUD. Given the theoretical support and evidence from animal models, the limited support for cue exposure may be attributable to methodological limitations (Conklin & Tiffany, 2002).

In sum, there is theoretical and empirical evidence supporting the use of CBT for treating SUD, particularly when used in combination with other treatments. Despite this support, individual differences appear to influence the effectiveness of CBT for treating SUD. For example, the presence of comorbid internalizing and externalizing psychopathology (e.g., Kushner, Thuras, Hanson, Brekke, & Sletten, 2005; Tomlinson, Brown, & Abrantes, 2004) in conjunction with low readiness to change (Gonzalez, Schmitz, & DeLaune, 2006) typically leads to a poorer outcome in CBT for SUD.

The goal of this chapter is to consider how CBT can be expanded to such diverse populations. We consider how CBT for SUD can be expanded to treat (a) those with comorbid psychopathologies, including anxiety, depression, and attention-deficit/hyperactivity disorder (ADHD), and (b) those at varying stages of readiness to change. We address the utility of using motivational techniques to increase readiness to change prior to beginning CBT treatment. To illustrate these two important factors in treatment refractoriness in CBT for SUD, toward the end of the chapter we examine a composite case example (Clift, 1986) drawn from the second author's clinical practice.

SUBSTANCE USE AND COMORBID DISORDERS: ADAPTING COGNITIVE–BEHAVIORAL THERAPY

Recently, Stewart and Conrod (2008b) presented an adaptation of Marlatt and Gordon's (1985; see also Marlatt & Donovan, 2005) cognitive–behavioral model of the relapse process in substance abusers. In the context of an edited book on the comorbidity of anxiety and SUD (Stewart & Conrod, 2008a), Stewart and Conrod's (2008b) adaptation of this classic cognitive–behavioral model was included to illustrate how the presence of a comorbid anxiety disorder could impact each of the components of the relapse pathway in Marlatt and Gordon's original model. Herein, we provide several illustrations of how this modified model (see Figure 10.1) might be applied to any mental health disorder that is comorbid with a SUD, provided that the two disorders are functionally interrelated.

Comorbid Anxiety Disorders

Let us first take the example of comorbid anxiety and SUD (see Stewart & Conrod, 2008b). The presence of a co-occurring anxiety disorder can influence which types of situations would be high-risk for relapse to substance use (see Figure 10.1, Step 1). For clients with comorbid anxiety disorders, high-risk situations for relapse involve contexts that the individual perceives as threatening. However, the precise situations that are perceived as threatening, and are thus likely to trigger substance misuse, vary across the anxiety disorders. For example, a client with social phobia is theorized to be at elevated risk of relapse to substance misuse in social performance or social interaction situations, or when anticipating such situations. In contrast, a client with co-occurring panic disorder with agoraphobia is theorized to be at elevated risk of relapse to substance misuse in situations in which feared arousal-related sensations are experienced and in which it might be difficult or embarrassing to escape in the event of a panic attack. Knowledge that a substance abusing client has a comorbid anxiety disorder helps the cognitive–behavioral clinician narrow in on the types of situations that are likely to place a client at risk of relapse to substance misuse. This can be advantageous to relapse prevention planning.

A comorbid anxiety disorder can also impact the second step in Marlatt and Gordon's (1985) cognitive–behavioral model of substance abuse relapse (see Figure 10.1, Step 2). Those with co-occurring anxiety disorders are theorized to be more likely to choose particular types of maladaptive coping responses to deal with the high-risk (i.e., threatening) situations for relapse to substance misuse. Given the established connection between anxiety pathology and the use of avoidant coping strategies (Barlow, 2002), substance misuse can be conceptualized as one example of a more general pattern of avoidance of feared situations among substance abusers with co-occurring anxiety disorders. Knowledge that a substance abusing client has a comorbid anxiety disorder will allow the cognitive–behavioral clinician to focus on the maladaptive coping strategies that are likely to be used to deal with high-risk situations (i.e., avoidant coping). For example, psychoeducation and behavioral experiments can be used to educate the client about the longer term negative consequences of avoidant coping and to alert the client to substance misuse as a form of avoidant coping. Skills training can also be used to equip the client with alternative and more active and adaptive (e.g., problem-focused) coping strategies.

The presence of a co-occurring anxiety disorder can also influence the third step in the cognitive–behavioral model of relapse (see Figure 10.1, Step 3). More specifically, the comorbid anxiety disorder can impact both self-efficacy and the particular beliefs held about the positive consequences that will likely result if alcohol is consumed in specific threatening (high-risk) situations. Across a variety of anxiety disorders that commonly co-occur with SUD, general tension reduction expectancies (i.e., beliefs that alcohol or drug use will result in reducing the aversive drive state of tension) may be especially important predictors of substance misuse (see Stewart & Conrod, 2008a). However, more specific positive outcome expectancies may hold in the case of individual anxiety disorders. For example, social facilitation expectancies may be especially important in predicting substance misuse among those with a social anxiety disorder (see Tran & Smith, 2008). Consistent with the idea that low self-efficacy in combination with strong positive outcome expectancies leads to substance misuse (see Figure 10.1, Steps 3–4), recent findings have shown that positive alcohol expectancies in the social realm interact with low self-efficacy to avoid heavy drinking in predicting alcohol misuse among those high in social anxiety (e.g., Gilles, Turk, & Fresco, 2006). Knowledge that a substance abusing client has a particular comorbid anxiety disorder can assist the cognitive–behavioral clinician in identifying the specific types of alcohol outcome expectancies that are likely to be activated in high-risk situations. This will allow for the use of cognitive–behavioral techniques such as expectancy challenge procedures (e.g., Darkes & Goldman, 1993). This knowledge about comorbid anxiety can also assist the clinician in identifying the types of situations in which the client is likely to encounter problems with his or her self-efficacy to refrain from heavy substance use. Again, this allows the clinician to better target therapy resources toward increasing self-efficacy beliefs in particular high-risk situations.

The combination of their sensitivities to high-risk situations involving threat, tendencies toward avoidant coping, tendencies to hold particular "risky" substance outcome expectancies such as tension reduction expectancies, and low self-efficacy to refrain from heavy substance use in situations they perceive as threatening makes those substance abusers with a co-occurring anxiety problem much more likely to engage in an initial lapse (see Figure 10.1, Step 4; for recent prospective evidence of earlier lapse to smoking among anxiety-sensitive smokers attending a standard smoking cessation program, see Zvolensky, Stewart, Vujanovic, Gavric, & Steeves, 2008).

Comorbid Mood Disorders

The presence of a comorbid mood disorder such as major depression can also impact each of the steps in the original Marlatt and Gordon (1985) cognitive–behavioral model of substance abuse relapse. First, the co-occurring mood disorder can influence the types of situations that are high-risk situations for relapse (see Figure 10.1, Step 1). For those with comorbid mood disorders, theoretically, these are situations that involve some type of loss (e.g., a loved one, a job) or perceived failure (e.g., not doing as well as one wanted on a test). Those with comorbid mood disorders are also theoretically more likely than substance abusers without comorbid mood disorders to choose ineffective coping responses to deal with the high-risk (i.e., loss or failure) situations for relapse (see Figure 10.1, Step 2). Characteristically, depressed individuals use maladaptive coping strategies such as social withdrawal and other attempts to numb pain, rather than active (e.g., problem-solving) coping strategies.

The presence of a comorbid mood disorder in a substance abusing client also provides the clinician with information specific to two aspects of a later step in Marlatt and Gordon's (1985) original model (see Figure 10.1, Step 3). Given that depression tends to be highly related to low self-efficacy in general, self-efficacy to refrain from heavy substance use in high-risk situations is likely to be low. Because depression involves both the presence of unpleasant affect (depressed mood) and the absence of positive affect (e.g., anhedonia), substance abusing clients with comorbid mood disorders are theoretically likely to experience the activation of both relief and reward substance outcome expectancies when in high-risk situations for substance relapse.

Together, their sensitivity to situations involving loss and failure, their coping through maladaptive strategies such as social withdrawal and attempts to escape pain, their generally low self-efficacy, and their heightened relief and reward outcome expectancies place substance abusers with comorbid depression at elevated risk of relapse to substance use. Further risk factors for this group are those that place them at elevated risk of having a lapse turn into a relapse (see Figure 10.1, Steps 4–7). Once a lapse has occurred, depressed substance abusers are particularly likely to experience excessive guilt about the lapse and to feel hopeless about overcoming their substance use problem (see Figure 10.1, Step 5). These reactions to the lapse support continued use among those with comorbid mood disorders. A recent study of those attempting to quit smoking supports this. In a daily diary study, Zvolensky et al. (2008) followed a large group of smokers for 2 weeks following a quit attempt, in the course of a structured tobacco cessation program. Although it was anxiety-sensitive smokers who were most likely to lapse to smoking (i.e., have a cigarette) over the 2-week interval, it was depressed smokers who were most likely to relapse (i.e., show a full return to smoking after the initial cessation attempt) over this same interval. Moreover, the effects of certain substances are likely to promote continued use among depressed substance abusers. Specifically, depressed substance abusers are theoretically more likely to notice and to appreciate (and may even be physiologically more sensitive to) the rumination dampening and/or analgesic effects of certain classes of substances of abuse (e.g., alcohol, opiates; see

Conrod, Pihl, Stewart, & Dongier, 2000). During the initial lapse, these effects would be experienced as highly reinforcing by a depressed substance abuser, again promoting escalated substance use following the initial lapse.

Comorbid Externalizing Disorders

Comorbidity of an externalizing disorder, such as ADHD, with an SUD can also heighten the risk of substance use relapse, according to Marlatt and Gordon's (1985) model. First, the presence of a co-occurring externalizing disorder may influence the types of situations that are high-risk for relapse (see Figure 10.1, Step 1). Brain-based links between ADHD and alcohol use disorders have been suggested, such that those with ADHD have dopaminergic-related deficits (i.e., lack of attention and impulse control) that are linked to disinhibited behavior (e.g., see Smith, Molina, & Pelham, 2002). However, there is evidence supporting an environmental interaction with this disinhibitory predisposition (e.g., Taylor, Iacono, & McGue, 2000). Given their impulsivity, those with co-occurring ADHD may be at particular risk of engaging in substance misuse in situations in which the rewards are immediate and the negative consequences are more distal (White et al., 1994). There is also some evidence of a mood link to substance use. Those with comorbid externalizing disorders may be at risk of substance misuse in situations that elicit a negative mood, such as boredom, frustration, or anxiety (Whalen, Jamner, Henker, Delfino, & Lozano, 2002); the presence of negative emotions may lead to disinhibition of control over their behavior. Recognizing that a substance abusing client has a comorbid externalizing disorder such as ADHD would allow the cognitive–behavioral clinician to identify these situational triggers for substance misuse. This may be incorporated into a behavioral plan that focuses on cue exposure and response prevention.

Co-occurrence of ADHD can also influence the second step in the cognitive–behavioral model (See Figure 10.1, Step 2). Impulsivity is central to risk of substance use (Molina & Pelham, 2003). With deficits in their ability to exert control over their immediate impulses (White et al., 1994), individuals with ADHD never have the opportunity to develop effective coping skills. Without alternative coping skills, those with ADHD may use substances to achieve the desired quick reward. This pattern becomes cyclical as substances are used in place of effective coping skills. What is key to this pattern is that those with ADHD do not focus on the long-term consequences of their behavior; rather, they attend to the large looming positive benefits. Central to treatment is teaching alternative coping skills. Arguably, teaching cognitive self-control may be difficult in this population (Pelham, Wheeler, & Chronis, 1998); however, there may be utility in teaching alternative behavioral coping responses. For example, teaching them to identify and walk away from specific high-risk situations may be helpful for a comorbid substance abuser with ADHD. Using contingency management strategies may also be effective. In this approach, individuals would be rewarded for not engaging in substance use. The reward would have to be large, meaningful to the individual, and comparable to the reward associated with substances. Given the characteristic impulsivity (e.g., desire for immediate reward) of this type of comorbid individual, this might involve self-reinforcement for resisting substance use by attending an action movie, for example.

ADHD comorbidity may also influence substance misuse through its effect on self-efficacy (see Figure 10.1, Step 3). As previously suggested, it is likely that these individuals have not developed effective coping skills. Thus, they may have a low self-efficacy for dealing with high-risk situations without engaging in impulsive behaviors, like substance use, that provide an immediate reward. Furthermore, individuals with impulsive disorders tend to do poorly in school, typically dropping out of formal education before their cohorts and, as a result, experience socioeconomic disadvantages (Moffitt, 1993). They may interpret this as further evidence that they are unable to handle conventional challenges effectively. This may result in their low self-efficacy that they can use anything other than maladaptive means to cope. Consistent with this, those with ADHD gravitate toward delinquent peers (Kaplan & Johnson, 1992), suggesting that they associate themselves with those for whom engaging in problem behaviors is normative. This low self-efficacy for coping with high-risk situations without using substances, combined with their overattention to the potential positive effects of substances (and the relative disregard to negative outcomes), can increase the risk of initiating substance use (see Figure 10.1, Step 4). SUD clients with comorbid ADHD may benefit from techniques that focus, in part, on improving self-efficacy. Using behavioral experiments in which the client has the opportunity to respond to a high-risk situation without engaging in substance use is important. Tracking successes may be particularly beneficial as clients build up their self-efficacy. Again, given the impulsiveness of substance use for those with ADHD, focusing on cognitive strategies to change outcome expectancies will likely be less fruitful than using behavioral strategies.

Substance Use Disorders and Comorbidity: Mutual Maintenance

We outlined in the previous sections how comorbid anxiety, depression, and ADHD can affect substance use. More specifically, these comorbid disorders influence several steps of the original Marlatt and Gordon (1985) cognitive–behavioral model, which increases the likelihood of lapsing and relapsing into a SUD. A final component added to this model by Stewart and Conrod (2008b; see Figure 10.1, Step 7) accounts for the reciprocal effect SUD has on comorbid disorders. This supports the mutual-maintenance hypothesis (e.g., Stewart & Conrod, 2008b), such that symptoms of anxiety, depression, and ADHD can all be maintained or exacerbated by continued substance use. For example, evidence has suggested that alcohol withdrawal

(Norton, Norton, Cox, & Belik, 2008), cigarette smoking (Breslau, Novak, & Kessler, 2004), and cocaine (Aronson & Craig, 1986) use are all potential precipitants of anxiety symptoms and panic attacks (Stewart & Conrod, 2008a). Psychoeducation regarding the longer term maintenance or even exacerbation of their mental health problems by substance misuse can be useful for some comorbid clients in helping them to increase their motivation to remain abstinent.

MOTIVATION TO CHANGE IN SUBSTANCE USE: EXPANDING COGNITIVE–BEHAVIORAL THERAPY TO INCLUDE MOTIVATIONAL ENHANCEMENT

As outlined at the beginning of this chapter, CBT is a well-supported form of treatment for SUD. Nonetheless, recovery rates are less than optimal, and compliance with CBT treatment procedures by substance abusers is often quite poor. If a client's readiness to change his or her substance use behavior is low, the outcome from CBT treatment is less than optimal (Gonzalez et al., 2006). This is concerning given that many SUD clients have low readiness to change their substance misuse, even when they present for treatment (Miller & Rollnick, 1991, 2002). This low readiness to change makes it unlikely that they will engage with an active treatment like CBT, which requires substantial commitment to pursuing change by the client (e.g., compliance with homework). In the terminology of the stages of change model (Prochaska & DiClemente, 1992), many clients presenting for CBT for an SUD are in the precontemplation stage (e.g., attending treatment session due to partner's ultimatum) or contemplation stage (e.g., just beginning to consider that they may have a substance problem) rather than the preparation or action stage needed for successful CBT.

Traditionally, practitioners have seen poor engagement with CBT treatment (e.g., failure to complete homework) as evidence of a client's resistance or noncompliance (Westra & Dozois, 2006). However, some have suggested that these behaviors reflect ambivalence about change (Engle & Arkowitz, 2006). Substance abusers are notoriously ambivalent about changing their use of alcohol and/or drugs (Miller & Rollnick, 1991, 2002). On the one hand, they are attracted to continued substance use for its many rewarding consequences (e.g., escape from worries, pleasurable high, relief from substance withdrawal). On the other hand, they see that there are severe negative consequences to their continued substance use (e.g., interpersonal conflicts, financial troubles, health complications). Traditionally, CBT does not consider or explicitly address this ambivalence. Yet, some argue that this ambivalence must be explored and resolved before the client will be ready for the heavy commitment required to engage with an active treatment like CBT (Miller & Rollnick, 1991). In terms of Prochaska and DiClemente's

(1992) model, the exploration and resolution of ambivalence would allow the client to move forward from the precontemplation or contemplation stage of change to the preparation or action stage. It is here that CBT skills training should be theoretically more useful because in the preparation or action stages clients are ready (or preparing) to actively adopt change-based strategies.

Using brief preparatory interventions as adjuncts to traditional CBT for SUD may help improve response rates and bolster clients' engagement with the therapy process, thereby enhancing compliance (Westra & Dozois, 2006). The idea of using brief preparatory interventions or "preludes" to increase response to subsequent psychotherapy was introduced as early as the 1960s (see Walitzer, Dermen, & Connors, 1999, for a review). Such prelude interventions have been considered as catalysts for enhancing clients' engagement with and response to existing effective treatments such as CBT.

Motivational interviewing (MI), developed by Miller and Rollnick (1991, 2002), has been identified as a particularly promising prelude treatment for SUD. MI is directed at exploring and resolving ambivalence about change and thereby increasing a client's readiness to change his or her problem behavior. Some have suggested that a combination of MI and CBT may be particularly promising for the treatment of SUD because the MI is directed at increasing motivation to change and resolving ambivalence, and CBT is directed at helping the client acquire the skills to achieve the desired changes in substance use (Arkowitz & Westra, 2004; Bux & Irwin, 2006).

MI has its origins in the humanistic, client-centered tradition (Miller & Rollnick, 1991). In MI, the therapist encourages clients to explore their own thoughts and feelings regarding the possibility of making a change in their substance use behavior. Although this might also be a task in CBT (e.g., decisional-balancing exercise looking at advantages and drawbacks of change vs. status quo), MI departs from traditional CBT in terms of the therapist's role with respect to change (Westra & Dozois, 2006). In CBT, the therapist takes the role of an advocate for change, whereas in MI, the therapist does not advocate for change, but instead helps clients become more effective advocates for their own change (Westra & Dozois, 2006). CBT and MI are similar in that both have a relatively directive component. However, the focus of this directive component differs across the two types of treatment. In MI, the directive component is oriented toward increasing client self-change statements. For example, MI uses techniques to steer the client toward talking more about change and less about staying with substance misuse. This technique is said to assist the client in committing to change. In contrast, in CBT, the directive component is oriented toward helping the client use cognitive and/or behavioral change strategies.

Existing data has suggested that such treatment preludes improve treatment attendance (for a review, see Walitzer et al., 1999). In addition, existing studies that have used brief courses of MI as preludes to other treatments have produced very promising outcomes in the SUD area (for a meta-analytic review, see Burke, Arkowitz, & Melanchola, 2003). The benefits of MI preludes in the treatment of SUD appeared to hold even when subsequent treatments were based on models and techniques quite different from MI, such as CBT (Burke et al., 2003). Moreover, there is evidence that MI is a more effective treatment when used as a prelude to CBT than when used as a stand-alone treatment (Burke et al., 2003). In short, MI has been shown to be a valuable treatment prelude to CBT in the SUD treatment domain.

CASE EXAMPLE

Joe was a 31-year-old single accountant who, at the time of presentation for treatment, was suffering from comorbid social phobia and alcohol dependence. In terms of readiness to change, he was somewhere between the preparation and action stage with his anxiety disorder (he had been reading about social anxiety and was attempting to engage in exposure to some of his feared social situations and was also considering other strategies, such as buying a yoga tape, to learn to unwind). In contrast, he was only at the contemplative stage for his SUD. On initial assessment, he was fairly unwilling to try to address his drinking at this time, because he saw his social anxiety as his primary problem. However, he did report having recently tried to cut back and then eliminate his misuse of alcohol, thus revealing that he had at least considered changing his drinking behavior.

A functional analysis of the relations between his two mental health disorders (Toneatto & Rector, 2008) revealed that the two disorders played a large role in mutually maintaining and exacerbating one another. For example, whenever he felt anxious about an upcoming social engagement (e.g., party, date), he typically used any coping response that eased his anxiety in the moment. For example, he often tried to avoid the event altogether (e.g., he would cancel or make an excuse about why he couldn't attend) or had a couple of drinks before going to the event. He believed that alcohol would act as an effective "social lubricant," allowing him to appear more outgoing and social. He had been engaging in this pattern of drinking to loosen up prior to feared social events since his college years. As this pattern had become ingrained, his beliefs in his own ability to handle social situations without the aid of coping drinking had substantially eroded. Joe reported that whenever he had his first drink before going out to a party, he felt immediate relief from his tension. He found that when drinking, he was not constantly focused on what others might be thinking of him. Joe also noted that even if he planned to have just one or two drinks to calm his social anxieties, he often ended up drinking quite a bit more than he intended once he went even slightly over his preset limit (i.e., limit violation effect).

These examples illustrate how the social anxiety prompted and maintained Joe's coping drinking. Further probing revealed that the problematic drinking also fed back to maintain and worsen his social anxieties. Joe found interacting with his boss very intimidating. His drinking hangovers were characterized by a great deal of physical tension, shakiness, and sweating. When he was hungover at work, Joe worried that his boss would notice these symptoms and evaluate him negatively. Joe also had a lot of anxieties around dating and typically self-medicated with alcohol before and during each date whenever possible. After each date, Joe would ruminate about the social blunders he had made due to alcohol intoxication, worsening his negative beliefs about his social skills and attractiveness to women. He was clearly caught in the vicious cycle often experienced by people with comorbid anxiety and SUD (Stewart & Conrod, 2008a).

Only a few months earlier, Joe had completed a course of CBT through the local addictions services that focused on his drinking. Although he had been quite reluctant to change his drinking behavior, he had nonetheless sought out the addictions services on the recommendation of staff at the local anxiety disorders clinic. Joe had sought treatment at the anxiety clinic 6 months earlier and had been informed that he would have to address his alcohol use problem first.

Joe reported that he learned behavioral and cognitive strategies to manage his drinking through the outpatient CBT program offered by addictions services. Through this program, Joe managed to cut back on his drinking and eventually become abstinent from alcohol. Although he found some of the skills he learned helpful, he did not receive any specific treatment to address his social anxiety or the relationship between his social phobia and his drinking. Upon completion of the addictions program, Joe's social anxiety progressively worsened. While he was waiting to be seen in the anxiety clinic, he experienced a couple of slips to heavy drinking triggered by high-risk feared social situations, followed by a full-blown relapse. Joe realized that he would be referred back to the addictions services before being seen at the anxiety clinic; thus, he decided to seek private treatment to learn to manage his social anxiety.

Because Joe's two problems were interrelated, an integrated treatment that addressed all of the components in the modified CBT model (see Figure 10.1) was indicated. Before proceeding to skills building, Joe's reluctance to change his drinking had to be addressed. Thus, the first step was to utilize a prelude of MI in an attempt to move Joe beyond the contemplation and into the preparation and action stages with respect to his drinking. Through the nonconfrontational and reflective context of MI, Joe began to see beyond the immediate self-medication function of his drinking and started to consider how his drinking was maintaining and even worsening his social anxiety. He ultimately made the decision that he would like to simultaneously tackle both his alcohol misuse and his social anxiety. The subsequent course of CBT followed the modified model for comorbidity (see Figure 10.1). This integrated treatment contained elements of empirically validated treatment for social phobia (Gruber & Heimberg, 1997) as well as empirically validated CBT for SUD (Marlatt & Donovan, 2005). These were not simply two empirically validated treatments delivered in parallel, which could be overwhelming for a complex client like Joe (Randall, Thomas, & Thevos, 2001). Instead, the basic elements of each were retained (e.g., exposure and cognitive restructuring for the social phobia treatment, examination of triggers for heavy drinking in the SUD treatment), and the interrelations of the symptoms of the two disorders were explicitly addressed in treatment (e.g., removal of drinking as a safety behavior during exposure treatment). Joe responded extremely well to both aspects of the treatment. The brief MI prelude increased his readiness to change his substance misuse. And the subsequent integrated CBT produced more lasting effects on reducing Joe's heavy drinking than had his previous course of CBT focused solely on his drinking. Finally, the simultaneous reduction in his social anxiety accomplished through the integrated CBT reduced Joe's risk of relapse to alcohol misuse. By addressing these two major sources of Joe's original CBT treatment refractoriness—namely, low readiness to change substance misuse at treatment outset and the presence of psychiatric comorbidity—a more effective version of CBT could be offered.

CONCLUSIONS

The scope of CBT for SUD has been substantially expanded in recent years through modifications to traditional CBT models, making it more suitable for hard-to-treat clients. Increased knowledge of the functional relationships between substance misuse and various comorbid mental health problems has allowed for modifications to traditional CBT models to better assist this severe group. Such modifications (e.g., Stewart & Conrod, 2008b) specify the pathways by which the comorbid disorder may elevate risk of relapse to substance misuse, as well as how substance misuse may maintain or exacerbate the comorbid mental health disorder. This modification to traditional CBT models allows for the development of more "integrated treatments" that simultaneously address both problems and that have been advocated for some time (e.g., Health Canada, 2001). Furthermore, there is an increased recognition of the impact client readiness to change has on CBT outcomes for those with SUD. This has led to incorporating motivational enhancement strategies with clients who begin treatment low in readiness to change. A particularly promising strategy appears to be the use of MI as a brief prelude to a more traditional course of CBT. This assists with engagement and retention, and consequently boosts the efficacy of CBT for a substantial number of substance-abusing clients.

REFERENCES

Abrams, D. B., & Niaura, R. S. (1987). Social learning theory of alcohol use and abuse. In H. Blane & K. Leonard (Eds.), *Psychological theories of drinking and alcoholism* (pp. 131–180). New York: Guilford Press.

Adlaf, E. M., Begin, P., & Sawka, E. (Eds.). (2005). *Canadian Addiction Survey (CAS): A national survey of Canadians' use of alcohol and other drugs: Prevalence of use and related harms: Detailed report.* Ottawa, Ontario, Canada: Canadian Centre on Substance Abuse.

American Psychiatric Association. (1994). *Diagnostic and statistical manual of mental disorders* (4th ed.). Washington, DC: Author.

Arkowitz, H., & Westra, H. A. (2004). Motivational interviewing as an adjunct to cognitive behavioral therapy for depression and anxiety. *Journal of Cognitive Psychotherapy, 18,* 337–350.

Aronson, T. A., & Craig, T. J. (1986). Cocaine precipitation of panic disorder. *The American Journal of Psychiatry, 143,* 643–645.

Bandura, A. (1977). *Social learning theory.* Englewood Cliffs, NJ: Prentice-Hall.

Bandura, A. (1997). *Self-efficacy: The exercise of control.* New York: Freeman.

Barlow, D. H. (2002). *Anxiety and its disorders: The nature and treatment of anxiety and panic* (2nd ed.). New York: Guilford Press.

Breslau, N., Novak, S. P., & Kessler, R. C. (2004). Daily smoking and the onset of psychiatric disorders. *Psychological Medicine, 34,* 323–333.

Burke, B. L., Arkowitz, H., & Menchola, M. (2003). The efficacy of motivational interviewing: A meta-analysis of controlled clinical trials. *Journal of Consulting and Clinical Psychology, 71,* 843–861.

Bux, D. A., & Irwin, T. W. (2006). Combining motivational interviewing and cognitive behavioral skills training for the treatment of crystal methamphetamine abuse/dependence. *Journal of Gay and Lesbian Psychotherapy, 10,* 143–152.

Carroll, K. M., Fenton, L. R., Ball, S. A., Nich, C., Frankforter, T. L., Shi, J., et al. (2004). Efficacy of disulfiram and cognitive behavior therapy in cocaine-dependent outpatients. *Archives of General Psychiatry, 61,* 264–272.

Clift, M. A. (1986). Writing about psychiatric patients: Guidelines for disguising case material. *Bulletin of the Menninger Clinic, 50,* 511–524.

Conklin, C. A., & Tiffany, S. T. (2002). Applying extinction research and theory to cue-exposure addiction treatments. *Addiction, 97,* 155–167.

Conrod, P. J., Pihl, R. O., Stewart, S. H., & Dongier, M. (2000). Validation of a system of classifying female substance abusers based on personality and motivational risk factors for substance abuse. *Psychology of Addictive Behaviors, 14,* 243–256.

Darkes, J., & Goldman, M. S. (1993). Expectancy challenge and drinking reduction: Experimental evidence for a mediational process. *Journal of Consulting and Clinical Psychology, 61,* 344–353.

Donovan, D. M., Kadden, R. M., DiClemente, C. C., & Carroll, K. M. (2002). Client satisfaction with three therapies in the treatment of alcohol dependence: Results from Project MATCH. *The American Journal on Addiction, 11,* 291–307.

Engle, D. E., & Arkowitz, H. (2006). *Ambivalence in psychotherapy: Facilitating readiness to change.* New York: Guilford Press.

Epstein, D. H., Hawkins, W. E., Covi, L., Umbricht, A., & Preston, K. L. (2003). Cognitive–behavioral therapy plus contingency management for cocaine use: Findings during treatment and across 12-month follow-up. *Psychology of Addictive Behaviors, 17,* 73–82.

Finney, J. W., & Monahan, S. C. (1996). The cost-effectiveness of treatment for alcoholism: A second approximation. *Journal of Studies on Alcohol, 57,* 229–243.

Gilles, D. M., Turk, C. L., & Fresco, D. M. (2006). Social anxiety, alcohol expectancies, and self-efficacy as predictors of heavy drinking in college students. *Addictive Behaviors, 31,* 388–398.

Gonzalez, V. M., Schmitz, J. M., & DeLaune, K. A. (2006). The role of homework in cognitive–behavioral therapy for cocaine dependence. *Journal of Consulting and Clinical Psychology, 74,* 633–637.

Greeley, J., & Oei, T. (1999). Alcohol and tension reduction. In K. E. Leonard & H. T. Blane (Eds.), *Psychological theories of drinking and alcoholism* (2nd ed., pp. 14–53). New York: Guilford Press.

Gruber, K., & Heimberg, R. G. (1997). A cognitive–behavioral treatment package for social anxiety. In W. T. Roth & I. D. Yalom (Eds.), *Treating anxiety disorders* (pp. 245–279). San Francisco: Jossey-Bass.

Hall, S. M., Muñoz, R. F., & Reus, V. I. (1994). Cognitive–behavioral intervention increases abstinence rates for depressive-history smokers. *Journal of Consulting and Clinical Psychology, 62,* 141–146.

Health Canada. (2001). *Best practices: Concurrent mental health and substance use disorders.* Retrieved February 2008, from http://www.hc-sc.gc.ca

Heart and Stroke Foundation. (2007). *Smoking statistics.* Retrieved February 2008, from http://www.heartandstroke.com

Kaplan, H. B., & Johnson, R. J. (1992). Relationships between circumstances surrounding initial drug use and escalation of drug use: Moderating effects of gender and early adolescent experiences. In M. Glantz & R. Pickens (Eds.), *Vulnerability to drug abuse* (pp. 299–358). Washington, DC: American Psychological Association.

Krishnan-Sarin, S., Duhig, A. M., McKee, S. A., McMahon, T. J., Liss, T., McFetridge, A., et al. (2006). Contingency management for smoking cessation in adolescent smokers. *Experimental and Clinical Psychopharmacology, 14,* 306–310.

Kushner, M. G., Thuras, P., Hanson, K. L., Brekke, M., & Sletten, S. (2005). Follow-up study of anxiety disorder and alcohol dependence in comorbid alcoholism treatment patients. *Alcoholism: Clinical and Experimental Research, 29,* 1432–1443.

Loeber, S., Croissant, B., Heinz, A., Mann, K., & Flor, H. (2006). Cue exposure in the treatment of alcohol dependence: Effects on drinking outcome, craving, and self-efficacy. *British Journal of Clinical Psychology, 45,* 515–529.

Maisto, S. A., Carey, K. B., & Bradizza, C. M. (1999). Social learning theory. In K. E. Leonard & H. T. Blane (Eds.), *Psychological theories of drinking and alcoholism* (2nd ed., pp. 106–163). New York: Guilford Press

Marissen, M. A. E., Franken, I. H. A., & Blanken, P. (2007). Cue exposure therapy for the treatment of opiate addiction: Results of a randomized controlled clinical trial. *Psychotherapy and Psychosomatics, 76,* 97–105.

Marlatt, G. A., & Donovan, D. M. (2005). *Relapse prevention: Maintenance strategies in the treatment of addictive behaviors* (2nd ed.). New York: Guilford Press.

Marlatt, G. A., & Gordon, J. R. (Eds.). (1985). *Relapse prevention.* New York: Guilford Press.

Miller, W. R., & Rollnick, S. (1991). *Motivational interviewing: Preparing people to change addictive behavior.* New York: Guilford Press.

Miller, W. R., & Rollnick, S. (2002). *Motivational interviewing: Preparing people for change* (2nd ed.). New York: Guilford Press.

Moffit, T. E. (1993). Life-course-persistent and adolescent-limited antisocial behavior: A developmental taxonomy. *Psychological Review, 100,* 674–701.

Molina, B. S. G., & Pelham, W. E., Jr. (2003). Childhood predictors of adolescent substance use in a longitudinal study of children with ADHD. *Journal of Abnormal Psychology, 112,* 497–507.

Monti, P. M., Kadden, R. M., Rohsenow, D. J., Cooney, N. L., & Abrams, D. B. (2002). *Treating alcoholic dependence: A coping skills training guide* (2nd ed.). New York: Guilford Press.

Niaura, R., Abrams, D. B., Shadel, W. G., Rohsenow, D. J., Monti, P. M., & Sirota, A. D. (1999). Cue exposure treatment for smoking relapse prevention: A controlled clinical trial. *Addiction, 94,* 685–695.

Norton, G. R., Norton, P. J., Cox, B. J., & Belik, S.-L. (2008). Panic spectrum disorders and substance use. In S. H. Stewart & P. J. Conrod (Eds.), *Anxiety and substance use disorders: The vicious cycle of comorbidity* (pp. 81–98). New York: Springer.

Oei, T. P. S., Lim, B., & Young, R. M. (1991). Cognitive processes and cognitive behavior therapy in the treatment of problem drinking. *Journal of Addictive Disorders, 10,* 63–80.

Pelham, W. E., Jr., Wheeler, T., & Chronis, A. (1998). Empirically supported psychosocial treatments for attention deficit hyperactivity disorder. *Journal of Clinical Child Psychology, 27,* 190–205.

Pomerleau, O. F., Fagerström, K. O., Marks, J. L., Tate, J. C., & Pomerleau, C. S. (2003). Development and validation of a self-rating scale for positive- and negative-reinforcement smoking: The Michigan Nicotine Reinforcement Questionnaire. *Nicotine and Tobacco Research, 5,* 711–718.

Prochaska, J. O., & DiClemente, C. C. (1992). The transtheoretical approach. In J. C. Norcross & M. R. Goldfried (Eds.), *Handbook of psychotherapy integration* (pp. 300–334). New York: Basic Books.

Project MATCH Research Group. (1997). Matching alcoholism treatments to client heterogeneity: Project MATCH posttreatment drinking outcome. *Journal of Studies on Alcohol, 58,* 7–29.

Project MATCH Research Group. (1998). Matching alcoholism treatments to client heterogeneity: Treatment main effects and matching effects on drinking during treatment. *Journal of Studies on Alcohol, 59,* 631–639.

Randall, C. L., Thomas, S., & Thevos, A. K. (2001). Concurrent alcoholism and social anxiety disorder: A first step toward developing effective treatments. *Alcoholism: Clinical and Experimental Research, 25,* 210–220.

Rawson, R. A., Gonzales, R., & Brethen, P. (2002). Treatment of methamphetamine use disorders: An update. *Journal of Substance Abuse Treatment, 23,* 145–150.

Rohsenow, D. J., Martin, R. A., & Monti, P. M. (2005). Urge-specific and lifestyle coping strategies of cocaine abusers: Relationships to treatment outcomes. *Drug and Alcohol Dependence, 78,* 211–219.

Sayette, M. A., Monti, P. M., Rohsenow, D. J., Gulliver, S. B., Colby, S. M., Sirota, A. D., et al. (1994). The effects of cue exposure on reaction time in male alcoholics. *Journal of Studies on Alcohol, 55,* 629–633.

Smith, B. H., Molina, B. S. G., & Pelham, W. E., Jr. (2002). The clinically meaningful link between alcohol use and attention deficit hyperactivity disorder. *Alcohol Research and Health, 26,* 122–129.

Stewart, S. H., & Conrod, P. J. (2005). Introduction to the special issue on state-of-the-art in cognitive–behavioral interventions for substance use disorders. *Journal of Cognitive Psychotherapy, 19,* 195–198.

Stewart, S. H., & Conrod, P. J. (Eds.). (2008a). *Anxiety and substance use disorders: The vicious cycle of comorbidity.* New York: Springer.

Stewart, S. H., & Conrod, P. J. (2008b). Anxiety disorder and substance use disorder co-morbidity: Common themes and future directions. In S. H. Stewart & P. J. Conrod (Eds.), *Anxiety and substance use disorders: The vicious cycle of comorbidity* (pp. 239–257). New York: Springer.

Substance Abuse and Mental Health Services Administration. (2007). Results from the 2006 National Survey on Drug Use and Health: National findings (NSDUH Series H-32, DHHS Publication No. SMA 07-4293). Rockville, MD: Author.

Taylor, J., Iacono, W. G., & McGue, M. (2000). Evidence for a genetic etiology of early-onset delinquency. *Journal of Abnormal Psychology, 109,* 634–643.

Tomlinson, K. L., Brown, S. A., & Abrantes, A. (2004). Psychiatric comorbidity and substance use treatment outcomes of adolescents. *Psychology of Addictive Behaviors, 18,* 160–169.

Toneatto, T., & Rector, N. (2008). Treating comorbid panic disorder and substance use disorder. In S. H. Stewart & P. J. Conrod (Eds.), *Anxiety and substance use disorders: The vicious cycle of comorbidity* (pp. 157–175). New York: Springer.

Tran, G. Q., & Smith, J. P. (2008). Co-morbidity of social phobia and alcohol use disorders: A review of psychopathology research findings. In S. H. Stewart &

P. J. Conrod (Eds.), *Anxiety and substance use disorders: The vicious cycle of comorbidity* (pp. 59–79). New York: Springer.

Walitzer, K. S., Dermen, K. H., & Connors, G. J. (1999). Strategies for preparing clients for treatment. *Behavior Modification, 23,* 129–151.

Waters, A. J., Shiffman, S., Sayette, M. A., Paty, J. A., Gwaltney, C. J., & Balabanis, M. H. (2003). Attentional bias predicts outcome in smoking cessation. *Health Psychology, 22,* 378–387.

Westra, H. A., & Dozois, D. J. A. (2006). Preparing clients for cognitive behavioral therapy: A randomized pilot study of motivational interviewing for anxiety. *Cognitive Therapy and Research, 30,* 481–498.

Whalen, C. K., Jamner, L. D., Henker, B., Delfino, R. J., & Lozano, J. M. (2002). The ADHD spectrum and everyday life: Experience sampling of adolescent moods, activities, smoking, and drinking. *Child Development, 73,* 209–227.

White, J. L., Moffitt, T. E., Caspi, A., Jeglum, D., Needles, D. J., & Stouthamer-Loeber, M. (1994). Measuring impulsivity and examining its relationship to delinquency. *Journal of Abnormal Psychology, 103,* 192–205.

Zvolensky, M. J., Stewart, S. H., Vujanovic, A., Gavric, D., & Steeves, D. (2008). *Anxiety sensitivity and anxiety and depressive symptoms in the prediction of early smoking lapse and relapse during smoking cessation.* Manuscript submitted for publication.

11

IMPULSE CONTROL DISORDERS

JON E. GRANT AND BRIAN L. ODLAUG

Impulse control disorders (ICDs) are characterized by the engagement in a rewarding behavior that is difficult to resist even though it may ultimately result in negative consequences. The formal ICDs include pathological gambling, trichotillomania, kleptomania, intermittent explosive disorder, and pyromania. Other ICDs that have not been included as formal disorders in the *Diagnostic and Statistical Manual of Mental Disorders* (*DSM–IV–TR*; 4th ed., text rev.; American Psychiatric Association, 2000) are currently classified as *not otherwise specified* and include compulsive buying, pathologic skin picking, and compulsive sexual behavior. These disorders are quite common in both adolescents and adults and are associated with significant morbidity and mortality (Grant & Potenza, 2007). Although data regarding psychosocial treatments of ICDs are relatively limited, both cognitive and behavioral interventions have shown promise in treating these disorders.

The purpose of this chapter is to detail the cognitive–behavioral strategies used to treat ICDs and to examine the factors associated with treatment response. Because rigorous research is particularly limited for pyromania, this chapter reviews the available research on the treatment of pathological gam-

This research was supported in part by a Career Development Award (JEG-K23 MH069754-01A1).

bling, trichotillomania, compulsive buying, kleptomania, intermittent explosive disorder, pathologic skin picking, and compulsive sexual behavior.

RELATIONSHIP OF IMPULSE CONTROL DISORDERS TO OBSESSIVE–COMPULSIVE DISORDER

ICDs are characterized by repetitive behaviors and impaired inhibition of these behaviors. The irresistible and uncontrollable behaviors characteristic of ICDs suggest a similarity to the frequently excessive, unnecessary, and unwanted rituals of obsessive–compulsive disorder (OCD). There are, however some clear differences between ICDs and OCD. For example, people with ICDs may report an urge or craving state prior to engaging in the problematic behavior and a hedonic quality during the performance of the behavior (Grant & Potenza, 2007). Individuals with OCD are also generally harm avoidant with a compulsive risk-aversive end point to their behaviors (Hollander, 1993), whereas individuals with ICDs are generally sensation seeking (Kim & Grant, 2001).

The pleasurable or rewarding aspects of ICDs, as well as the sensation-seeking personality of individuals with ICDs, have necessitated cognitive–behavioral strategies for ICDs that are distinct from those used in OCD. Certain ICDs (e.g., trichotillomania, pathologic skin picking) share substantial clinical similarities to OCD, and treatment approaches may borrow largely from the exposure response-prevention techniques used to treat OCD. However, other ICDs (e.g., pathological gambling, compulsive buying) exhibit striking differences from OCD, and these differences have necessitated novel cognitive–behavioral strategies (e.g., imaginal desensitization, relapse prevention). Of course, there may be subtypes of each ICD that are more or less like OCD. The subtyping of ICDs and the question of whether certain cognitive–behavioral therapies (CBTs) may work preferentially for certain subtypes await further research.

PATHOLOGICAL GAMBLING

Pathological gambling is characterized by persistent and recurrent maladaptive patterns of gambling behavior. It has been described as a chronic, relapsing condition that affects from 0.9% to 1.6% of the U.S. population (National Opinion Research Center, 1999). Psychosocial problems are common among pathological gamblers, including significant financial and marital problems, reduced quality of life, bankruptcy, divorce, incarceration, and impaired functioning (Grant & Kim, 2001). To fund the gambling addiction or to atone for losses resulting from past gambling, many pathological gamblers resort to engaging in illegal behavior, such as stealing, embezzlement, and writing bad checks (Potenza, Steinberg, McLaughlin, Rounsaville, & O'Malley, 2000). Suicide attempts are also common and have been reported in 17% of persons in treatment for pathological gambling (Petry & Kiluk, 2002).

Although the history of gambling treatment extends over several decades, there is a surprising lack of reliable knowledge of what constitutes effective treatment for this disorder. According to a critical review of the literature on the treatment of pathological gambling (Toneatto & Ladouceur, 2003), the interventions falling within the cognitive–behavioral spectrum have good empirical support at present.

Cognitive–Behavioral Therapy for Pathological Gambling

The majority of the psychosocial treatment literature for pathological gambling has focused on cognitive and behavioral therapy techniques. In general, the cognitive approach includes psychoeducation, increased awareness of irrational cognitions, and cognitive restructuring. Behavioral therapy (BT) generally includes identification of gambling triggers and the development of nongambling sources to compete with the reinforcers associated with gambling. There have been 15 published randomized trials of CBT for pathological gambling.

Cognitive Therapy

Three controlled studies have examined how changing the cognitions of pathological gambling can lead to improvement in overall symptoms. In one study of 40 participants, individual cognitive therapy (CT) plus relapse prevention resulted in reduced gambling frequency and increased perceived self-control over gambling at 12 months when compared with a wait-list control group (Sylvain, Ladouceur, & Boisvert, 1997). A replication study of CT plus relapse prevention in 88 participants also produced improvement in gambling symptoms compared with a wait-list group at 3 months that was maintained for 12 months (Ladouceur et al., 2001).

Group CT was tested against a wait-list control condition in 71 participants with pathological gambling (Ladouceur et al., 2003). Groups met weekly for 10 weeks and each session was 2 hours. After 10 sessions, 88% of those in group CBT no longer met criteria for pathological gambling, compared with 20% in the wait-list condition. At 24-month follow-up, 68% of the original sample still did not meet criteria for pathological gambling.

Although both individual and group cognitive therapies have shown early promise in treating pathological gambling, rates of treatment discontinuation are high (up to 47%). In addition, the studies of CT have not yet determined the optimal number of sessions needed to improve and maintain gambling symptoms.

Behavioral Therapy

Behavioral approaches have also been examined in three controlled studies. In the first study, researchers reported significant reduction in gambling behaviors in a comparison of imaginal desensitization (i.e., participants were taught relaxation and then instructed to imagine experiencing and resisting triggers to gambling) with traditional aversion therapy in the randomized treatment of 20 compulsive gamblers (McConaghy, Armstrong, Blaszczynski, & Allcock, 1983). Both therapies had positive outcomes, but the group assigned to imaginal desensitization was more effective in reducing gambling urges and behavior.

In another study by McConaghy, Armstrong, Blaszczynski, and Allcock (1988), 20 inpatient participants were randomized to receive either imaginal desensitization or imaginal relaxation in 14 sessions over a 1-week period. Both groups improved at posttreatment; however, therapeutic gains were not maintained by either group at a 12-month follow-up (McConaghy et al., 1988).

In a larger study of 120 participants randomly assigned to aversion therapy, imaginal desensitization, in vivo desensitization, or imaginal relaxation, participants assigned to imaginal desensitization reported better outcomes at 1 month and up to 9 years later (McConaghy, Blaszczynski, & Frankova, 1991). This latter study, however, failed to follow up on approximately half of the participants.

Although imaginal desensitization has yielded promising results in the treatment of pathological gambling, the outcome data are limited. In addition, the studies have not been replicated by an independent investigator, and there is no data on the how many sessions are associated with greatest benefit.

Cognitive–Behavioral Therapy

Most research studies have recognized that both distorted cognitions and behaviors need to be addressed in pathological gambling. CBT aims to link awareness of one's thoughts to their behaviors. Cognitive restructuring is used to improve control over gambling urges and the negative emotions associated with gambling. In addition, CBT uses strategies to directly modify behaviors and develop skills in social communications, assertiveness, and adaptive behavioral coping.

A randomized study of CBT in slot-machine playing pathological gamblers assigned participants to one of four groups: (a) individual stimulus control and in vivo exposure with response prevention, (b) group cognitive restructuring, (c) a combination of a and b, and (d) a wait-list control (Echeburúa, Baez, & Fernández-Montalvo, 1996). At 12 months, rates of abstinence or minimal gambling were higher in the individual treatment (69%) compared with group cognitive restructuring (38%) and the combined treatment (38%). The same investigators further assessed individual and group relapse prevention for completers of a 6-week individual treatment program. At 12 months, 86% of those receiving individual relapse prevention and 78% of those in group relapse prevention had not relapsed, compared with 52% with no follow-up (Echeburúa, Fernández-Montalvo, & Baez, 2001).

Melville, Davis, Matzenbacher, and Clayborne (2004) described two studies that used a three-topic mapping system (targeting understanding randomness, problem solving, and relapse prevention) to improve outcome. In the first study, 13 participants were assigned to either 8 weeks of group CBT, group CBT with the mapping-enhanced treatment, or a wait-list group. In the second study, 19 participants were assigned to a mapping group or a wait-list group for 8 weeks. For those participants who were in the CBT with mapping group, significant improvement was maintained both posttreatment and at 6-month follow-up. In addition, the second study, which included measures for comorbid depression and anxiety, found that both pathological gambling symptoms and depression and anxiety scores decreased significantly for the CBT with mapping group compared with the control group (Melville et al., 2004).

Milton, Crino, Hunt, and Prosser (2002) compared CBT (i.e., psychoeducation, cognitive restructuring, problem-solving skills, and relapse prevention) with CBT combined with interventions designed to improve treatment compliance (interventions included positive reinforcement, identifying barriers to change, and applying problem-solving skills) in 40 participants using eight sessions of manualized, individual therapy. Of the CBT plus interventions group, 65% completed treatment, whereas only 35% of the CBT alone group did so. At 9-month follow-up, there was no difference in outcome between treatments, although both produced clinically significant change.

Petry et al. (2006) examined an eight-session manualized form of CBT in which 231 participants were randomized to weekly sessions with an individual counselor, to the therapy in the form of a workbook, or to referral to Gamblers Anonymous (Petry et al., 2006). Although all groups reduced their gambling, those participants assigned to individual therapy or the self-help workbook reduced gambling behaviors to a greater degree than did those referred to Gamblers Anonymous.

In a study examining cognitive motivational behavior therapy (CMBT), a method that combines gambling-specific CBT with motivational interviewing (MI) techniques to aid in resolving treatment ambivalence and to subsequently improve retention rates, 9 men received manualized treatment compared with a control group of 12 men who received treatment as usual (TAU). All 9 participants (100%) in the CMBT group completed treatment versus 8 (67%) in the TAU group. Significant improvements in the number of *DSM–IV–TR* pathological gambling criteria met and South Oaks Gambling Screen scores were observed through 12-month follow-up for the CMBT group (Wulfert, Blanchard, & Freidenberg, 2006).

Brief Interventions and Motivational Interviewing

Brief interventions using CBT approaches have also been examined for pathological gambling. Brief treatments are designed to use less professional resources or time than face-to-face interventions. Brief interventions may include single-session interventions, workbooks, or bibliotherapy. MI is often used in brief interventions. Motivation is empathic and uses the client's strengths to enhance self-efficacy regarding change in behavior.

In one study of brief interventions, Dickerson, Hinchy, and England (1990) randomly assigned 29 participants to either workbook or to workbook plus a single in-depth interview. The workbook included CBT and motivational enhancement techniques. Both groups reported significant reductions in gambling at 6 months.

A separate study assigned 102 gamblers to a CBT workbook, a workbook plus a telephone motivational enhancement intervention, or a wait-list group. Rates of abstinence at 6 months did not differ among groups, although the frequency of gambling and money lost gambling were lower in the motivational intervention group (Hodgins, Currie, & el-Guebaly, 2001). Compared with the workbook alone, those gamblers assigned to the motivational intervention and workbook reduced gambling throughout a 2-year follow-up period; however, 77% of the entire follow-up sample were still rated as improved at the 24-month assessment (Hodgins, Currie, el-Guebaly, & Peden, 2004).

Another study conducted by Diskin (2006) compared a single-session motivational-interviewing module for pathological gamblers. Half of the sample was randomized to receive MI plus a self-help workbook, whereas the other half received the workbook and spoke with an interviewer about their gambling for 30 minutes. At 12-month follow-up, those who received the MI plus workbook gambled less and spent less money than the workbook-alone group (Hodgins & Holub, 2007).

A study using a relapse-prevention-based bibliotherapy compared 169 participants who had recently quit gambling. Participants were randomized to receive either a summary booklet that detailed all relapse prevention information available (single mailing group, *n* = 85) or the same booklet and seven additional informational booklets mailed over the course of the next 12 months (repeated mailing group, *n* = 84; Hodgins, Currie, el-Guebaly, & Diskin, 2007). At the 12-month assessment, those persons in the repeated mailing group reported using the strategies to prevent relapse; however, only 44% of the overall sample reported having not gambled over the 3 months prior to the 12-month assessment.

Conclusions

Although CBT appears quite promising for the treatment of pathological gambling, there are several limitations to the current body of knowledge. First, the studies have generally lacked a large enough sample for adequate statistical power. One exception is the CBT study by Petry et al. (2006) that was adequately powered at the time of enrollment. Second, no manualized CBT treatment has been examined in a confirmatory study by another independent investigator, and most published studies have relatively small sample sizes. Third, with the exception of the Hodgins et al. (2001) study, CBT studies for pathological gambling have generally lacked published therapist adherence and competence measures. Fourth, although CBT treatments appear effective for pathological gambling, few studies have systematically compared interventions or examined whether combinations of treatments are more beneficial. In addition, no study has examined whether certain individuals with pathological gambling would benefit differentially from specific CBT treatments. Fifth, although CBT studies have shown that both brief interventions and longer term therapy are potentially effective, no study has yet examined the optimal duration of CBT. Finally, there are limited data concerning the effectiveness of CBT for pathological gambling participants with co-occurring psychiatric conditions.

TRICHOTILLOMANIA

Trichotillomania is characterized by repetitive hair pulling that causes noticeable hair loss and results in clinically significant distress or functional impairment (American Psychiatric Association, 2000). Clinically significant hair pulling has been found in 0.6% to 3.4% of college students surveyed (Christenson, Pyle, & Mitchell, 1991), but only 65% of individuals with trichotillomania have ever sought treatment for the disorder (Woods et al., 2006). Trichotillomania appears to be more common in females (93% of a recent sample of 1,697 participants; Woods et al., 2006). Significant social and occupational disability is common, with 35% of individuals reporting daily interference with job duties and 47% reporting avoidance of social situations such as dating or participating in group activities (Woods et al., 2006).

Cognitive–Behavioral Therapy for Trichotillomania

Psychosocial treatment data for trichotillomania has been relatively limited, with only five controlled studies published to date. In each published study, however, some form of CBT has been examined. The strongest evidence appears currently to support habit-reversal therapy as the most effective first-line treatment for trichotillomania (Bloch et al., 2007).

In the first study using CBT techniques, 34 individuals with chronic hair pulling were randomized to receive either habit-reversal training (*n* = 19) or negative practice (*n* = 15; Azrin, Nunn, & Frantz, 1980). A single 2-hour session of individual therapy was used. The habit-reversal training included competing reaction training (i.e., hand clenching for 3 minutes), awareness training, identifying response precursors, identifying habit-prone situations, relaxation training, prevention training, habit interruption, positive attention, self-recording (i.e., participants were given notebooks to record each hair-pulling incident), display of improvement, social support, and annoyance review. Negative practice involved standing in front of a mirror and acting out the motions of hair pulling without doing any damage. Habit reversal resulted in a 91% reduction in hair-pulling symptoms when evaluated at 4-month follow-up and proved to be twice as effective as negative practice in reducing pulling frequency.

Habit reversal has been modified for other studies and compared with medication. Twenty-three participants with trichotillomania were treated with either nine weekly sessions of CBT (a combination of habit reversal, stimulus control, and a stress management; *n* = 7), clomipramine (up to 250 mg/d; *n* = 10), or placebo (*n* = 6). CBT significantly reduced the severity of trichotillomania symptoms compared with clomipramine and placebo over the 9 weeks of the study. No long-term follow-up was reported to determine whether treatment gains were maintained (Ninan, Rothbaum, Marsteller, Knight, & Eccard, 2000).

Van Minnen, Hoogduin, Keijsers, Hellendbrand, and Hendriks (2003) examined six sessions (12 weeks) of BT compared with fluoxetine (up to 60 mg/d) or a wait-list control group in the treatment of trichotillomania. The manualized BT consisted of stimulus control, stimulus-response interventions, and response consequences. Forty-three participants were enrolled, and 40 (14 in behavior therapy, 11 in the fluoxetine group, and 15 in the wait-list group) completed the study. Posttreatment assessment demonstrated that the BT group improved significantly more than either the fluoxetine or wait-list group. A 2-year follow-up of the same patients, however, showed that symptom improvement did not last (Keijsers et al., 2006).

In another controlled study of trichotillomania, researchers used acceptance and commitment therapy/habit-reversal training (ACT/HRT), a CBT technique that combines habit-reversal techniques with components designed to eliminate or reduce negative private experiences such as urges or emotional states like depression that contribute to the pulling behavior (Woods, Wetterneck, & Flessner, 2005). The 12 participants who completed the 10 sessions of ACT/HRT reported significantly greater improvement in hair-pulling symptoms compared with those assigned to the wait-list group (*n* = 13). Also, the ACT/HRT group reported a 58% reduction in the number of hairs pulled per day compared with a 28% increase in the wait-list group. Participants in the ACT/HRT group maintained this improvement at 3-month follow-up (Woods et al., 2005).

Only one study has examined combination treatment of CBT and pharmacotherapy versus either treatment alone. Forty-two participants were enrolled in a 12-week double-blind trial of sertraline compared with placebo. Those who failed to respond were enrolled in a two-session behavioral intervention (consisting of habit-reversal training, cognitive restructuring, and relapse prevention). Those participants enrolled in the dual modality treatment demonstrated significantly greater improvement than those in either single modality (sertraline or habit reversal; Dougherty, Loh, Jenike, & Keuthen, 2006).

Group CBT therapy has also been used in the treatment of trichotillomania. In a study of 24 trichotillomania participants, group BT ($n = 12$) was compared with group supportive therapy ($n = 12$). The eight-session BT group focused on psychoeducation, awareness training, stimulus control, competing response training, relaxation training, CT, self-monitoring, motivation, and relapse prevention. Participants were required to complete weekly homework assignments and discuss progress with the group. The focus of the supportive therapy group was having group members interact with one another and share their experiences of hair pulling with the group. Following treatment, the BT group showed significant reductions in trichotillomania symptoms compared with the support therapy group. Follow-up at 1 month, 3 months, and 6 months, however, showed a significant worsening of treatment gains for the BT group (Diefenbach, Tolin, Hannan, Maltby, & Crocetto, 2006).

Conclusions

Although there are many case reports on effective treatments for trichotillomania, the data from controlled trials are sparse. The one treatment that has shown potential promise in treating trichotillomania is habit-reversal therapy, or some modification thereof. The manualized treatments using habit reversal, however, have not been examined in a confirmatory study by an independent investigator. Although habit reversal appears promising in the short term, there are no controlled trials examining the long-term effects of this treatment.

COMPULSIVE BUYING

Although not specifically recognized in the *DSM–IV–TR* as an impulse control disorder, the following diagnostic criteria have been proposed for *compulsive buying*: (a) a preoccupation with buying (characterized by either an irresistible, intrusive, and/or senseless preoccupation with buying or buying more than one can afford, buying unneeded items, or shopping for longer durations of time than originally intended) and (b) the buying preoccupation results in marked distress, interferes with social or occupational functioning, and causes financial problems (McElroy, Keck, Pope, Smith, & Strakowski, 1994). Pleasurable feelings during and immediately following a shopping binge are common for compulsive shoppers but are quickly replaced by feelings of guilt, shame, and embarrassment. The rates of compulsive buying were examined using a random-sample survey of 2,513 adults in the United States. In this sample, 5.8% of adults screened positive for compulsive buying (Koran, Faber, Aboujadoude, Large, & Serpe, 2006). The items purchased are usually given away, returned to the stores, or go unused.

Cognitive–Behavioral Therapy for Compulsive Buying

Although recent research has found that compulsive buying rates in the United States may be as high as 5.8% (Koran et al., 2006), very little research has focused on the treatment of this disorder. Several case reports have suggested that possible effective psychotherapeutic interventions might include exposure and response prevention, and supportive or insight-oriented psychotherapy (McElroy et al., 1994), but there have been no studies of individual psychosocial interventions in compulsive buying.

Only one controlled trial study using group CBT has been published. In that study, Mitchell, Burgard, Faber, Crosby, and de Zwaan (2006) compared 12 sessions of group CBT ($n = 28$) to wait-list ($n = 11$) over a period of 10 weeks in a total of 39 adult female participants. Participants were required to attend 2 sessions in the 1st week and then 1 session a week for the remaining 8 weeks of the program. A workbook with homework assignments, which included readings and self-monitoring assessments, was completed by participants between sessions. A 6-month follow-up was also conducted for those in the treatment group, and a 3-month follow-up for those in the wait-list group was conducted prior to receiving treatment. Of the 28 participants in the treatment group, 21 completed the program. Four of the 11 participants in the wait-list control group dropped out prior to any follow-up assessment. Forty-three percent of the 21 participants in the treatment group reported complete remission of compulsive shopping symptoms 4 weeks after treatment, and 59% (10/17) reported the same improvement at the 6-month follow-up. No significant improvement was noted in the wait-list group.

Conclusions

There is scant evidence concerning effective treatment for compulsive buying. On the basis of available data, group CBT treatment may be effective for compulsive buying but larger, longer studies are needed.

KLEPTOMANIA

Kleptomania is characterized by repetitive, uncontrollable stealing of items not needed for their personal use (American Psychiatric Association, 2000). Kleptomania typically has its onset in early adulthood or late adolescence (McElroy, Pope, Hudson, Keck, & White, 1991) and has shown rates of 8.8% and 7.8% in adolescent and adult psychiatric populations, respectively (Grant, Levine, Kim, & Potenza, 2005; Grant, Williams, & Potenza, 2007). Legal consequences are common and can result in significant guilt, shame, and poor quality of life (Grant & Kim, 2002; Presta et al., 2002). Suicide attempts are also high in those with kleptomania and have been reported in 24.3% of participants (McElroy et al., 1991). The stolen items are often given or thrown away or hoarded (McElroy et al., 1991).

Cognitive–Behavioral Therapy for Kleptomania

To date, there have been no controlled clinical trials of psychosocial interventions for the treatment of kleptomania. Case studies, however, have shown that CBT is a potentially promising treatment for kleptomania. One case discusses a man who was able to reduce the frequency of his shoplifting after undergoing seven sessions of covert sensitization combined with exposure and response prevention over a 4-month period. In addition, the man went to stores and was asked to imagine that the store manager was observing him. The young man reduced his stealing behavior, although his urges to steal went unchanged (Guidry, 1969).

In other cases of covert sensitization, a young woman underwent five weekly sessions wherein she was instructed to practice covert sensitization whenever she had urges to steal. She was then able to go 14 months with only a single lapse in behavior and with no reported urges to steal (Gauthier & Pellerin, 1982). A 77-year-old woman responded well to both a self-imposed ban on shopping and covert sensitization (McNeilly & Burke, 1998).

Similarly, another woman was instructed to have increasing nausea when tempted to steal with imagery of vomiting associated with actual stealing (Glover, 1985). After four sessions over 8 weeks, the woman was able to go with only a single lapse in behavior over the next 19 months. In a similar case, aversive breath holding in combination with diary keeping of urges to steal and six weekly sessions of therapy resulted in significantly reduced stealing frequency (Keutzer, 1972).

Imaginal desensitization in fourteen 15-minute sessions over 5 days resulted in complete remission of symptoms for a 2-year period for two participants (McConaghy & Blaszczynski, 1988). One case involved a woman treated weekly for 5 months to assist her in finding alternative sources of excitement, pleasure, and self-fulfillment. She was able to report a 2-year period of remitted symptoms (Gudjonsson, 1987).

Conclusions

No controlled trials of psychosocial interventions have been reported in kleptomania. The current research is therefore based solely on case reports. Although there is some evidence supporting CBT in the treatment of kleptomania, those data are also severely limited. The research on treatment outcome in kleptomania contrasts sharply with the quantity and quality of studies in other impulse control disorders. This may be attributable to the low prevalence of kleptomania and to clinical difficulties in treating individuals involved in illegal activities. There is, however, substantial need for systematic studies of the treatment of this disorder. Given the existing data, it is not possible to construct evidence-based clinical recommendations regarding psychosocial treatment for this disorder.

INTERMITTENT EXPLOSIVE DISORDER

Intermittent explosive disorder is characterized by recurrent, significant outbursts of aggression, often leading to assaultive acts against people or property that are disproportionate to outside stressors and not better explained by another psychiatric diagnosis (American Psychiatric Association, 2000). Individuals suffering from intermittent explosive disorder regard their behavior as distressing and problematic (McElroy, Soutulo, Beckman, Taylor, & Keck, 1998). Outbursts are generally short lived (usually less than 30 minutes in duration) and frequent (multiple times per month). Legal and occupational difficulties are common (McElroy et al., 1998). Recent research has suggested that intermittent explosive disorder may be common with 6.3% of a community sample meeting lifetime criteria for the disorder (Coccaro, Schmidt, Samuels, & Nestadt, 2004).

Cognitive–Behavioral Therapy for Intermittent Explosive Disorder

Although case reports have suggested that insight-oriented psychotherapy and BT may be beneficial, there are no published controlled psychological treatment studies for intermittent explosive disorder (IED). Controlled trials of participants with significant anger and aggression, however, have been described in the literature. Deffenbacher, Huff, Lynch, Oetting, and Salvatore (2000) examined the use of group therapy combining relaxation training with CBT techniques compared with relaxation training alone and an assessment-only group for self-reported high-anger drivers. Both the relaxation-only and relaxation-plus CBT therapy groups demonstrated improvement on driving anger but not general trait anger. When the study was replicated using drivers with higher levels of anger, trait anger improved in both treatment groups (Deffenbacher, Filetti, Lynch, Dahlen, & Oetting, 2002), suggesting that relaxation training alone may be a viable treatment option for such aggression.

Another study of 30 aggressive drivers (70% male) examined the use of group CBT (4 weeks) versus symptom monitoring (6 weeks). Ten of the participants met criteria for IED. The CBT component combined relaxation training, coping skills, cognitive strategies, and education about aggressive driving and its impact on others. The CBT group showed significant improvement at both posttreatment and at 2-month follow-up on measures of aggressive driving. Participants with IED, however, did not improve significantly. More intensified treatment may be necessary for those drivers with IED (Galovski & Blanchard, 2002).

Conclusions

Appropriate treatments for intermittent explosive disorder have yet to be developed. On the basis of the limited studies that have examined aggressive behavior, relaxation therapy in conjunction with CT presents as a possible treatment; however, extensive controlled clinical trials are necessary.

PATHOLOGIC SKIN PICKING

Pathologic skin picking, a condition characterized by the repetitive or compulsive picking of skin that causes tissue damage, has an estimated prevalence of 2% to 4% in collegiate and dermatological populations (Gupta, Gupta, & Haberman, 1987; Keuthen et al., 2000). Individuals with pathologic skin picking report significant shame and embarrassment associated with the behavior, which results in social, occupational, and familial impairment (Arnold, Auchenbach, & McElroy, 2001). Most often, those with pathologic skin picking pick their face, but other body parts such as the legs, arms, torso, and hands may be the focus of their picking and may consume several hours of each day (Odlaug & Grant, 2007). Significant medical complications such as scarring and infections can result from the behavior (Odlaug & Grant, 2007).

Cognitive–Behavioral Therapy for Pathologic Skin Picking

Although pathologic skin picking appears to be a fairly common disorder, treatment research for the behavior is relatively nonexistent. There is only one formal study of psychotherapy for pathologic skin picking. In a study examining habit reversal compared with wait-list, 19 participants with pathologic skin picking were randomly assigned (Teng, Woods, & Twohig, 2006). Habit reversal consisted of standard self-monitoring and competing responses. Those assigned to habit reversal were able to significantly reduce picking behavior compared with those assigned to wait-list and to maintain those gains for 3 months.

A small case series of CBT also demonstrated promise for treating pathologic skin picking. In one report, three participants were treated with a combination of habit reversal and other CBT techniques (competing response, stimulus control, stress-regulation skills, awareness training, self-monitoring, emotion regulation training, psychoeducation, and cognitive-restructuring; Deckersbach, Wilhelm, Keuthen, Baer, & Jenike, 2002). After a total of four weekly, 60-minute sessions, one participant had complete remission of picking behavior and only mild urges to pick, and the improvement was maintained for 2 months. Another participant reported remission of picking for nearly 3 years following CBT. The third participant, who had comorbid body dysmorphic disorder, underwent seven weekly, 60-minute sessions and reported fewer than three picking episodes per day following treatment (cf. baseline of 20 episodes per day; Deckersbach et al., 2002).

Conclusions

Pathologic skin picking has received a very limited amount of treatment research. Although habit reversal has shown benefit in treating this behavior, further controlled trials are necessary. Because of the preliminary success of habit reversal and because of similarities between picking and trichotillomania, habit-reversal techniques may prove particularly beneficial in the treatment of pathologic skin picking.

COMPULSIVE SEXUAL BEHAVIOR

Compulsive sexual behavior (CSB) is described as excessive or uncontrolled sexual thoughts or behavior that lead to marked distress, causing consequences to social, occupational, legal, and/or financial aspects of the person's life (Black, Kehrberg, Flumerfelt, & Schlosser, 1997). A range of both nonparaphilic (e.g., pornography, sexual promiscuity, masturbation) and paraphilic (i.e., sexual sadism, exhibitionism, voyeurism, and fetishes) sexual behavior that has become excessive and out of the person's control characterize the disorder. Although the exact prevalence is unknown, the rate of CSB in adults is estimated to range from 3% to 6% (Coleman, 1992).

Cognitive–Behavioral Therapy for Compulsive Sexual Behavior

Although case reports have discussed the possible benefits of CBT for compulsive sexual behavior, only one study has been published. The study examined the efficacy of group CBT for gay and bisexual men with compulsive sexual behavior (Quadland, 1985). The group therapy was effective in reducing targeted sexual behaviors.

Conclusions

Extensive research has yet to be conducted in the area of compulsive sexual behavior treatment. Although group therapy is a promising treatment option, controlled trials have not been conducted.

CASE EXAMPLE

Blake, a 38-year-old married man with a graduate-level education, presented for treatment of both pathological gambling and compulsive shopping. He endorsed a history of alcohol abuse with abstinence for 3 years. Blake described "constant" urges to gamble and, when unable to gamble, reported engaging in uncontrolled shopping binges. Conversely, Blake often found his desire to gamble was increased when he was presented with the large debts from his shopping. He believed that gambling would result in money to pay the bills. Although he reports that both gambling and shopping produced "rush" or "thrill" for him, he also acknowledged that the debt ($30,000 in credit cards) and lack of control over his behavior resulted in shame, guilt, and depression. Blake also endorsed frequent thoughts of suicide.

Weekly CBT was implemented for a period of 12 weeks, during which time the therapist worked to identify Blake's specific gambling and shopping triggers. MI was used to address the ambivalence of stopping a "thrilling" behavior. His illusion of control over gambling, and cognitive distortions about money and the probabilities of winning money from gambling, were all identified and subsequently challenged. BT focused on replacing the prior behaviors with other stimulating, healthy activities. The final session focused on relapse prevention strategies and identifying both high-risk situations and coping strategies so that a relapse could be prevented. Because of his significant financial problems, Blake also saw a financial counselor who helped him establish a payment plan for his debts. Following 12 weeks of weekly therapy, Blake reported that his behaviors were well controlled. Blake continued to see his therapist once every month for the next year. He reported minimal intrusive thoughts to engage in the behavior and rated himself as improved in both his gambling and shopping urges and behavior.

CLINICAL APPROACH TO TREATMENT

Because the triggers, as well as the consequences, of ICD behaviors differ markedly among patients, clinicians need to individually tailor CBT treatment. To do this, it is important that the clinicians assess for all co-occurring disorders using valid and reliable diagnostic tools. Focusing treatment on one ICD alone without addressing other co-occurring conditions may affect treatment outcome. For example, if treatment focused on Blake's gambling (in the previous case example) without awareness of how his gambling and compulsive buying interacted, long-term outcomes for both disorders may be jeopardized. Also, because suicidal thoughts are quite common among individuals with ICDs (Hodgins, Mansley, & Thygesen, 2006; McElroy et al., 1991), a suicidal-risk assessment needs to be performed at initial evaluation and periodically throughout treatment. On the basis of this risk assessment, the clinician may need to implement other interventions, such as emergency care, until the individual is stabilized.

Motivation for change should be addressed with the patient at the initial visit. Many aspects of ICD may result in lack of motivation to reduce or stop the behaviors. These behaviors are characterized by a hedonic quality— individuals find these behaviors rewarding or stimulating to some extent. For many people, their real desire is to prevent the negative consequences of the behavior, not necessarily the behaviors themselves. For example, many individuals with pathological gambling want to stop losing but may not want to stop gambling. Motivation interviewing may be particularly helpful in addressing the inherent ambivalence underlying these behaviors.

Because of the illegal nature of certain ICDs (e.g., kleptomania), the perceived immoral aspects of other ICDs (e.g., compulsive sexual behavior), and the shame associated with other disorders (e.g., pathological gambling, trichotillomania, pathologic skin picking), patients may feel apprehensive about, or minimize, their symptoms. It is important for the therapist to establish a nonjudgmental atmosphere wherein the patient can feel free to discuss the extent of his or her behaviors and any complicating factors that may interfere with therapy (e.g., legal repercussions). Involving a significant other in the therapy may aid in the process of full disclosure, as well as create additional support for the patient, but needs to be addressed on an individual basis.

In addition to the standard CBT techniques in the previously described studies, people with ICDs (such as Blake) may need some additional treatments to address legal or financial problems. Given the possible legal repercussions of certain ICDs (e.g., kleptomania, pathological gambling) and the significant financial difficulties of other ICDs (e.g., compulsive buying, pathological gambling), referral to legal and financial counseling may also be necessary. CBT techniques may also address the catastrophic thinking that often accompanies legal and financial problems.

Group therapy or self-help groups such as Gamblers Anonymous, Shoplifters Anonymous, Sexaholics Anonymous, and Shopaholics Anonymous may be helpful in cases in which the patient feels that he or she is the only person dealing with the particular behavior or that no one understands his or her struggle.

Because shame, embarrassment, and guilt are common in individuals with ICDs, therapy needs to acknowledge the individual's strengths as well as analyzing and identifying the individual's weaknesses (Hodgins & Peden, 2008). For example, a patient who is trained in relaxation techniques and possesses good problem-solving skills would not require those two skills incorporated into a treatment plan. This can serve not only to eliminate areas of treatment that are unnecessary but also to show the patient that he or she is capable of success (Hodgins & Holub, 2007). The clinician should work with the patient to identify these strengths as well as obstacles to treatment success.

PREDICTORS OF TREATMENT RESPONSE

Although several CBT studies have been conducted in the area of ICDs, a very limited number of those studies identified or addressed predictors of treatment success. The data supporting which factors predict treatment response are very limited; however, some early indications emerge from the studies.

Social Support Associated With Improved Treatment Outcome

One study of 29 gamblers found that those who initially presented with the ideation of a successful outcome and reported using social support systems such as a spouse, friend, or counselor had more successful gambling symptom reductions (Dickerson et al., 1990). Social support may be especially beneficial for patients who report having very few social contacts outside of engaging in the ICD behavior. A goal of increasing social support through family and friends and introducing other enjoyable activities may be considered for such a patient (Hodgins & Peden, 2008).

Co-Occurring Disorders Complicate Treatment Compliance

Although treatment studies in ICDs have generally excluded participants with comorbid psychiatric disorders, there is evidence that these disorders need to be addressed if the ICD is to be successfully treated. Alcohol or drug abuse, for example, has been found in 30% to 50% of pathological gamblers (Lesieur & Rosenthal, 1991; Ramirez, McCormick, Russo, & Taber, 1983) and correlates with high rates of treatment dropout and relapse (Echeburúa et al., 2001). Milton et al. (2002) studied CBT response in 40 participants with pathological gambling. They found that comorbid problem drinking, drug use, and duration of gambling disorder were predictors of poor treatment compliance. Evidence has suggested that substance use can adversely affect cognitive processes, leading to poor judgment and increased risk taking (Baron & Dickerson, 1999). Substance use might also increase risk taking by restricting attention to only the most salient and immediate cues, leading to less regard for the actual odds of a gamble and past gambling losses (Steele & Josephs, 1988). One study found that alcohol intake was associated with greater spending on gambling activities and with gambling problems (Smart & Ferris, 1996).

In the case of trichotillomania, Keijsers et al. (2006) found that higher depressive symptoms at pretreatment screening negatively affected treatment outcome at 2-year follow-up. The authors recommended that depressive symptoms be addressed prior to the implementation of treatment. This finding is consistent with the literature on OCD, a disorder related in some ways to ICDs. Co-occurring major depression in patients with OCD has been found to be a significant predictor of poor treatment outcome (Steketee, Chambless, & Tran, 1999). Although the predictive role of depression in the treatment of other ICDs has not been systematically evaluated, the fact that untreated depression may complicate or worsen treatment outcome makes intuitive sense. Because of the intensive nature of CBT, it may be difficult for a clinically depressed patient to complete homework assignments or show up for weekly appointments. Although the data regarding co-occurring disorders is sparse, early data suggest that clinicians should assess the co-occurrence of other disorders and their severity prior to developing a treatment plan.

Duration and Severity of Symptoms Predict Worse Outcome

One study of men hospitalized for the treatment of their pathological gambling found that more severe gambling symptoms prior to CBT treatment significantly predicted poorer treatment success at follow-up (McCormick & Taber, 1988).

In a study of 40 pathological gambling participants, Sylvain et al. (1997) compared treatment completers with those who either refused treatment or dropped out of treatment prematurely. They found that the refuser/dropout group started gambling and developed gambling problems at an earlier age compared with the completer group.

FACTORS THAT INFLUENCE TREATMENT DECISIONS

Even knowing the evidence for various treatment options of ICDs, multiple factors may influence which treatment option is chosen for a particular patient. First, many clinicians are simply unaware of these disorders. Therefore, if a clinician is referring a patient for CBT, it may be difficult to find someone with experience in treating the behavior. This problem can be minimized by having a list of providers who know about these disorders and can provide treatment.

Second, there are no clear recommendations of treatment for the clinician to follow. For example, it is unclear how many sessions of CBT are most helpful for a particular ICD. These gaps in knowledge make it difficult to inform patients about what their care may entail and what expectations they may have.

Third, patients with ICDs exhibit high rates of placebo response in treatment studies. Clinicians need to understand that for many patients with these behaviors, just telling the clinicians about their problem may help substantially at first. This initial robust response, however, may cause the clinician to believe that his or her treatment approach is successful. Clinicians should carefully monitor the patients for several months and not assume they will continue to do well.

Fourth, patients with ICDs often do not follow recommendations or follow through with treatment. The treatment data show that dropout rates are high for most patients with ICDs. This may be due to two factors: (a) Patients often believe that they are doing better than in fact they are and therefore see treatment as unnecessary, and (b) patients do not have an instantaneous response and therefore do not stay with treatment. Both of these concerns may be minimized by providing psychoeducation about the illness, the expectations of treatment, and the need to stay in treatment.

CONCLUSIONS AND FUTURE DIRECTIONS

The systematic study of treatment for ICDs is in its infancy. With few studies published, it is not possible to make treatment recommendations with a substantial degree of confidence. Nonetheless, CBT offers promise for the effective treatment of many of the ICDs. For example, CBT and imaginal desensitization both appear beneficial for pathological gambling, and habit-reversal therapy has shown some benefit for trichotillomania.

Clinicians, however, should be aware of the limitations of treatment knowledge in this area. Most published studies have used relatively small sample sizes, are of limited duration, and involve possibly nonrepresentative clinical groups (e.g., those without co-occurring psychiatric disorders). In addition, response measures have varied across studies, in part because the definition of *response* in many of these disorders remains debated. Heterogeneity of treatment samples may also complicate identification of effective treatments. At present, issues such as the duration of CBT cannot be sufficiently addressed with the available data. Identification of factors related to treatment response will help inform future studies and advance treatment strategies for these disorders.

REFERENCES

American Psychiatric Association. (2000). *Diagnostic and statistical manual of mental disorders* (4th ed., text rev.). Washington, DC: Author.

Arnold, L. M., Auchenbach, M. B., & McElroy, S. L. (2001). Psychogenic excoriation: Clinical features, proposed diagnostic criteria, epidemiology and approaches to treatment. *CNS Drugs, 15*, 351–359.

Azrin, N. H., Nunn, R. G., & Frantz, S. E. (1980). Treatment of hairpulling (trichotillomania): A comparative study of habit reversal and negative practice training. *Journal of Behavior Therapy and Experimental Psychiatry, 11*, 13–20.

Baron, E., & Dickerson, M. (1999). Alcohol consumption and self-control of gambling behavior. *Journal of Gambling Studies, 15*, 3–15.

Black, D. W., Kehrberg, L. L., Flumerfelt, D. L., & Schlosser, S. S. (1997). Characteristics of 36 participants reporting compulsive sexual behavior. *The American Journal of Psychiatry, 154*, 243–249.

Bloch, M. H., Landeros-Weisenberger, A., Dombrowski, P., Kelmendi, B., Wegner, R., Nudel, J., et al. (2007). Systematic review: Pharmacological and behavioral treatment for trichotillomania. *Biological Psychiatry, 62*, 839–846.

Christenson, G. A., Pyle, R. L., & Mitchell, J. E. (1991). Estimated prevalence of trichotillomania in college students. *Journal of Clinical Psychiatry, 52*, 415–417.

Coccaro, E. F., Schmidt, C. A., Samuels, J. F., & Nestadt, G. (2004). Lifetime and 1-month prevalence rates of intermittent explosive disorder in a community sample. *Journal of Clinical Psychiatry, 65*, 820–824.

Coleman, E. (1992). Is your patient suffering from compulsive sexual behavior? *Psychiatric Annals, 22*, 320–325.

Deckersbach, T., Wilhelm, S., Keuthen, N. J., Baer, L., & Jenike, M. A. (2002). Cognitive–behavior therapy for self-injurious skin picking. *Behavior Modification, 26*, 361–377.

Deffenbacher, J. L., Filetti, L. B., Lynch, R. S., Dahlen, E. R., & Oetting, E. R. (2002). Cognitive–behavioral treatment of high-anger drivers. *Behaviour Research and Therapy, 40*, 895–910.

Deffenbacher, J. L., Huff, M. E., Lynch, R. S., Oetting, E. R., & Salvatore, N. F. (2000). Characteristics and treatment of high-anger drivers. *Journal of Counseling Psychology, 47*, 5–17.

Dickerson, M., Hinchy, J., & England, S. L. (1990). Minimal treatments and problem gamblers: A preliminary investigation. *Journal of Gambling Studies, 6*, 87–102.

Diefenbach, G. J., Tolin, D. F., Hannan, S., Maltby, N., & Crocetto, J. (2006). Group treatment for trichotillomania: Behavior therapy versus supportive therapy. *Behavior Therapy, 37*, 353–363.

Diskin, K. M. (2006). *Effect of a single session motivational intervention on gambling.* Unpublished doctoral dissertation, University of Calgary, Calgary, Alberta, Canada.

Dougherty, D. D., Loh, R., Jenike, M. A., & Keuthen, N. J. (2006). Single modality versus dual modality treatment for trichotillomania: Sertraline, behavioral therapy, or both? *Journal of Clinical Psychiatry, 67*, 1086–1092.

Echeburúa, E., Baez, C., & Fernández-Montalvo, J. (1996). Comparative effectiveness of three therapeutic modalities in psychological treatment of pathological gambling: Long term outcome. *Behavioural and Cognitive Psychotherapy, 24,* 51–72.

Echeburúa, E., Fernández-Montalvo, J., & Baez, C. (2001). Predictors of therapeutic failure in slot-machine pathological gamblers following behavioural treatment. *Behavioural and Cognitive Psychotherapy, 29,* 379–383.

Galovski, T. E., & Blanchard, E. B. (2002). The effectiveness of a brief psychological intervention on court-referred and self-referred aggressive drivers. *Behaviour Research and Therapy, 40,* 1385–1402.

Gauthier, J., & Pellerin, D. (1982). Management of compulsive shoplifting through covert sensitization. *Journal of Behavior Therapy and Experimental Psychiatry, 13,* 73–75.

Glover, J. H. (1985). A case of kleptomania treated by covert sensitization. *British Journal of Clinical Psychology, 24,* 213–214.

Grant, J. E., & Kim, S. W. (2001). Demographic and clinical features of 131 adult pathological gamblers. *Journal of Clinical Psychiatry, 62,* 957–962.

Grant, J. E., & Kim, S. W. (2002). Clinical characteristics and associated psychopathology of 22 patients with kleptomania. *Comprehensive Psychiatry, 43,* 378–384.

Grant, J. E., Levine, L., Kim, D., & Potenza, M. N. (2005). Impulse control disorders in adult psychiatric inpatients. *The American Journal of Psychiatry, 162,* 2184–2188.

Grant, J. E., & Potenza, M. N. (2007). Treatments for pathological gambling and other impulse control disorders. In P. E. Nathan & J. M. Gorman (Eds.), *A guide to treatments that work* (3rd ed., pp. 561–577). New York: Oxford University Press.

Grant, J. E., Williams, K. A., & Potenza, M. N. (2007). Impulse control disorders in adolescent psychiatric inpatients: Co-occurring disorders and sex differences. *Journal of Clinical Psychiatry, 68,* 1584–1592.

Gudjonsson, G. H. (1987). The significance of depression in the mechanism of "compulsive" shoplifting. *Medicine, Science and the Law, 27,* 171–176.

Guidry, L. S. (1969). Use of a covert punishing contingency in compulsive stealing. *Journal of Behavior Therapy and Experimental Psychiatry, 6,* 169.

Gupta, M. A., Gupta, A. K., & Haberman, H. F. (1987). The self-inflicted dermatoses: A critical review. *General Hospital Psychiatry, 9,* 45–52.

Hodgins, D. C., Currie, S., & el-Guebaly, N. (2001). Motivational enhancement and self-help treatments for problem gambling. *Journal of Counseling and Clinical Psychology, 69,* 50–57.

Hodgins, D. C., Currie, S., el-Guebaly, N., & Diskin, K. M. (2007). Does providing extended relapse prevention bibliotherapy to problem gamblers improve outcome? *Journal of Gambling Studies, 23,* 41–54.

Hodgins, D. C., Currie, S., el-Guebaly, N., & Peden, N. (2004). Brief motivational treatment for problem gambling: A 24-month follow-up. *Psychology of Addictive Behaviors, 18,* 293–296.

Hodgins, D. C., & Holub, A. (2007). Treatment of problem gambling. In G. Smith, D. C. Hodgins, & R. J. Williams (Eds.), *Research and measurement issues in gambling studies* (pp. 371–397). Burlington, MA: Elsevier.

Hodgins, D. C., Mansley, C., & Thygesen, K. (2006). Risk factors for suicide ideation and attempts among pathological gamblers. *American Journal of Addiction, 15*, 303–310.

Hodgins, D. C., & Peden, N. (2008). Cognitive–behavioral treatment for impulse control disorders. *Revista Brasileira de Psiquiatria, 30*(Suppl. 1), S31–S40.

Hollander, E. (1993). Obsessive–compulsive spectrum disorders: An overview. *Psychiatric Annals, 23*, 355–358.

Keijsers, G. P., van Minnen, A., Hoogduin, C. A., Klaassen, B. N., Hendriks, M. J., & Tanis-Jacobs, J. (2006). Behavioural treatment of trichotillomania: Two-year follow-up results. *Behaviour Research and Therapy, 44*, 359–370.

Keuthen, N. J., Deckersbach, T., Wilhelm, S., Hale, E., Fraim, C., Baer, L., et al. (2000). Repetitive skin-picking in a student population and comparison with a sample of self-injurious skin-pickers. *Psychosomatics, 41*, 210–215.

Keutzer, C. S. (1972). Kleptomania: A direct approach to treatment. *British Journal of Medical Psychology, 45*, 159–163.

Kim, S. W., & Grant, J. E. (2001). Personality dimensions in pathological gambling disorder and obsessive–compulsive disorder. *Psychiatry Research, 104*, 205–212.

Koran, L. M., Faber, R. J., Aboujaoude, E., Large, M. D., & Serpe, R. T. (2006). Estimated prevalence of compulsive buying behavior in the United States. *The American Journal of Psychiatry, 163*, 1806–1812.

Ladouceur, R., Sylvain, C., Boutin, C., Lachance, S., Doucet, C., & Leblond, J. (2003). Group therapy for pathological gamblers: A cognitive approach. *Behaviour Research and Therapy, 41*, 587–596.

Ladouceur, R., Sylvain, C., Boutin, C., Lachance, S., Doucet, C., Leblond, J., et al. (2001). Cognitive treatment of pathological gambling. *The Journal of Nervous and Mental Disease, 189*, 774–780.

Lesieur, H. R., & Rosenthal, R. J. (1991). Pathological gambling: A review of the literature. *Journal of Gambling Studies, 7*, 5–39.

McConaghy, N., Armstrong, M. S., Blaszczynski, A., & Allcock, C. (1983). Controlled comparison of aversive therapy and imaginal desensitization in compulsive gambling. *The British Journal of Psychiatry, 142*, 366–372.

McConaghy, N., Armstrong, M. S., Blaszczynski, A., & Allcock, C. (1988). Behavior completion versus stimulus control in compulsive gambling: Implications for behavioral assessment. *Behavior Modification, 12*, 371–384.

McConaghy, N., & Blaszczynski, A. (1988). Imaginal desensitization: A cost-effective treatment in two shop-lifters and a binge-eater resistant to previous therapy. *Australian and New Zealand Journal of Psychiatry, 22*, 78–82.

McConaghy, N., Blaszczynski, A., & Frankova, A. (1991). Comparison of imaginal desensitisation with other behavioural treatments of pathological gambling: A two- to nine-year follow-up. *The British Journal of Psychiatry, 159*, 390–393.

McCormick, R. A., & Taber, J. I. (1988). Attributional style in pathological gamblers in treatment. *Journal of Abnormal Psychology, 97,* 368–370.

McElroy, S. L., Keck, P. E., Pope, H. G., Jr., Smith, J. M., & Strakowski, S. M. (1994). Compulsive buying: A report of 20 cases. *Journal of Clinical Psychiatry, 55,* 242–248.

McElroy, S. L., Pope, H. G., Hudson, J. I., Keck, P. E., Jr., & White, K. L. (1991). Kleptomania: A report of 20 cases. *The American Journal of Psychiatry, 148,* 652–657.

McElroy, S. L., Soutullo, C. A., Beckman, D. A., Taylor, P., Jr., & Keck, P. E., Jr. (1998). *DSM–IV* intermittent explosive disorder: A report of 27 cases. *Journal of Clinical Psychiatry, 59,* 203–210.

McNeilly, D. P., & Burke, W. J. (1998). Stealing lately: A case of late-onset kleptomania. *International Journal of Geriatric Psychiatry, 13,* 116–121.

Melville, C. L., Davis, C. S., Matzenbacher, D. L., & Clayborne, J. (2004). Node-link-mapping-enhanced group treatment for pathological gambling. *Addictive Behaviors, 29,* 73–87.

Milton, S., Crino, R., Hunt, C., & Prosser, E. (2002). The effect of compliance-improving interventions on the cognitive–behavioural treatment of pathological gambling. *Journal of Gambling Studies, 18,* 207–229.

Mitchell, J. E., Burgard, M., Faber, R., Crosby, R. D., & de Zwaan, M. (2006). Cognitive behavioral therapy for compulsive buying disorder. *Behaviour Research and Therapy, 44,* 1859–1865.

National Opinion Research Center. (1999). *Gambling impact and behavior study: Report to the National Gambling Impact Study Commission.* Retrieved October 1, 2007, from http://www.norc.uchicago.edu/new/gamb-fin.htm

Ninan, P. T., Rothbaum, B. O., Marsteller, F. A., Knight, B. T., & Eccard, M. B. (2000). A placebo-controlled trial of cognitive–behavioral therapy and clomipramine in trichotillomania. *Journal of Clinical Psychiatry, 61,* 47–50.

Odlaug, B. L., & Grant, J. E. (2007). Clinical characteristics and medical complications of pathologic skin picking. *General Hospital Psychiatry, 30,* 61–66.

Petry, N. M., Ammerman, Y., Bohl, J., Doersch, A., Gay, H., Kadden, R., et al. (2006). Cognitive–behavioral therapy for pathological gamblers. *Journal of Consulting and Clinical Psychology, 74,* 555–567.

Petry, N. M., & Kiluk, B. D. (2002). Suicidal ideation and suicide attempts in treatment-seeking pathological gamblers. *The Journal of Nervous and Mental Disease, 190,* 462–469.

Potenza, M. N., Steinberg, M. A., McLaughlin, S. D., Rounsaville, B. J., & O'Malley, S. S. (2000). Illegal behaviors in problem gambling: An analysis of data from a gambling helpline. *Journal of the American Academy of Psychiatry and the Law, 28,* 389–403.

Presta, S., Marazziti, D., Dell'Osso, L., Pfanner, C., Pallanti, S., & Cassano, G. B. (2002). Kleptomania: Clinical features and comorbidity in an Italian sample. *Comprehensive Psychiatry, 43,* 7–12.

Quadland, M. C. (1995). Compulsive sexual behavior: Definition of a problem and an approach to treatment. *Journal of Sex & Marital Therapy, 11,* 121–132.

Ramirez, L. F., McCormick, R. A., Russo, A. M., & Taber, J. I. (1983). Patterns of substance abuse in pathological gamblers undergoing treatment. *Addictive Behaviors, 8,* 425–428.

Smart, R. G., & Ferris, J. (1996). Alcohol, drugs and gambling in the Ontario adult population. *Canadian Journal of Psychiatry, 41,* 36–45.

Steele, C. M., & Josephs, R. A. (1988). Drinking your troubles away: II. An attention-allocation model of alcohol's effects on psychological stress. *Journal of Abnormal Psychology, 97,* 196–205.

Steketee, G., Chambless, D., & Tran, G. Q. (1999). Effects of Axis I and II comorbidity on behavior therapy outcome for obsessive–compulsive disorder and agoraphobia. *Comprehensive Psychiatry, 42,* 76–86.

Sylvain, C., Ladouceur, R., & Boisvert, J.-M. (1997). Cognitive and behavioral treatment of pathological gambling: A controlled study. *Journal of Consulting and Clinical Psychology, 65,* 727–732.

Teng, E. J., Woods, D. W., & Twohig, M. P. (2006). Habit reversal as a treatment for chronic skin picking: A pilot investigation. *Behavior Modification, 30,* 411–422.

Toneatto, T., & Ladouceur, R. (2003). Treatment of pathological gambling: A critical review of the literature. *Psychology of Addictive Behaviors, 42,* 92–99.

van Minnen, A., Hoogduin, K. A., Keijsers, G. P., Hellenbrand, I., & Hendriks, G. J. (2003). Treatment of trichotillomania with behavioral therapy or fluoxetine: A randomized, waiting-list controlled study. *Archives of General Psychiatry, 60,* 517–522.

Woods, D. W., Flessner, C. A., Franklin, M. E., Keuthen, N. J., Goodwin, R. D., Stein, D. J., et al. (2006). The Trichotillomania Impact Project (TIP): Exploring phenomenology, functional impairment, and treatment utilization. *Journal of Clinical Psychiatry, 67,* 1877–1888.

Woods, D. W., Wetterneck, C. T., & Flessner, C. A. (2005). A controlled evaluation of acceptance and commitment therapy plus habit reversal for trichotillomania. *Behaviour Research and Therapy, 44,* 639–656.

Wulfert, E., Blanchard, E. B., & Freidenberg, B. M. (2006). Retaining pathological gamblers in cognitive behavior therapy through motivational enhancement. *Behavior Modification, 30,* 315–340.

12

SEXUAL PROBLEMS

PETER J. DE JONG, JACQUES VAN LANKVELD,
AND HERMIEN J. ELGERSMA

This chapter begins with a discussion about the problems associated with classifying and defining sexual dysfunctions and illustrates that the present classification is not a very helpful starting point for making (differential) diagnoses and selecting proper treatment options. We therefore argue that it is important to reconsider the current conceptualization of the sexual dysfunctions and to focus on underlying mechanisms and transdiagnostic processes rather than on symptoms when considering the various treatment options. To elucidate factors that may lead to refractoriness of sexual problems, we focus on vaginistic complaints because refractory cases seem the rule rather than the exception in the context of vaginismus. In this main section we first illustrate that apparently refractory cases may often be the result of a suboptimal match of the problem conceptualization and the design of the intervention technique. Subsequently, we argue (and illustrate) on the basis of an initially refractory case that considering the role of disgust may be another important lead to improve currently available treatment options.

SEXUAL DYSFUNCTIONS:
PROBLEMS WITH CURRENT CLASSIFICATION

Sexual dysfunctions are defined as persistent or recurrent sexual problems that interfere with normal performance and cause distress for the individual and his or her partner (e.g., McAnulty & Burnette, 2004). There are no data available from large-scale epidemiological studies such as the Epidemiological Catchment Area study (Simons & Carey, 2001), so there is no reliable information regarding the actual prevalence of sexual disorders in the general population. Meanwhile, survey studies have indicated that sexual problems are very common. For example, results of the National Health and Social Life Survey (using face-to-face interviews; Laumann, Paik, & Rosen, 1999) showed that 31% of men and 43% of women indicated having a sexual dysfunction over the previous 12 months (see also Rosen & Landmann, 2003).

As we argue in this section, there are considerable problems associated with the present *Diagnostic and Statistical Manual of Mental Disorders* (*DSM–IV–TR*; 4th ed., text rev.; American Psychiatric Association, 2000) classification of disorders of desire, arousal, orgasm, and pain. These problems associated with classifying and defining sexual dysfunctions do not render the present classification as a very solid starting point for making (differential) diagnoses or for selecting proper treatment options. In the remainder of this section, we therefore first critically discuss the current conceptualization of the sexual dysfunctions and focus on the importance of taking the underlying mechanisms rather than symptoms as the starting point when diagnosing individuals' sexual problems and considering the various treatment options.

The current categories of sexual dysfunctions as described in the *DSM–IV–TR* closely follow Kaplan's (1974) three stage model of the sexual response cycle consisting of desire, excitement, and orgasm. Accordingly, dysfunctions are defined on the basis of problems involving desire (i.e., hypoactive sexual desire disorder, sexual aversive disorder), excitement (i.e., female sexual arousal disorder, male erectile disorder), and orgasm (i.e., female orgasmic disorder, male orgasmic disorder; premature ejaculation). As an additional category, the *DSM–IV–TR* refers to sexual pain disorders including dyspareunia and vaginismus.

There is, however, increasing consensus that this classification is unsatisfactory (e.g., Basson et al., 2003; Meston & Bradford, 2007), and doubts may be raised whether the present differentiation is adequate as a basis for understanding the mechanisms involved in the sexual problems as well as for selecting the best available treatment options. Perhaps most important, the underlying model assumes a linear pattern of sequential stages, starting with desire leading to increased arousal culminating in orgasm. Yet, one may question whether that is an accurate conceptualization of the sexual response cycle. For example, it is conceivable that under particular conditions (e.g., in the context of direct genital stimulation by the partner), elicited arousal precedes rather than follows a state of desire. Accordingly, complaints related to lack of desire may in fact reflect arousal problems or problems related to inaccurate/ineffective sexual stimulation. In addition, as a more general drawback of a classification on the basis of particular symptoms, similar symptoms may be the result of different underlying mechanisms, whereas similar mechanisms may result in different symptoms.

To illustrate this point, the *DSM–IV–TR* classifies dyspareunia as one of the sexual pain disorders, and it is broadly defined as genital pain associated with sexual activity that causes distress or interpersonal difficulty. However, it is doubtful whether these symptoms call for a separate category of dysfunctions. For example, it is conceivable that, in fact, low arousal rather than pain is at the heart of the problem. That is, genital pain may have been caused by attempts of penetration in the absence of sufficient arousal (e.g., due to heightened friction because of lack of lubrication). These painful experiences in turn may have resulted in fearful preoccupations with sexual activities. Obviously, such fear of sexual pain will logically oppose the generation of sexual arousal and responsive desire in contexts that may give rise to sexual intercourse. Accordingly, these women may enter a vicious circle in which low arousal reciprocally reinforces the generation of genital pain. In such cases, focusing on pain via pain management or on fear of pain via exposure may not be very helpful to the extent that the problems are actually due to low arousal.

The high comorbidity between sexual pain disorders and hyposexual desire disorder (HSDD) in clinical practice adds further to the suspicion that low sexual arousal disorder (LSAD) may be involved in the etiology of genital pain problems. It is interesting that there is not only a close connection between sexual pain disorders and low sexual arousal but also a high comorbidity between low sexual arousal and HSDD. Building on this, it is tempting to conclude that most of the sexual dysfunctions may essentially reflect disruptions in sexual arousal.

The problems related to the classification of dysfunctions are complicated further by the criteria that are described in the *DSM* to define the various sexual dysfunctions. For example, the *DSM–IV–TR* lists dyspareunia as distinct from lack of lubrication. However, it is virtually impossible to assess reliably whether indeed this is the case. First, under controlled lab conditions, the subjective degree of lubrication has been shown to be largely dissociated from the actual degree of lubrication, which renders self-reports a questionable source of information in this respect (e.g., Laan & Everaerd, 1995; Laan, van Driel, & van Lunsen, 2003). Second, the cause of genital pain (e.g., low arousal and lack of lubrication) may not be implicated in the maintenance of the symptoms.

As another example, the key criterion for the diagnosis of vaginismus is a recurrent or persistent involuntary spasm of the musculature of the outer third of the vagina that interferes with intercourse (American Psychiatric Association, 2000). This criterion is of limited use in clinical practice because it is obviously very difficult to reliably assess this feature in the consulting room. Even more important, recent research casts doubts whether such spasms occur at all in women suffering from vaginistic complaints (Reissing,

Yitzchak, Khalifé, Cohen, & Amsel, 2004). On the basis of this type of problem, a recent international consensus committee proposed the following revised criteria for vaginismus: "Persistent difficulties to allow vaginal entry of a penis, a finger, and/or object, despite the women's expressed wish to do so," and "there is a variable involuntary pelvic muscle contraction, (phobic) avoidance and anticipation/fear/experience of pain. Structural or other physical abnormalities must be ruled out/addressed" (Basson et al., 2003, p. 226). Yet, although these modified criteria may more accurately reflect the actual symptoms and may be helpful for improving the reliability of the diagnosis, one may still wonder why vaginismus should be classified as a sexual pain disorder given that pain is not a defining feature and again whether these symptoms require a separate diagnostic entity. To the extent that pain is critically involved, it is unclear how (and why) one should differentiate between vaginismus and dyspareunia. In such cases, vaginistic complaints may be best conceptualized as a chronic pain disorder (cf. Vlaeyen & Linton, 2000), perhaps with low sexual arousal as the underlying problem. When fear and phobic avoidance rather than pain are critically involved, the vaginistic complaints can perhaps best treated as a specific phobia of penetration rather than as a separate type of sexual pain disorder (e.g., Crespo & Fernández-Velasco, 2004; ter Kuile, 2007). Accordingly, this may be considered as an example of how two different nosological entities may share the same key symptom (i.e., difficulty of penetration).

All in all, the problems associated with classifying and defining sexual dysfunctions indicate that the present classification is not a very helpful starting point for making (differential) diagnoses and selecting proper treatment options. So it seems important to reconsider the current conceptualization of the sexual dysfunctions and to focus on underlying mechanism and transdiagnostic processes rather than on symptoms when considering the various treatment options.

Low (or disrupted) sexual arousal is an important candidate for being a common factor underlying many of the dysfunctions described in the *DSM–IV–TR*, such as hypoactive sexual desire disorder, sexual arousal disorder, and sexual pain disorders. Theory-grounded conceptualizations of how low arousal may be involved in these particular sexual problems may not only shed light on the particular etiological mechanisms but may also provide a helpful starting point for selecting interventions. Clearly, various different factors may eventually result in disruptions of sexual arousal.

First of all, people may simply be unaware of how to become aroused; they may lack relevant communicative skills and/or have insufficient knowledge about their own and/or their partner's anatomy. Accordingly, sexual education, directed masturbation, and learning communication skills are often implied as important components of current cognitive–behavioral therapy (CBT). Second, people may lack the motivation for attempting to become sexually aroused. One prominent reason for being unwilling or uninterested in becoming aroused may be the lack of reinforcing sexual experiences. If so, then sexual education and sexual (sensate focus) exercises still appear indicated. However, lack of interest may also follow from a completely different source, such as dysfunctional beliefs of the type "it is wrong if a woman enjoys sex" (cf. Nobre & Pinto-Gouveia, 2006). Obviously, this would also require a completely different approach, with the focus on challenging beliefs that undermine sexual desire. Third, anxiety and fearful preoccupations may disrupt the generation of sexual arousal. The consequences of fear in terms of phenomenological symptoms may vary considerably and logically depend on the actual focus of people's fear. For example performance anxiety in men may direct attention away from sexual cues and may elicit concerns related to attaining and maintaining an erection, which both logically interfere with the generation of sexual arousal (e.g., Janssen & Everaerd, 1993). Performance anxiety may also lower sexual arousal via enhancing self-focused attention (i.e., seeing oneself through the eyes of the other), which in turn may elicit self-evaluative concerns related to sexual (un)attractiveness (cf. van Lankveld & van den Hout, 2004).

Fearful preoccupations may also focus on catastrophic consequences associated with penetration (e.g., "It will not fit," "It will elicit unbearable pain"; e.g., ter Kuile et al., 2007). Apart from undermining the generation of sexual arousal, these types of concerns may also elicit defensive contractions of the pelvic floor muscles that are characteristic of vaginistic complaints. In addition, attempted intercourse under these conditions may give rise to genital pain. Repeated attempts may even cause chronic vulvar irritation and infections and eventually lead to avoidance of sex or even sexual aversion.

Current psychological theories and empirical research related to sexual dysfunctions focus predominantly on emotional and cognitive processes linked to fear and pain (e.g., Payne, Binik, Amsel, & Khalifé, 2005). Therefore, current cognitive–behavioral interventions often include some form of fear reduction exercises (e.g., exposure and/or cognitive restructuring) and pain management techniques (e.g., van Lankveld et al., 2006). Recent research has suggested that disgust may also be involved in sexual dysfunctions. Clearly, disgust seems an obvious candidate when it comes to undermining sexual arousal/desire (e.g., de Jong & Peters, 2008).

Disgust is seen as a defensive mechanism that has evolved to protect the organism from contamination by pathogens present in the environment (Curtis, Aunger, & Rabie, 2004). Accordingly, disgust is focused on the intersection between the body and the environment and concentrates on the skin and body apertures (Rozin, Nemeroff, Horowitz, Gordon, & Voet, 1995). The mouth and vagina/penis are the body parts with the highest subjective disgust sensitivity. Given the central role of these organs in the context of sexual behavior, together with the fact that bodily products (e.g., saliva, sweat, semen) and odors are among the strongest disgust elicitors (Rozin & Fallon, 1987), it is not very difficult to envisage that feelings of disgust and disgust-related appraisals may arise during sex, which in turn may disrupt the development of sexual arousal.

It is also conceivable that disgust elicits defensive reflexes that may interfere with sexual behaviors. From its function to protect the organism from contamination, disgust may give rise to reflexes that are associated with the expulsion of potentially hazardous pathogens from the body. Accordingly, disgust may elicit retching during oral sex or French kissing. In addition, disgust may give rise to defensive contractions of the pelvic floor muscles. Increased activity of these muscles will enhance the friction between penis and vulvar or anal skin, eventually giving rise to genital pain during intercourse, or adding to the impossibility of having intercourse (or anal sex) altogether. These types of aversive experiences may not only disrupt sexual arousal but also seriously detract from sexual satisfaction. In its turn lack of sexual satisfaction may undermine sexual desire and/or lead to active avoidance of sexual activities. It may also give rise to fearful preoccupations concerning the interpersonal consequences of retching during sexual activities or of the impossibility of having intercourse (i.e., beliefs such as "If penetration is impossible, I will lose my sexual attractiveness"), which in turn may undermine the generation of sexual arousal.

EFFECTIVE TREATMENT

As outlined in the previous section, it is questionable whether the currently defined sexual dysfunctions reflect meaningful diagnostic entities. The current classification does not provide a straightforward starting point for understanding the underlying mechanisms of people's sexual complaints or for making a selection among the available treatment options. Moreover, in sheer contrast with the enormous number of books on sex therapy and successful case reports, randomized controlled trials (RCTs) in the domain of sexual dysfunctions are extremely scarce. Obviously, this further hampers a proper scientific judgment of the efficacy of current treatment strategies and obstructs rational guidance of selecting treatment options. Yet, in the previous section we also showed that there are convincing similarities between sexual problems and other disorders such as anxiety disorders. As the treatment of anxiety disorders is firmly rooted in research, evidence-based interventions that have been developed in the context of the anxiety disorders may provide important leads for selecting (or designing) interventions in the area of sexual dysfunctions. Meanwhile, it is generally assumed that most sexual problems associated with disrupted sexual arousal can be successfully treated by a mixture or selection of sexual education, sensate focus exercises, directed masturbation, and challenging dysfunctional beliefs (for a short overview of current psychological interventions, see Heiman, 2002).

FACTORS THAT MAY LEAD TO POOR TREATMENT RESPONSE

Although CBT techniques integrating elements of more traditional sex therapies based on the work of Masters and Johnson (1970) are widely used and generally considered very effective, it should be acknowledged that the supportive evidence is carried mainly by clinical impression and clinical case reports. This is an important restriction because the few RCTs that are available in the literature shed a completely different light on the effectiveness of currently available treatment options (e.g., van Lankveld et al., 2006). Lack of theory-grounded and rigorously tested conceptualizations of the symptoms together with suboptimal selection and/or implementation of intervention techniques may play an important role here. The selection of the intervention procedure, the implementation of the intervention, as well as the rationale that is provided to the patient are all components that directly follow from the conceptualization of the complaints, and all may heavily impact on treatment success.

For example, in routine clinical practice (at least in the Netherlands), vaginismus is often approached as an essentially somatic problem. A commonly used intervention technique involves inserting a pelotte of increasing size. This gradual dilation procedure can be theoretically framed as an attempt to habituate the reflective contraction of the circumvaginal musculature in response to attempts of penetration. However, such an approach does not match with the notion that vaginismus may reflect fear of pain or fear of penetration. For example, the logical approach when conceptualizing vaginismus as fear of penetration would be to design an intervention that not so much aims at habituation but at extinction (or refutation) of a dysfunctional predictive relationship between a conditioned and an unconditioned stimulus (e.g., see Hofmann, 2008). As extinction of fear is known to be highly cue- and context specific, it may not come as a surprise that pelotte therapy is not very effective in reducing vaginistic complaints.

Another factor that may help explain refractory cases is considering the role of disgust. Thus far, disgust has been largely overlooked as a potentially relevant factor in sexual problems. Disgust may nevertheless be a critical factor in the etiology and maintenance of the various sexual dysfunctions. For example, current feelings of disgust and disgust-related appraisals will logically oppose the generation of sexual arousal and may thus contribute to problems associated with reduced sexual arousal (e.g., erection problems) as well as to male/female orgasmic disorder. Focusing exclusively on fearful preoccupations (e.g., performance anxiety) or sexual skills may not succeed in solving problems connected to low sexual arousal if disgust-related concerns are critically involved. In addition to current feelings, anticipated feelings of disgust will logically motivate sexual avoidance and withdrawal, whereas cognitive biases may further confirm the negative appreciation of sex. Accordingly, the unattended presence of disgust-related preoccupations may also interfere with traditional sex therapies in the context of hypoactive sexual desire disorder, sexual arousal disorders, or sexual aversive disorder.

It is important that disgust may be elicited not only by offensive stimuli but also by particular (sexual) behaviors. It has been argued that the defensive mechanism of disgust, which originally evolved to prevent the body from contamination by pathogens, is extended to behaviors that remind us of our animal nature (Rozin, Haidt, & McCauley, 1999). This disgust-mediated rejection of our animal nature is argued to serve a defensive function by maintaining the hierarchical division between humans and animals via distancing the self from animals and animal properties (Haidt, McCauley, & Rozin, 1994). Because sexual behaviors are highly suggestive of our underlying animal nature, they may well elicit disgust to guard the human–animal border and may thus give rise to avoidant strategies interfering with functional sexual behaviors. This type of disgust-relevant appraisals may, for example, be involved in orgasmic disorders, because orgasm involves a sudden loss of voluntary control. Disgust-induced reluctance of "letting go" may thus block sexual arousal. In instances in which these types of appraisals are involved, directed masturbation alone (e.g., Heiman, LoPiccolo, & Palladini, 1988) may not be successful in treating orgasmic disorder.

A third category of disgust that may be of relevance for understanding particular resistant cases is sociomoral disgust (Rozin et al., 1999). This type of disgust is argued to be linked to the protection and internalization of (sub)culture-based rules and is elicited by behaviors that apparently violate such rules (Rozin et al., 1999). For example, a woman who has grown up in a strict heterosexual peer group may react with disgust when finding out that her daughter is having sex with another woman, because her daughter's behavior violates the heterosexual standard of the mother's reference group. When people have acquired strict moral rules concerning sexual behaviors, these rules may have strong influence on their emotional responding toward particular sexual behaviors and may thus contribute to the generation and/or maintenance of sexual complaints (e.g., Koukounas & McCabe, 1997; Stark et al., 2005).

On the basis of research in the context of anxiety showing that people tend to infer danger from experienced anxiety (e.g., "If I feel anxious, there must be danger"; Arntz, Rauner, & van den Hout, 1995), one could speculate that elicited feelings of disgust may also further confirm the importance of adhering to certain sociomoral rules via a similar form of emotional reasoning along the lines of "If I feel disgusted, it must be an inappropriate behaviour" (cf. Rachman, 2004, p. 1252). Making these kinds of emotion-based inferences will logically further inhibit individuals' motivation to get involved in these particular disgust-eliciting sexual behaviors and/or motivate people to refrain from sex altogether. In support of the notion that the experience of disgust may indeed bolster already internalized sociomoral rules, there is evidence that experimentally augmenting feelings of disgust can increase the severity of moral judgments (Wheatley & Haidt, 2005). People might not always be aware of the relationship between the transgression of moral rules and the experience of disgust. However, when moral disgust is involved in generating sexual problems, neglecting these types of moral disgust relevant representations may obviously hamper treatment efficacy. Tailoring CBT to challenge individuals' restricted moral values may be required in these cases to eventually alleviate their sexual problems.

Because sexual problems may also occur as a by-product of other psychological or physiological dysfunctions, it is important to be aware of potential comorbid psychological disorders and medical conditions. For example, substance misuse or panic disorder may cause (or contribute to) erectile dysfunction. In a similar vein, depression or generalized anxiety disorder may result in lowered sexual desire and lowered sexual arousability (other examples of same symptoms, different mechanisms; for experimental evidence, see Kuffel & Heiman, 2006). In such cases, sexuality-focused treatments are obviously bound to be unsuccessful. Comorbid problems may also complicate the treatment of sexual problems if particular components are shared by both disorders such as (moral) disgust and/or contamination-related preoccupations in individuals also suffering from obsessive–compulsive problems.

People's physiological makeup is also a crucial element that may moderate treatment success but may also guide the selection of treatment options. For example, factors involved in sexual arousal and/or desire may differ between pre- and postmenopausal women (e.g., Rosen, Taylor, Leiblum, & Bachmann, 1993). In addition, hormonal disturbances (e.g., due to endocrine disorders such as diabetes) may have a profound influence on all components of the sexual response cycle. Finally, most people (patients as well as therapists) are unaware of the potentially profound impact that frequently prescribed drugs such as antihypertensives, anxiolytics, and antidepressants may have on sexual arousal, erectile function, and sexual desire (for an overview, see McAnulty & Burnette, 2004, p. 409). All in all, before selecting a particular treatment option, thorough assessment is required to get detailed insight into the sexual problems, potentially comorbid complaints, medication use, and medical history.

THE CASE OF VAGINISMUS AND GENITAL PAIN

To elucidate factors that may lead to refractoriness of sexual problems, we eventually decided to focus on vaginistic complaints. This was done for various reasons. Most important, there is clinical consensus that the majority of other sexual problems (e.g., erectile dysfunction, HSDD, LSAD, sexual aversion disorder) can be adequately addressed by traditional sex therapy together with cognitive techniques to challenge dysfunctional beliefs, although directed masturbation for preorgasmic disorder and CBT for erectile dysfunction are the only interventions in the area of sexual dysfunctions that meet the stringent criteria (of the American Psychological Association task force on the promotion and dissemination of psychological procedures; Meston & Bradford, 2007) of being a "well-established" treatment. Despite case studies reporting that CBT interventions can also be highly successful in vaginismus, the clinical impression is that, in general, vaginismus reflects a rather refractory sexual problem.

Consistent with this, a recent RCT showed that only a very small minority (18%) of patients who received a widely applied CBT for vaginismus eventually reported successful intercourse (van Lankveld et al., 2006). It would seem, therefore, that refractory cases seem the rule rather than the exception in the context of vaginismus, and the room for improvement of the current treatment seems quite dramatic. Such improvement may be expected from a more precise (and comprehensive) conceptualization of the presented symptoms as well as of factors that may act in a way to maintain or even enhance this sexual problem. In addition, reconsidering the current selection, framing, as well as implementation of intervention techniques may provide important leads to more optimally target the mechanisms of change.

The ingredients in common CBT for vaginismus that were also used in the RCT are quite heterogeneous and include sexual education, sensate focus exercises, relaxation exercises, gradual exposure to vaginal touching and penetration, and cognitive restructuring. As part of the sexual education, the therapist explains the biological and psychological mechanisms that are assumed to be involved in the origin and maintenance of vaginismus. Anatomical and functional aspects of the pelvic floor are illustrated with drawings of the vulva, relevant pelvic floor muscles, and bone structures involved. Next, instructions are given for progressive (Jacobson, 1938) and suggestive relaxation (Schultz & Luthe, 1959) exercises. The therapist encourages the woman to practice on a daily basis and to monitor progress using a diary. The therapist further asks the male partner to encourage his female partner to actually comply with this regimen. Exercises initially focus on general relaxation. After having mastered this technique, the woman continues with pelvic floor relaxation exercises. Following this, the therapist introduces gradual exposure under relaxation and provides detailed homework assignments following a stepwise procedure on the basis of a personalized hierarchy. The assignments include visual self-inspection of the vagina (by using a mirror) and touching the vagina (without penetration) by herself and by her partner; vaginal insertion of one finger, then two fingers, then one finger of the partner during which the woman guided the partner's hand, then two fingers; insertion of plastic dilator; touching entry with erect penis; and vaginal insertion of erect penis. In an attempt to gradually replace the anxiety response with a lust response, each step in the hierarchy is initially performed with an exclusive focus on relaxation that can be optionally followed by using a stronger focus on sexual arousal (along the lines of Masters and Johnson's, 1970, instruction for the sensate focus exercises). As a final component, the therapist teaches how to identify irrational beliefs (e.g., "My vaginal entry is just too tight") and how to convert these beliefs into more rational ones following a rational emotive therapy type procedure. The woman is encouraged to first attempt the use of these new beliefs while performing a relevant step of the hierarchy on an imagery level and to make flash cards to prompt rational beliefs. In the RCT, the treatment was delivered in group format (6–9 women) and comprised 10 sessions (2 hours each). Partners did not attend the group sessions.

Only a small minority of the women who were treated following this widely used, well-defined, and protocol-driven intervention reached their treatment goal (i.e., successful intercourse). Several factors might have been responsible for the apparent refractoriness of the women's symptoms. Perhaps most important, the present approach did (could) not control for response prevention. However, if anxiety reduction (i.e., extinction of the conditioned fear response upon attempts of penetration) is the relevant mechanism of change, response prevention is a critical component. The maintaining influence of avoidance and escape behaviors of the woman herself as well as of her partner should be thoroughly explained before the start of treatment. In addition, it seems important to take measures in order to prevent avoidance (or safety) behaviors from undermining the efficacy of the homework exposure assignments. It might therefore be necessary to initially carry out the exposure exercises in the presence of a therapist.

In addition, taking a fear of penetration perspective points to the importance of "functional" exposure and of behavioral experiments that are designed as an ultimate test of the (in)validity of the individual's critical catastrophical concern. This requires a careful construction of the exercise and thorough discussion concerning the exact outcome that would be accepted by the woman as falsification of the dysfunctional outcome expectancies. The present gradual exposure might be considered as a rather indirect, nonspecific, and therefore inefficient way to gather evidence to correct the woman's catastrophical views. Furthermore, cue and context specificity seem of critical importance for successful extinction. Yet, in the present setup no control was possible regarding the partner's commitment or the way in which the partner assisted during the exposure exercises. Another major issue concerns the impact of the relaxation exercises on the efficacy of the present intervention. Relaxation exercises and physiotherapy to train the pelvic floor musculature are currently common practices. However, first, it seems questionable whether relaxation skills that have been learned outside the relevant context can be successfully applied during sexual situations that may give rise to attempts of having intercourse. Second, and even more important, it might well be that applying relaxation during the exposure exercises undermines their efficacy as a fear-extinction procedure. Relaxation will logically interfere with the activation of the fear network, which is generally considered as a necessary prerequisite for incorporating corrective information.

It is interesting that during the last World Congress of Behavioral and Cognitive Therapies in Barcelona, Spain, Moniek ter Kuile (2007) presented results of a newly designed treatment for vaginismus that incorporated many of the elements discussed in this section. Most important, she explicitly framed the intervention as a fear-extinction procedure conceptually similar to exposure in vivo of specific phobias (e.g., de Jong, Vorage, & van den Hout, 2000; Öst, 1989). Accordingly, the women received a treatment rationale in which the focus was on exposing themselves to the phobic situations. In line with the alleged critical importance of response prevention, the initial exposure exercises were carried out in the clinic in the presence of the therapist, who coached the women in a way to prevent avoidance and escape behaviors. In addition, the partner was always present during the treatment sessions. This was important with respect to the cue and context specificity of the in-clinic exposure, but it also allowed the therapist to coach and instruct the partner concerning his role during the homework assignments. In the initial part of treatment, the role of the partner was mainly to help in confronting the phobic (penetration) situations. Gradually, the partner was expected to become more actively involved in the home exercises (e.g., vaginal insertion of one and two fingers, touching of the vaginal entry with the erect penis, vaginal insertion of the erect penis).

To add focus and limit the opportunity to avoid completing the homework assignments, the main part of this intervention was concentrated within 1 week. Depending on the degree of progress, a maximum of three treatment sessions were scheduled in that week with homework assignments following each session working through a personalized fear hierarchy. To create optimal conditions for completing homework assignments and maintaining commitment to the intervention, the couples were advised to take a week off from work. After the prolonged exposure sessions in the 1st week, three follow-up sessions were scheduled over a period of 6 weeks. This allowed the therapist to tackle possible factors that obstruct treatment efficacy such as more covert or subtle avoidance strategies and to modify/extend the homework assignments in a way to further enhance treatment success.

The straightforward conceptualization of the complaints in terms of fear avoidance, the increased focus on extinction as the mechanism of change, together with optimizing the design of the exercises (prolonged in vivo exposure in the relevant context gradually reaching cue specificity) as well as the implementation with emphasis on response prevention appeared highly effective in improving treatment efficacy. All five women who complied with this treatment procedure (one woman stopped treatment at Session 2 because she decided that she did not want to have intercourse with her partner) reported successful intercourse at posttreatment, compared with none of these women after the wait-list control period. Clearly this favorable outcome supports the notion that vaginistic complaints can be effectively conceptualized as a specific phobia. In addition, this apparently dramatic gain in treatment efficacy points to the importance of a rigorous theory-grounded conceptualization of the symptoms together with theory-driven design and implementation of the intervention technique. Perhaps treatment can be even more efficient if the exposure procedure is more explicitly framed and designed as a test of the validity of the central catastrophical belief (e.g., Craske & Mystkowski, 2006). In addition, recent work has suggested that distraction during exposure may further improve the efficacy of exposure as an extinction procedure. Distraction during exposure (e.g., some kind of backward counting task) may prevent the activation and initial strengthening of dysfunctional fear associations, whereas concurrent visual focus on the feared stimulus (e.g., via a mirror) provides the necessary input of corrective information that erodes the fear network (for a more extensive discussion of this option, see Johnstone & Page, 2004).

We have illustrated that a suboptimal match of problem conceptualization and design of intervention technique might give rise to apparently refractory cases. In the next section, we describe a case that was selected to illustrate that it might be helpful to consider the role of disgust as one of the factors that may be involved in the origin and maintenance of sexual problems involving low (or disrupted) arousal and genital pain.

CASE EXAMPLE

Sara was 22 years of age at the time of referral and had had a relationship with her boyfriend for 6 years. Since the previous year, they had been living together. She was a hairdresser and ran a salon in their house. Right from the start of their sexual relationship (5 years prior), she suffered from coital pain during intercourse. In the beginning of their relationship, there were unproblematic instances of successful intercourse. During that period, she was infected by vaginal mildew (Candida albicans). The infection was successfully treated by the practitioner, and pain and itching outside sexual situations disappeared. However, pain during intercourse remained. Prior to initiating treatment, Sara was examined by a gynecologist, who did not find a somatic cause for the genital pain. For the prior 6 months, Sara and her boyfriend stopped attempts at having intercourse. They anticipated that any attempt would be painful. In the past, they abruptly interrupted their sexual activities at the moment pain emerged, and under such circumstances they both felt very disappointed. They experienced great difficulties with discussing this issue and sometimes were quiet and avoided contact for several days before they again carefully approached each other and tried to make sexual contact. Attempts at having intercourse became increasingly infrequent, and other ways of having sex were not in their repertoire. They were very fond of each other and did not consider breaking up because of the pain complaints and the increasing absence of a sexual relationship.

Sara described their most recent attempt at having sex. Her boyfriend always took the initiative for physical contact. She was always a bit reluctant and often experienced some hesitance in interrupting her daily activities to fit sex into her routine. She usually reciprocated his advances, though, mainly because of pity for her boyfriend (e.g., "The previous time we had sex was already so long ago," "I am deficient and doing my partner short"). From the moment that it became clear that mere physical contact would lead to sex and they started to unclothe, she became increasingly anxious, and her fear of pain increased. She did not feel well and became very nervous, with stomach pain evident as well as intestinal unease, sometimes followed by an attack of diarrhea. She would usually carry on and accept attempts at penetration. At the first sign of pain, she would stop abruptly and start weeping.

Sara had been previously treated by a sex therapist, who proposed physiotherapy for training the pelvic floor muscles combined with sensate focus therapy according to treatment described by Masters and Johnson (1970). After 10 sessions of physiotherapy, she was still not able to apply relaxation, in general or with respect to her pelvic floor muscles. The physiotherapist subsequently advised her to explore potentially relevant psychological aspects that might be involved and, if indicated, to continue with physiotherapy afterward. On the basis of this advice, she started group therapy that followed a CBT program. She started with mirror exercises and was instructed to inspect and visually explore her vagina. During the intake, she admitted that she actually had never done such a thing before. During the next group session, she explained that she did not complete the exercise because she felt too afraid. She also avoided completing the first-stage sensate focus exercises, during which the sexual organs are not allowed to be touched, mainly by avoiding precise arrangements with her boyfriend. During the following weeks, they were too busy with other activities and obligations, or it came too late to their minds and at least one of them was too tired, so they did not engage in any efforts at sexual activity. Sara had difficulty listening to other participants who did carry out exercises and report on their progress. She indicated that she felt her problem would never be solved, and she could not imagine that her problem would subside. She cried during the group session and indicated that she considered terminating therapy. If attention was focused on Sara, she would dwell on minor matters and tell extensive associative stories that touched on various subjects without necessarily dealing with the sexual issues that had led to treatment.

The therapist asked her to provide a very detailed description of how she approached the mirror exercise to get more precise insight into the factors that lead to avoidance. In the context of an imagination exercise, she was asked to describe the situation, what she perceived, what she felt, and what kind of thoughts emerged. She eventually stated that she felt strongly inhibited in examining her sexual organ because it looked ugly and disgusting.

As a homework assignment, she was instructed to again do the mirror exercise and to carefully register what she actually considered disgusting and what kinds of thoughts or memories popped into her mind while doing the exercises. She was also instructed to carefully study a book containing photos of vaginas.

She stated that she could hardly look at her vagina. Here are some illustrative comments Sara offered in describing her genital area:

> "It is a tangle of pledges, slime, and secretions; it is ugly and can
>   not be kept clean."
> "It stinks, although I am too far off to actually smell it myself."
> "When I had this infection, it also smelled very badly."
> "Sperm of my partner stinks and is sticky; that is also disgusting.
> "If there is sperm on my body, I should not touch it."

When discussing these registrations in the group session, it appeared that the majority of women recognized these feeling of disgust but also had concurrent thoughts and feelings that were not aversive. During cognitive restructuring, Sara received suggestions for alternative thoughts from the other group members that had some appeal to her. She further said, "I realize now that I have explicitly outspoken my thoughts and feelings [so much] that they sound strange to me. It is strange that I have these kinds of thoughts; I think they are inaccurate."

During a thought-challenge procedure, she arrived at the following alternative thoughts:

> "My vagina did smell when I had this infection, yet the infection
>   is gone, and it now smells completely normal."
> "My vagina looks normal. The pledges are a normal part of my
>   organ that protects my vagina."
> "The presence of vaginal fluids is a normal response of the body to
>   keep the vagina clean."
> "Lubrication in response [to] sexual arousal is a healthy response
>   of my body to prevent painful penetration during intercourse."
> "Vaginal fluids and sperm are healthy body products."

She was instructed to rehearse the new thoughts and to again carry out the mirror exercises. She also planned to touch and penetrate her vagina with a finger, to smell the fluid on her finger, and to wait to wash her hands until the fluid had completely dried up. The next exercise involved touching sperm of her partner, to feel its composition by rubbing the sperm between two fingers, and again to wait to wash her hands until the sperm had dried completely.

During the next session, she reported some success in completing the exercises. She had successfully completed the mirror exercises and had several times smelled her own vaginal fluid and waited to wash her hands until the fluid was dried. In the next couple of weeks, she continued to complete the therapeutic exercises with her partner's sperm. Penetration exercises became increasingly more successful. Without experiencing pain, she was able to insert two fingers, either her own or those of her boyfriend. After 2 more weeks, she reported successful intercourse in the absence of pain.

According to the original conceptualization, genital pain was caused by two factors: inflated tension of the pelvic floor muscles and lack of lubrication due to insufficient arousal that were both reinforced by fear of pain. The modified conceptualization also implicated disgust and disgust-induced avoidance as a major factor in disrupting the generation of sexual arousal. This led to designing homework assignments targeting feelings of disgust and disgust-related preoccupations that eventually appeared successful in solving the refractory symptoms.

CONCLUSIONS AND FUTURE DIRECTIONS

There is increasing consensus that the present *DSM–IV–TR* classification into disorders of desire, arousal, orgasm, and pain is unsatisfactory. The present differentiation seems adequate neither as a lead for understanding the mechanisms involved in the sexual problems nor for selecting the best available treatment options. It seems, therefore, important to reconsider the current conceptualization of the sexual dysfunctions and to focus on underlying mechanism and transdiagnostic processes when considering the various treatment options (cf. Harvey, Watkins, Mansell, & Shafran, 2004). In addition, there is a clear need for well-controlled treatment outcome research to rigorously assess the viability of current treatment options. This type of research is important not only because it examines whether the current treatment of sexual problems deserves the qualification "well established," but also because it helps to improve the currently available treatment arsenal and to further limit the occurrence of refractory cases.

It is important not only to improve the efficacy of current treatment options but also to inform people that sexual problems are very common and to explain to them what the effective interventions are and where to find them. There seems to be a substantial discrepancy between the estimated prevalence of sexual problems and the number of individuals who actually seek treatment. So it appears that in many cases, effective treatment does not reach the target population, resulting in a lot of silent suffering. One reason why people may not apply for treatment might be that health care institutions are not sufficiently accessible for these types of complaints. In addition, people may be reluctant to share their sexual problems with other people including health care providers. Internet-based interventions may therefore prove a welcome addition when compared with the more traditional treatment options, because Internet-based interventions are easily accessible and allow for relatively anonymous contact with the therapists. Both characteristics may well lower the threshold for applying for help.

Finally, it might be profitable when designing more effective treatments to consider the role of disgust in sexual behavior. Current psychological views roughly consider sexual dysfunction as a consequence of a negative emotional reaction to erotic stimulation (e.g., Barlow, 1986; Janssen & Everaerd, 1993). Although disgust seems an obvious candidate for being one of these negative emotional reactions interfering with healthy sexual behavior and/or sexual pleasure, current theories and empirical research predominantly focus on emotional and cognitive processes related to fear and pain (e.g., Payne et al., 2005), whereas the reference to disgust is mainly anecdotal (e.g., Carnes, 1998; Kaneko, 2001). In a similar vein, current cognitive behavioral interventions often include some form of fear reduction exercises (exposure/cognitive restructuring) and pain management techniques, whereas interventions targeted at reducing or neutralizing disgust-related feelings, appraisals, and/or action tendencies are virtually absent in the literature.

Disgust may nevertheless be a critical factor in the generation and maintenance of sexual problems (e.g., see de Jong & Peters, 2008, for a review), and considering the role of disgust may provide fresh clues that may help improve the available interventions. For example, a disgust conceptualization of sexual dysfunctions would suggest that it might be worthwhile in CBT to add a focus on contamination-related preoccupations and to include exposure exercises aimed at reducing the contamination potency of sexual products (cf. de Jong et al., 2000). So-called conceptual reorientation is another mechanism that may act to reduce disgust responses (Rozin & Fallon, 1987). This notion refers to the phenomenon that the disgust response can disappear when, for example, a person discovers that what he or she thought was rotting milk is actually yogurt. Such a cognitive switch may also be of relevance in the context of sexual complaints. For example, a meaningful proportion of people with sexual complaints might never have had a close and detailed look at their own sex organs or at those of their sex partner. Homework assignments to get a more elaborated and accurate view of the sex organs and their responding to the various stages of the sexual response cycle may, for example, contribute to a reorientation of a penis from being an atrocious, uncontrollable, attacking, dirty monster toward the conception of the penis as a cute, caring body part that can share love and sexual pleasure with a loved sex partner; or from an ugly bunch of pubic hair to a mysterious camouflage of a "holy" secret place; or an ugly mesh of folds to a nicely designed protection of a beautiful though vulnerable organ, and so forth.

To the extent that moral disgust is involved, it might be helpful to use CBT-like techniques to facilitate changing a dysfunctional conception of sex as being dirty, sinful, and immoral acts into a more functional (and arousing) conception of sex. Finally, disgust responses can weaken via extinction or habituation; for example, when someone is consistently placed into close contact with the disgusting item, disgust will gradually subside (e.g., when cleaning toilets is part of your job, the aversion toward dirty toilets gradually declines). Yet individuals suffering from disgust-relevant sexual dysfunctions will usually avoid opportunities that would provide for the extinction or habituation of the disgust response. They are likely to use all kinds of strategies, such as distracting attention, withdrawing from particular behaviors, or avoiding sustained contact with particular sexual products. It might therefore be useful to arrange homework assignments to help clients force themselves to tolerate close and sustained/prolonged direct physical contact with disgusting stimuli. It may be most efficient to arrange these assignments in a gradual manner (disgust hierarchy) from stimuli/situations that are only mildly disgusting/aversive to stimuli/situations that are maximally disgusting. Future efforts to further develop and test interventions targeted at reducing disgust-related feelings and appraisals may lead to welcome theory-derived contributions to the available psychological intervention techniques.

REFERENCES

American Psychiatric Association. (2000). *Diagnostic and statistical manual of mental disorders* (4th ed., text rev.). Washington, DC: Author.

Arntz, A., Rauner, M., & van den Hout, M. A. (1995). "If I feel anxious, there must be danger": Ex-consequential reasoning in inferring danger in anxiety disorders. *Behaviour Research and Therapy, 33,* 917–925.

Barlow, D. H. (1986). The causes of sexual dysfunction: The role of anxiety and cognitive interference. *Journal of Consulting and Clinical Psychology, 54,* 140–148.

Basson, R. (2002). Are our definitions of women's desire, arousal and sexual pain disorders too broad and our definition of orgasmic disorder too narrow? *Journal of Sex & Marital Therapy, 28,* 289–300.

Basson, R., Leiblum, S., Brotto, L., Derogatis, L., Foucroy, J., Fugl-Meyer, K., et al. (2003). Definitions of women's sexual dysfunction reconsidered: Advocating expansion and revision. *Journal of Psychosomatic Obstetrics and Gynecology, 34,* 221–229.

Carnes, P. J. (1998). The case for sexual anorexia: An interim report on 144 patients with sexual disorders. *Sexual Addiction & Compulsivity, 5,* 293–309.

Craske, M. G., & Mystkowski, J. L. (2006). Exposure therapy and extinction: Clinical studies. In M. G. Craske, D. Hermans, & D. Vansteenwegen (Eds.), *Fear and learning: From basic processes to clinical implications* (pp. 217–233). Washington, DC: American Psychological Association.

Crespo, M. E. O. C., & Fernández-Velasco, R. (2004). Cognitive–behavioural treatment of a case of vaginism and phobic about pelvic examination. *Psychology in Spain, 8*, 106–121.

Curtis, V., Aunger, R., & Rabie, T. (2004). Quantative evidence that disgust evolved to protect from risk of disease. *Proceedings of the Royal Society: Biological Letters, 271*(Suppl. 4), S131–S133.

de Jong, P. J., & Peters, M. L. (2008). Sex and the sexual dysfunctions: The role of disgust and contamination sensitivity. In B. Olatunji & D. McKay (Eds.), *Disgust and its disorders: Theory, assessment, and treatment implications* (pp. 253–270). Washington, DC: American Psychological Association.

de Jong, P. J., Vorage, I., & van den Hout, M. A. (2000). Counterconditioning in the treatment of spider phobia: Effects on disgust, fear, and valence. *Behaviour Research and Therapy, 38*, 1055–1069.

Haidt, J., McCauley, C., & Rozin, P. (1994). Individual differences in sensitivity to disgust: A scale sampling seven domains of disgust elicitors. *Personality and Individual Differences, 16*, 701–713.

Harvey, A., Watkins, E., Mansell, W., & Shafran, R. (2004). *Cognitive behavioral processes across psychological disorders: A transdiagnositic approach to research and treatment.* Oxford, England: Oxford University Press.

Heiman, J. R. (2002). Psychological treatments for female sexual dysfunction: Are they effective and do we need them? *Archives of Sexual Behavior, 31*, 445–450.

Heiman, J. R., LoPiccolo, J., & Palladini, D. (1988). *Becoming orgasmic: A sexual and personal growth program for women.* Upper Sadle River, NJ: Prentice Hall.

Hoffmann, S. G. (2008). Cognitive processes during fear acquisition and extinction in animals and humans: Implications for exposure therapy of anxiety disorders. *Clinical Psychology Review, 28*, 199–210.

Jacobson, E. (1938). *Progressive relaxation.* Chicago: University of Chicago Press.

Janssen, E., & Everaerd, W. (1993). Determinants of male sexual arousal. *Annual Review of Sex Research, 4*, 211–245.

Johnstone, K. A., & Page, A. C. (2004). Attention to phobic stimuli during exposure: The effect of distraction on anxiety reduction, self-efficacy and perceived control. *Behaviour Research and Therapy, 42*, 585–600.

Kaneko, K. (2001). Penetration disorder: Dyspareunia exists on the extension of vaginismus. *Journal of Sex & Marital Therapy, 27*, 153–155.

Kaplan, H. S. (1974). *The new sex therapy: Active treatment of sexual dysfunctions.* New York: Brunner/Mazel.

Koukounas, E., & McCabe, M. (1997). Sexual and emotional variables influencing sexual response to erotica. *Behaviour Research and Therapy, 35*, 221–231.

Kuffel, S. W., & Heiman, J. R. (2006). Effects of depressive symptoms and experimentally adopted schemas on sexual arousal and affect in sexually healthy women. *Archives of Sexual Behaviour, 35*, 163–177.

Laan, E., & Everaerd, W. (1995). Determinants of female sexual arousal: Psychophysiological theory and data. *Annual Review of Sex Research, 6*, 32–76.

Laan, E., van Driel, E., & van Lunsen, R. H. W. (2003). Seksuele reakties van vrouwenmet een seksuele opwindingsstoornis op visuele seksuele stimuli [Sexual responses in response to visual stimuli in women suffering from sexual arousal disorder]. *Tijdschrift voor Seksuologie, 27,* 1–13.

Laumann, E. O., Paik, A., & Rosen, R. C. (1999). Sexual dysfunction in the United States: Prevalence and predictors. *JAMA, 281,* 537–544.

Masters, W. H., & Johnson, V. E. (1970). *Human sexual inadequacy.* Boston: Little, Brown.

McAnulty, R. D., & Burnette, M. M. (2004). *Exploring human sexuality, making healthy decisions.* Boston: Pearson.

Meston, C. M., & Bradford, A. (2007). Sexual dysfunctions in women. *Annual Review of Clinical Psychology, 3,* 233–256.

Nobre, P. J., & Pinto-Gouveia, J. (2006). Dysfunctional sexual beliefs as vulnerability factors for sexual dysfunction. *Journal of Sex Research, 43,* 68–75.

Öst, L.-G. (1989). One-session treatment for specific phobias. *Behaviour Research and Therapy, 27,* 1–7.

Payne, K. A., Binik, Y. M., Amsel, R., & Khalifé, S. (2005). When sex hurts, anxiety and fear orient attention towards pain. *European Journal of Pain, 9,* 427–436.

Rachman, S. (2004). Fear of contamination. *Behaviour Research and Therapy, 42,* 1227–1255.

Reissing, E. D., Yitzchak, B. M., Khalifé, S. M. D., Cohen, D. M. D., & Amsel, R. M. A. (2004). Vaginal spasm, pain and behavior: An empirical investigation of the diagnosis of vaginismus. *Archives of Sexual Behavior, 33,* 1, 5–17.

Rosen, R. C., & Laumann, E. O. (2003). The prevalence of sexual problems in women: How valid are comparisons across studies? Commentary on Bancroft, Loftus, and Long's (2003) "Distress about sex: A national survey of women in heterosexual relationships." *Archives of Sexual Behavior, 32,* 209–211.

Rosen, R. C., Taylor, J. F., Leiblum, S. R., & Bachmann, G. A. (1993). Prevalence of sexual dysfunction in women: Results of a survey study of 329 women in an outpatient gynecological clinic. *Journal of Sex & Marital Therapy, 19,* 171–188.

Rozin, P., & Fallon, A. E. (1987). A perspective on disgust. *Psychological Review, 94,* 23–41.

Rozin, P., Haidt, J., & McCauley, C. R. (1999). Disgust: The body and soul emotion. In T. Dalgleish & M. Power (Eds.), *Handbook of cognition and emotion* (pp. 429–445). Chichester, England: Wiley.

Rozin, P., Nemeroff, C., Horowitz, M., Gordon, B., & Voet, W. (1995). The borders of the self: Contamination sensitivity and potency of the body apertures and other body parts. *Journal of Research in Personality, 29,* 318–340.

Schultz, J. H., & Luthe, W. (1959). *Autogenic training.* New York: Grune & Stratton.

Simons, J. S., & Carey, M. P. (2001). Prevalence of sexual dysfunctions: Results from a decade of research. *Archives of Sexual Behavior, 30,* 177–219.

Stark, R., Schienle, A., Girod, C., Walter, B., Kirsch, P., Blecker, C., et al. (2005). Erotic and disgust-inducing pictures: Differences in the hemodynamic responses of the brain. *Biological Psychology, 70,* 19–29.

ter Kuile, M. M. (2007, July). *Exposure in vivo in the treatment of primary vaginismus: A replicated single-case experimental design*. Paper presented at the V World Congress of Behavioural & Cognitive Therapies, Barcelona, Spain.

ter Kuile, M. M., van Lankveld, J. J. D. M., de Groot, E., Melles, R., Neffs, J., & Zandbergen, M. (2007). Cognitive–behavioral therapy for women with lifelong vaginismus: Process and prognostic factors. *Behaviour Research and Therapy, 45,* 359–373.

van Lankveld, J. J. D. M., ter Kuile, M. M., de Groot, H. E., Melles, R., Nefs, J., & Zandbergen, M. (2006). Cognitive–behavioral therapy for women with lifelong vaginismus: A randomized waiting-list controlled trial of efficacy. *Journal of Clinical and Consulting Psychology, 74,* 168–178.

van Lankveld, J. J. D. M., & van den Hout, M. A. (2004). Increasing neutral distraction inhibits genital but not subjective sexual arousal of sexually functional and dysfunctional men. *Behaviour Research and Therapy, 33,* 549–559.

Vlaeyen, J. W. S., & Linton, S. J. (2000). Fear-avoidance and its consequences in chronic musculoskeletal pain: A state of the art. *Pain, 85,* 317–332.

Wheatley, T., & Haidt, J. (2005). Hypnotic disgust makes moral judgments more severe. *Psychological Science, 16,* 780–784.

13

INSOMNIA

ALLISON G. HARVEY

Insomnia is a chronic condition that involves difficulty getting to sleep, difficulty maintaining sleep, and/or waking in the morning not feeling restored. It is prevalent, reported by approximately 10% of the population (Ancoli-Israel & Roth, 1999). The consequences are severe and include functional impairment, work absenteeism, impaired concentration and memory, increased use of medical services (Roth & Ancoli-Israel, 1999), and increased risk of accidents (Ohayon, Caulet, Philip, Guilleminault, & Priest, 1997). Given the prevalence and associated impairments, the cost to society is enormous (Martin, Aikens, & Chervin, 2004).

In the context of this volume on refractory cases, this chapter addresses two broad domains. First, common factors that can lead to poor response when implementing cognitive–behavioral therapy for insomnia (CBT-I) are highlighted. Second, in light of accruing empirical evidence suggesting that sleep disturbance is a key, yet underrecognized, mechanism across a range of psychological disorders, we address the potential for adapting CBT-I to assist in the treatment of refractory cases of depression, bipolar disorder, attention-deficit/hyperactivity disorder (ADHD), and a wide range of other conditions. In addition, given the evidence indicating a critical function for sleep in mood/emotion regulation and for learning and problem solving (Kryger, Roth, & Dement, 2005), in discussing future directions, we raise the potential for developing a "transdiagnostic" sleep intervention. The goal would be to not only treat the insomnia but also improve symptoms associated with the comorbid psychological disorder.

DIAGNOSTIC CRITERIA

There are three main classification systems for sleep disorders: the second edition of the International Classification of Sleep Disorders (ICSD-2; American Academy of Sleep Medicine, 2005), the Research Diagnostic Criteria (RDC; Edinger et al., 2004), and the *Diagnostic and Statistical Manual of Mental Disorders* (*DSM–IV–TR*; 4th ed., text rev.; American Psychiatric Association, 2000). In this section, we focus on the *DSM–IV–TR* criteria; however, readers are encouraged to consult the ICSD-2 manual and RDC criteria for further information about other nosologies commonly used in both clinical and research settings.

Within the *DSM–IV–TR*, a diagnosis of insomnia may be given when there is a subjective complaint of trouble falling asleep, staying asleep, or obtaining restorative sleep. Additionally, these difficulties must be associated with daytime impairment and must not be better accounted for by another medical or psychiatric condition. Because insomnia can be associated with a wide range of medical illnesses and mental health conditions, the *DSM–IV–TR* distinguishes between *primary* and *secondary* insomnia, with the latter referring to cases in which the sleep difficulty is thought to be caused by a medical illness, psychological disturbance, medication, or substance. However, a recent National Institutes of Health State of the Science conference (National Institutes of Health, 2005) concluded that the term *secondary* should be replaced with *comorbid* on the basis of evidence that insomnia constitutes a risk factor for the development of certain disorders and contributes to relapse in others and also to the maintenance of a wide range of disorders (Harvey, 2001; Perlis et al., 2006; Smith, Huang, & Manber, 2005).

DESCRIPTION OF COGNITIVE–BEHAVIORAL THERAPY FOR INSOMNIA

The primary goal of CBT-I is to reverse the cognitive and behavioral processes involved in maintaining sleep disturbance. A second important goal is to teach coping techniques that patients can use in instances of residual sleep difficulty. CBT-I is currently considered the treatment of choice for insomnia. It is a multicomponent treatment that typically comprises one or more of the following components: stimulus control, sleep restriction, sleep hygiene, paradoxical intention, relaxation therapy, imagery training, and cognitive restructuring for unhelpful beliefs about sleep. Each of these components is described in the following sections.

Stimulus Control

The rationale for stimulus control procedures lies in the notion that insomnia is a result of conditioning that occurs when the bed becomes associated with inability to sleep. As described by Bootzin, Epstein, and Wood (1991), stimulus control requires patients (a) to set a regular sleep schedule with a consistent waking time and no daytime naps, (b) to only go to bed and stay in bed when sleepy and when sleep is imminent (this requires the individual to leave the bed if unable to fall asleep and to return to bed only when feeling very sleepy), and (c) to eliminate all sleep-incompatible activities (e.g., upsetting conversations, problem solving, and watching television) from the bedroom.

Sleep Restriction

Sleep restriction therapy, as developed by Spielman, Saskin, and Thorpy (1987), rests on the general premise that time in bed should be limited to maximize the sleep drive and so that the association between the bed and sleeping is strengthened. It begins with a reduction of time spent in bed so that time in bed is equivalent to the time the patient estimates he or she spends sleeping. Thus, for instance, if an individual thinks he or she gets approximately 6 hours of sleep per night but usually spends about 2 additional hours trying to get to sleep, the sleep restriction therapy would begin by limiting the individual's time spent in bed to 6 hours. This initial reduction in time spent in bed is intended to heighten a person's homeostatic sleep drive (Perlis & Lichstein, 2003). Following this restriction, sleep gradually becomes more efficient. Then, time spent in bed is gradually increased to reach an optimal sleep efficiency. *Sleep efficiency* is defined as total sleep time divided by time in bed, multiplied by 100. The goal is to increase sleep efficiency to more than 85%.

Sleep Hygiene

Information about sleep and sleep-incompatible behaviors and the daytime consequences of sleep disturbance is given to inform patients of basic steps they can take to improve their sleep. This component aims to identify and reduce the use of sleep-incompatible routines. Factors typically addressed in sleep hygiene interventions include alcohol, tobacco, caffeine use, diet, exercise, and the bedroom environment (Morin & Espie, 2003). Although sleep hygiene education is typically included as one component of CBT-I, its use as the sole intervention in treating insomnia has not been empirically supported (Morin et al., 2006).

Paradoxical Intention

In paradoxical intention, patients are instructed to stay awake for as long as possible. The aim is to reduce performance anxiety related to getting to sleep (e.g., Espie & Lindsay, 1985). Paradoxical intention aims to replace the tendency to actively try to get to sleep that is often used by individuals struggling with insomnia. Because using an active focus and strategy to induce sleep is actually generally sleep incompatible (Espie, 2002), paradoxical intention places patients in the role of passive observer, thereby decreasing anxiety and increasing the likelihood of sleep onset.

Relaxation Therapy

Patients are taught to implement a variety of relaxation exercises while in the therapy session. They are then encouraged to practice these exercises as much as they can between sessions, but the emphasis is on practice during the day (as opposed to using them only at night in an effort to get to sleep). Practice is essential and is often aided by making a tape of the relaxation instructions that the patient can use at home. Morin and Espie (2003) made a number of recommendations to maximize the effectiveness of relaxation therapy. Specifically, among the available relaxation techniques, they suggested a focus on imagery, breathing exercises, and the release of muscle tension. Additionally, Morin and Espie noted that although patients are generally receptive to relaxation therapy, it is important for them to understand that relaxation serves to set a context in which sleep is more likely to occur as opposed to functioning as a sleeping medication.

Cognitive Therapy and Restructuring

This component of CBT-I, often administered in one session, involves altering faulty beliefs about sleep by education and discussion about sleep requirements, the biological clock, and the effects of sleep loss on sleep–wake functions (e.g., Edinger, Wohlgemuth, Radtke, Marsh, & Quillian, 2001a). This approach is distinct from an intervention we refer to later in which the entire treatment is focused on reversing cognitive-maintaining processes (Harvey, Sharpley, Ree, Stinson, & Clark, 2007). An empirical question that remains to be answered is whether combining CBT-I and the cognitive therapy (CT) intervention would improve overall outcome.

Evidence for the Effectiveness of Cognitive–Behavioral Therapy for Insomnia

In a recent review, the Standards of Practice Committee of the American Academy of Sleep Medicine found CBT-I to be highly effective and to have sustainable gains over long-term follow-up of up to 24 months in adult and older adult samples (Morin et al., 2006). This review used the American Psychological Association (APA) criteria for well-supported empirically based treatments (Chambless & Hollon, 1998) and concluded that these criteria are met by stimulus control, paradoxical intention, relaxation, sleep restriction approaches, and the administration of multiple components in the form of CBT-I. The sleep hygiene intervention alone has not been found to be effective as a treatment for insomnia. CT for insomnia is a promising new approach; however, randomized controlled trials are still required before APA criteria for an empirically supported treatment are met.

FACTORS ASSOCIATED WITH POOR TREATMENT RESPONSE

Phase Delay

A tendency toward a delay in the circadian phase, such that sleep onset does not occur until the early hours of the morning, can contribute to diminished treatment response to CBT-I. This is particularly common in adolescents and young adults. The literature for treating delayed phase is small. Exposure to bright light looks promising, although the optimal timing and dose of the exposure remain to be established (Hoban, 2004). More simply, such procedures as gradual advances in bedtime and wake-up times (say by 15 minutes a day), avoiding daytime napping, and maintaining consistency on the weekend are recommended. Or, when the bedtime is very late, it may be easier to institute successive delays in bedtime. The reason that moving in this direction may be favorable is that the circadian cycle naturally runs over 24 hours Hence, delays that capitalize on the natural tendency for the circadian system to run over 24 hours may be more easily achieved than advances in bedtime (Dahl, 1992).

Worry

It is well documented that people with insomnia lie in bed worrying about a range of topics, including not being able to get to sleep (Harvey, 2000; Wicklow & Espie, 2000). Cognitive models of insomnia suggest that worry activates the sympathetic nervous system (the so-called fight-or-flight response), thereby triggering physiological arousal and distress. This combination of worry, arousal, and distress spirals the individual into a state of heightened anxiety that is antithetical to falling asleep and staying asleep (Espie, 2002; Harvey, 2002). In support, there is convergent empirical evidence suggesting that worrying while trying to get to sleep serves to maintain insomnia (Harvey, 2005b). A new topic, just starting to attract research attention, relates to the finding that some thought control strategies, such as thought suppression, are important contributors to the maintenance of worry in insomnia patients (Bélanger, Morin, Gendron, & Blais, 2005; Harvey, 2003a; Harvey & Payne, 2002; Ree, Harvey, Blake, Tang, & Shawe-Taylor, 2005). Accordingly, for some insomnia patients, an intervention to reduce worry and establish helpful strategies for managing unwanted thoughts may be critical.

Following CT for other disorders, we begin the intervention for worry by defining negative automatic thoughts (NATs) and then teaching the patient to monitor, identify, and evaluate them (Beck, 1995). Patients are asked to choose sleep-related NATs as examples to work on, although we suggest that the procedure for worrisome thoughts is helpfully applied to any topic. Themes that emerge from the patient observing and recording their NATs are then used to detect unhelpful beliefs that serve to maintain the insomnia. These can be tested with an individualized behavioral experiment (Ree & Harvey, 2004). This procedure alone is rarely sufficient for managing worry among patients with insomnia. Hence, several other approaches are required, three of which we briefly describe in the following sections (for a fuller description, see Harvey, 2005b).

Assessing How the Patient Attempts to Manage Worry While Trying to Get to Sleep

Typically, patients report trying to stop worrying by "blanking my mind" or "trying to stop all thoughts" (for a questionnaire that assesses thought management strategies, see Ree et al., 2005). For these patients, it can be helpful to conduct a behavioral experiment within the session to demonstrate the adverse consequences of thought suppression. For example, we use Wegner and Schneider's (1989) white bear experiment in which the patient is asked to close his or her eyes and try to suppress all of his or her thoughts relating to white bears (the therapist does this, too). After a few minutes, the patient is asked to stop and share how successful the suppression attempts were (or more typically, were not!). This provides a stunning demonstration of the counterproductive nature of thought control and is a springboard to discussing alternative thought management strategies such as letting the thoughts come (i.e., the opposite of suppression) or gently redirecting attention to interesting and engaging imagery. Then, for homework during the subsequent week, one or more individualized behavioral experiments are devised in which the patient tries out the various alternative thought control strategies.

Identifying Why Questions

On the basis of work by Watkins and Baracaia (2001), we listen for patients asking themselves *why* questions (e.g., Why am I not sleepy? Why are my thoughts racing? Why do I always feel so sleepy?). These questions often become evident either (a) during the initial case formulation when the thoughts the patient is having when trying to get to sleep are elicited or (b) when the content of worry episodes is unpacked. *Why* questions rarely have definite answers. Hence, asking them tends to lead to more distress. For example, if a person were to ask "Why can't I control my sleep?" the chances are that he or she would not find a simple, definite answer and would end up feeling as if there were no solution to the problem, heightening anxiety and distress.

Identifying Positive Beliefs About Worrying

We also assess whether the patient holds positive beliefs about worrying in bed. The importance of positive beliefs about worry is drawn from the generalized anxiety disorder literature that suggests that pathological worry may be at least partly maintained because the individual believes that worry will lead to positive consequences (see Wells, 1995). To help identify positive beliefs, we ask our patients to complete a questionnaire that lists a range of positive and negative beliefs about worry (Harvey, 2003b). Examples of positive beliefs about worry include "Worrying while trying to get to sleep helps me get things sorted out in my mind" and "Worrying is a way to distract myself from worrying about even more emotional things I don't want to think about." If we discover that patients hold these beliefs, we use Socratic questioning and behavioral experiments to examine and test their validity.

Daytime Distress and Impairment

CBT-I focuses on nighttime symptoms and processes and does not directly address daytime impairment (Riedel & Lichstein, 2000). This is surprising given that there are well-established daytime consequences of chronic insomnia. Specifically, during the day people with insomnia report decreased ability to accomplish daily tasks and more sleepiness, tiredness, and difficulty functioning socially. They also report impaired concentration and memory problems. In addition, work absenteeism, increased use of medical services, and self-medication with either over-the-counter medications or alcohol are common among individuals with insomnia (Roth & Ancoli-Israel, 1999). Other studies have reported the daytime consequences of insomnia to include increased anxiety and depression, poor self-esteem, and social withdrawal (Alapin et al., 2000). These impairments adversely affect interpersonal, social, and occupational functioning (Rombaut, Maillard, Kelly, & Hindmarch, 1990). Moreover, there is empirical evidence that daytime processes may be independent of nighttime processes (Neitzert Semler & Harvey, 2005).

Despite the reliable and durable changes reported on several sleep parameters following treatment for insomnia, to date there is very limited evidence that treatment improves daytime functioning (Means, Lichstein, Epperson, & Johnson, 2000). This is, in part, because few trials have included measures of daytime functioning as outcome measures.

Accordingly, some patients may require a specific intervention for daytime distress. The seeds of this approach are in the process of being developed and tested (Harvey, 2005a; Ree & Harvey, 2004), such as "energy generating" experiments and surveys of friends and family to normalize that some daytime tiredness and lapses in attention and memory are experienced by everyone, even good sleepers. In an open trial, this approach was associated with improvement in daytime impairment (Harvey et al., 2007).

Unhelpful Beliefs About Sleep

Following the pioneering work of Morin, Stone, Trinkle, Mercer, and Remsberg (1993), the evidence that patients with insomnia hold more unhelpful and inaccurate beliefs about sleep, relative to individuals without insomnia, continues to accrue. Also, the finding that reducing unhelpful beliefs about sleep is associated with better treatment outcome (Edinger, Wohlgemuth, Radtke, Marsh, & Quillian, 2001b; Morin, Blais, & Savard, 2002) highlights their importance to the treatment of insomnia.

In CBT-I, unhelpful beliefs about sleep are typically corrected through education about sleep. When unhelpful beliefs are resistant to education, we suggest devising an individualized behavioral experiment (Ree & Harvey, 2004; Tang & Harvey, 2006). *Behavioral experiments* are "planned experiential activities, based on experimentation or observation, that [arise from a] formulation of the problem, and their primary purpose is to obtain new information which . . . [includes] contributing to the development and verification of the cognitive formulation" (Bennett-Levy et al., 2004, p. 8). To give one example, for patients who continue to believe that "even 1 night of poor sleep substantially impairs my daytime functioning," an individualized behavioral experiment is collaboratively devised and conducted toward the end of treatment. We do this experiment toward the end of the treatment because that is when the patient feels that he or she has developed an ability to manage the daytime consequences of a poor night, and we time it so that the patient will not be engaging in any activities known to be adversely affected by sleepiness (e.g., driving) during the following day.

This experiment involves actually choosing to have 1 "poor night" of sleep (e.g., choosing to sleep 6.5 hours for a patient who believes he or she needs 8 hours). It has typically been done by the patient by accident on several occasions (i.e., those sessions when a patient has come in and said, "You know, I only slept 6 hours last night, and I actually feel OK today"). However, these experiences still haven't always fundamentally changed the belief that "I need 8 hours of sleep every single night in order to cope" and may even have been dismissed as a fluke or attributed to some other occurrence (e.g., "I coped because I drank a lot of coffee"). So by actually choosing to sleep less, for just 1 night, the patient has the opportunity to learn that getting less than the ideal amount of sleep 1 night is not necessarily devastating to next-day performance and often leads to improvement the following night. Before attempting this experiment, the patient decides whether to go to bed later, set the alarm earlier, or some combination of both.

We plan interesting and engaging activities for the patient to do during this time to stay awake and ensure the experiment is memorable. For example, those who choose to wake earlier in the morning might decide to have a leisurely breakfast in bed or take more time reading the morning newspaper. Care should be exercised to not choose a night prior to a day when the patient is driving or would be at risk if he or she is sleepy and to only attempt this experiment when the patient feels that he or she has developed an ability to manage the daytime consequences of a poor night of sleep. With a careful rationale, planning, and support (e.g., phone calls), most patients will give this experiment a try, and the results provide a compelling and memorable refutation of the belief that "even 1 night of poor sleep substantially impairs my daytime functioning." Perhaps paradoxically, by reducing fear of poor sleep, the potential to obtain more sleep of better quality can be markedly increased.

Comorbid Sleep Disorder

In the pretreatment assessment, questions should be asked to screen for comorbid sleep disorders. The possibility that a comorbid sleep disorder is present should be revisited if the patient does not respond to CBT-I. Specifically, consideration should be given to referring the patient for a full night of polysomnography. *Polysomnography* involves placing surface electrodes on the scalp and face to measure electrical brain activity (electroencephalogram), eye movement (electro-oculogram), and muscle tone (electromyogram). The data obtained are used to classify each epoch of data by sleep stage. The addition of monitors of breathing and leg movements enable an assessment of comorbid sleep disorders. The most important of these are briefly detailed next.

In *sleep apnea*, transient closure of the upper airway during sleep is associated with disruption to sleep. The nighttime symptoms can include snoring, pauses in breathing during sleep, shortness of breath during sleep, choking during sleep, headaches on waking, difficulty getting breath, or breathlessness on waking. The adverse outcomes include daytime sleepiness and cardiovascular problems.

The symptoms of *restless leg syndrome* are a sensation of an urge to move the limbs (usually legs) and a feeling of restlessness because of sensations in the limbs (usually legs). The sensations start or get worse when resting, relaxing, or first going to bed. A clear circadian pattern must be present.

The hallmark feature of *periodic limb movement disorder* is repetitive episodes of limb movements during sleep, usually the legs. The movements are associated with a partial or full awakening.

Narcolepsy is a disorder characterized by excessive sleepiness. Episodes of short uncontrollable naps during the day are typical. Often the nap is associated with cataplexy (i.e., loss of muscle tone triggered by strong emotion), sleep paralysis, or hypnogogic hallucinations.

Comorbid Psychological Disorder

This section addresses the potential for adapting treatments for insomnia to assist refractory cases of psychiatric disorders in which insomnia is comorbid. Insomnia can occur as the sole presenting problem or as a condition that is comorbid with another psychological disorder. Indeed, there is evidence that insomnia is highly comorbid across a range of disorders (Benca, Obermeyer, Thisted, & Gillin, 1992). In the past there has been a tendency to assume that insomnia is secondary to a so-called primary disorder (e.g., depression, anxiety). However, it is now widely agreed that perceiving insomnia to be merely epiphenomenal to the comorbid disorder is unwise. Prominent among the reasons are the following. First, the evidence indicates that insomnia is a risk factor for, and can be causal in, the development and/or maintenance of the comorbid disorder (Harvey, 2001; McCrae & Lichstein, 2001). Second, substantial evidence is accruing to suggest that insomnia that is comorbid with another psychological or medical disorder does not necessarily remit with the treatment of the so-called primary disorder (Smith et al., 2005). Third, there is convincing evidence of a bidirectional relationship between daytime mood and symptoms and nighttime sleep whereby a vicious cycle of symptoms and mood disturbance interfere with sleep, and the effects of sleep deprivation at night exacerbate daytime symptoms and mood (e.g., Harvey, in press). For reviews of this evidence, see Smith et al. (2005), who discussed a range of psychological disorders, and Dahl and Lewin (2002), who focused on adolescents, and Harvey et al., who focused on bipolar disorder (Harvey, Mullin, & Hinshaw, 2006) and the anxiety disorders (Harvey, Hairston, Gruber, & Gershon, in press).

Another assumption that has dominated the field until recently is that insomnia that is comorbid with another mental health condition or medical disorder cannot be successfully treated if the primary condition with which it was associated is not treated first. Although it is certainly true that cases of comorbid insomnia present additional challenges, recent evidence has suggested that insomnia does respond to treatment when it is treated with CBT-I, even if the psychological or medical disorder is not under control. For example, in a comparison of CBT-I with an active control condition in a sample of older adults suffering from a range of chronic illnesses (such as osteoarthritis and pulmonary disease), CBT-I was associated with a significant improvement in 8 out of 10 sleep measures compared with the control condition (Rybarczyk, Lopez, Schelble, & Stepanski, 2005). In a review of this small but growing literature, Smith et al. (2005) concluded that treatment effects are generally moderate to large for CBT-I administered to patients who have insomnia that is comorbid with a medical or psychological disturbance and are comparable to treatment effects in primary insomnia, although Smith et al. added the caveat that CBT-I may need to be adapted for certain disorders. An example of this is provided later in this chapter for a patient with bipolar disorder.

In summary, the available evidence indicates great potential for adapting CBT-I for patients who have insomnia that is comorbid with another psychological disorder. There is considerable excitement and optimism in the field centering on the possibility that improving sleep will not only improve quality of life but may also reduce symptoms associated with the comorbid problem. If this potential is realized, this direction will provide a novel treatment target for refractory cases of depression, bipolar disorder, ADHD, and a wide range of other conditions in which sleep disturbance is a feature. Future research is needed to determine whether there is potential to develop a transdiagnostic sleep intervention that is relevant across psychological disorders, or if disorder-specific sleep interventions that are unique to particular syndromes are required.

BACKGROUND TO CASE EXAMPLE

Bipolar disorder is a common, severe, and chronic disorder, ranked in the Top 10 leading causes of disability worldwide. Although there have been significant and important advances in treatments, the risk of relapse remains high. Thus, there is an urgent need to uncover the mechanisms that trigger relapse and to then use this information to develop new adjunctive interventions that reverse the influence of the identified mechanisms, thereby substantially reducing risk of relapse.

Sleep disturbance is a core symptom of bipolar disorder. During mania, there is a reduced need for sleep. During depression, people suffer insomnia or hypersomnia (Hudson et al., 1992). Our research has shown that sleep disturbance is common even when patients with bipolar disorder are interepisode (Harvey, Schmidt, Scarna, Semler, & Goodwin, 2005). Yet, relative to the interepisode phase, sleep disturbance escalates just before an episode and worsens further during an episode (Barbini, Bertelli, Colombo, & Smeraldi, 1996; Jackson, Cavanagh, & Scott, 2003; Wehr, Sack, & Rosenthal, 1987).

There is evidence suggesting that sleep disturbance contributes to emotional lability and relapse in bipolar disorder. First, among patients with bipolar disorder, sleep disturbance is the most common prodrome of mania and the sixth most common prodrome of depression (Jackson et al., 2003). A *prodrome* is a symptom that appears before an episode. Second, experimentally induced sleep deprivation is associated with the onset of hypomania or mania in a proportion of patients (Colombo, Benedetti, Barbini, Campori, & Smeraldi, 1999; Kasper & Wehr, 1992; Leibenluft, Albert, Rosenthal, & Wehr, 1996; Wehr et al., 1987; Wu & Bunney, 1990). Third, bipolar disorder is a disorder of emotion regulation (Hyman, 2000). Accruing evidence in the basic sleep research literature has suggested that sleep has a key mood regulatory function (Cartwright, Luten, Young, Mercer, & Bears, 1998; Perlis & Nielsen, 1993) and that there is a dose–response relationship between sleep deprivation and mood disturbance the next day in healthy participants (Dinges et al., 1997; Pilcher & Huffcutt, 1996; Van Dongen, Maislin, Mullington, & Dinges, 2003). Finally, at the neural systems level, circuits involved in emotion regulation and circuits involved in sleep regulation interact in bidirectional ways (e.g., Saper, Cano, & Scammell, 2005).

In sum, this evidence converges on the hypothesis that sleep disturbance may be one causal pathway that leads to relapse in bipolar disorder (Goodwin & Jamison, 1990; Wehr et al., 1987). The case of Jerry presented in the next section explores the possibility raised by this evidence that an intervention could be developed to target the sleep disturbance and not only improve quality of life but reduce the risk of, or contribute to the prevention of, episodes. The sleep problem described was considered refractory given that several medication approaches had been tried and failed over the years.

CASE EXAMPLE

Jerry had just dropped out of his 3rd year as an undergraduate because of episodes of mania and depression. He was diagnosed with bipolar disorder when he was 16 years old. Jerry not only experienced insomnia between episodes, but also his sleep substantially worsened approximately 2 weeks prior to a relapse. Moreover, during a manic episode Jerry found it very difficult to get to and maintain sleep. Multiple sleep medications had been tried over several years. These treatments were unsuccessful because of side effects (particularly daytime sedation). Jerry was aware of the damage each episode caused in his life, and he had encoded that sleep disturbance was an early warning signal of an impending episode. Hence, he had developed a significant fear of poor sleep and was constantly worried about his sleep. He no longer had a social life in the evening and would go to bed early most nights (9:30 p.m.) in an attempt to ensure a good night of sleep. He would nap during the day to try to guarantee he was getting enough sleep. Some days he would not get out of bed at all. Jerry believed that he should aim to get over 10 hours of sleep a day to avoid episodes of mania and depression, and that if he didn't get 10 hours he would become worried and preoccupied with his sleep.

Given that stimulus control and sleep restriction can entail short-term sleep deprivation (for a week or 2) and that Jerry's history indicated that significant sleep loss triggers an episode, administration of standard CBT-I seemed unwise. Hence, an adapted treatment was administered that empha-sized targeting unhelpful beliefs about sleep (e.g., "I must get 10 hours of sleep per night or else I will have an episode") and worry about sleep.

In addition, daily sleep diaries kept for 14 days identified several addi-tional targets of intervention. On weekdays, although Jerry reported getting into bed by 9:30 p.m., he often did not fall to sleep until 1 a.m. or 2 a.m. He reported spending hours in bed awake and worrying about not being able to get to sleep. On 2 or 3 nights per week, he would give up staying in bed and would go over to the computer in his bedroom and use the Internet. On weekends, without the need to attend lectures the next day, he would stay up watching movies or using the Internet, typically getting into bed at 1 a.m. Hence, other targets of intervention were the tendency toward a delayed sleep phase (i.e., a natural rhythm of preferring to go to bed late and wake up late), regularizing the sleep–wake schedule to diminish the difference be-tween weekday and weekends, and the reduction of Internet use at bedtime or in the middle of the night. This began with Jerry receiving information about sleep and circadian rhythms and how to manage his tendency toward a phase delay (outlined earlier in this chapter). And we brainstormed practical strategies for establishing a more regular sleep–wake cycle (e.g., aiming to go to bed at 11 p.m. rather than 9:30 p.m.). Another target was to correct un-helpful sleep-related habits (e.g., Internet use when unable to sleep) while developing new healthy sleep habits and to maintain these new healthier habits (e.g., personal writing or reading). In addition, because bright light exposure in the morning helps to counter phase delay in the circadian rhythm, Jerry was encouraged to obtain morning exposure to bright light (e.g. out-door sunshine, bright artificial light), and daytime naps and caffeine use were discouraged.

This intervention was effective in reducing Jerry's worry about sleep and stabilizing his sleep–wake cycle. In addition, during the period of follow-up he did not have any episodes of mania or depression and his mood was relatively stable.

CONCLUSIONS AND FUTURE DIRECTIONS

This chapter focused on the most common sleep disorder, namely, chronic insomnia. We have provided a description of the disorder and an overview of the current treatment of choice (CBT-I), and we have high-lighted a number of issues associated with poor treatment response along with suggestions as to how to manage these issues. A focus has been on the potential for developing a transdiagnostic sleep intervention. The goal would be not only to treat the insomnia but also to improve symptoms associated with the comorbid psychological disorder. This may be possible given the accumulating evidence indicating a critical function for sleep in mood/emotion regulation and for learning and problem solving (Kryger et al., 2005) and the evidence that insomnia is not epiphenomenal to other psychiatric disorders but is an important (yet underrecognized) mechanism.

Although we spend approximately one third of our lives sleeping, sleep is a relatively new topic of scientific study. As such, there are myriad mysteries and questions about the function of sleep and sleep disorders that are yet to be answered. Several of these have already been raised. In closing this chapter, we outline two additional domains for future research.

First, there is evidence for the efficacy and effectiveness of CBT-I for both adults and older adults. What about adolescents? What about children? What about toddlers and infants? We know that sleep varies substantially across the age range and may be particularly critical given the importance of sleep to optimal learning (Walker, Brakefield, Morgan, Hobson, & Stickgold, 2002; Yoo, Hu, Gujar, Jolesz, & Walker, 2007). Hence, an important direction for the future is treatment development efforts for sleep problems in infancy, children, and youth.

Second, although there is no doubt that CBT-I is an effective treatment (Morin et al., 2006), the field is not at a point at which patients can be offered a maximally effective psychological treatment as indicated by (a) the significant subset of patients who do not improve following CBT-I (19%–26%), (b) the average overall improvement being in the range of 50% to 60% (Morin, Culbert, & Schwartz, 1994; Murtagh & Greenwood, 1995), and (c) the fact that only a minority of patients reach a high-end state (i.e., become good sleepers; Harvey & Tang, 2003). Several ongoing treatment development efforts await testing in RCTs (e.g., Harvey et al., 2007; Heidenreich, Tuin, Pflug, Michal, & Michalak, 2006).

REFERENCES

Alapin, I., Fichten, C. S., Libman, E., Creti, L., Bailes, S., & Wright, J. (2000). How is good and poor sleep in older adults and college students related to daytime sleepiness, fatigue, and ability to concentrate? *Journal of Psychosomatic Research*, *49*, 381–390.

American Academy of Sleep Medicine. (2005). *International classification of sleep disorders (ICSD): Diagnostic and coding manual* (2nd ed.). Westchester, IL: Author.

American Psychiatric Association. (2000). *Diagnostic and statistical manual of mental disorders* (4th ed., text rev.). Washington, DC: Author.

Ancoli-Israel, S., & Roth, T. (1999). Characteristics of insomnia in the United States: Results of the 1991 National Sleep Foundation Survey: I. *Sleep, 22*(Suppl. 2), S347–353.

Barbini, B., Bertelli, S., Colombo, C., & Smeraldi, E. (1996). Sleep loss, a possible factor in augmenting manic episode. *Psychiatry Research, 65*, 121–125.

Beck, J. (1995). *Cognitive therapy: Basics and beyond.* New York: Guilford Press.

Bélanger, L., Morin, C. M., Gendron, L., & Blais, F. C. (2005). Presleep cognitive activity and thought control strategies in insomnia. *Journal of Cognitive Psychotherapy, 19,* 17–27.

Benca, R. M., Obermeyer, W. H., Thisted, R. A., & Gillin, J. C. (1992). Sleep and psychiatric disorders: A meta-analysis. *Archives of General Psychiatry, 49,* 651–668.

Bennett-Levy, J., Butler, G., Fennell, M. J. V., Hackmann, A., Mueller, M., & Westbrook, D. (2004). *The Oxford handbook of behavioural experiments.* Oxford, England: Oxford University Press.

Bootzin, R. R., Epstein, D., & Wood, J. M. (1991). Stimulus control instructions. In P. J. Hauri (Ed.), *Case studies in insomnia* (pp. 19–28). New York: Plenum Press.

Cartwright, R., Luten, A., Young, M., Mercer, P., & Bears, M. (1998). Role of REM sleep and dream affect in overnight mood regulation: A study of normal volunteers. *Psychiatry Research, 81,* 1–8.

Chambless, D. L., & Hollon, S. D. (1998). Defining empirically supported theories. *Journal of Consulting and Clinical Psychology, 1,* 7–18.

Colombo, C., Benedetti, F., Barbini, B., Campori, E., & Smeraldi, E. (1999). Rate of switch from depression into mania after therapeutic sleep deprivation in bipolar depression. *Psychiatry Research, 86,* 267–270.

Dahl, R. E. (1992). Child and adolescent sleep disorders. In D. Kaufmann (Ed.), *Child and adolescent neurology for the psychiatrist* (pp. 169–194). Baltimore, MD: Williams & Wilkins.

Dahl, R. E., & Lewin, D. S. (2002). Pathways to adolescent health sleep regulation and behavior. *Journal of Adolescent Health, 31,* 175–184.

Dinges, D. F., Pack, F., Williams, K., Gillen, K. A., Powell, J. W., Ott, G. E., et al. (1997). Cumulative sleepiness, mood disturbance, and psychomotor vigilance performance decrements during a week of sleep restricted to 4–5 hours per night. *Sleep, 20,* 267–277.

Edinger, J. D., Bonnet, M. H., Bootzin, R. R., Doghramji, K., Dorsey, C. M., Espie, C. A., et al. (2004). Derivation of research diagnostic criteria for insomnia: Report of an American Academy of Sleep Medicine Work Group. *Sleep, 27,* 1567–1596.

Edinger, J. D., Wohlgemuth, W. K., Radtke, R. A., Marsh, G. R., & Quillian, R. E. (2001a). Cognitive behavioral therapy for treatment of chronic primary insomnia: A randomized controlled trial. *JAMA, 285,* 1856–1864.

Edinger, J. D., Wohlgemuth, W. K., Radtke, R. A., Marsh, G. R., & Quillian, R. E. (2001b). Does cognitive–behavioral insomnia therapy alter dysfunctional beliefs about sleep? *Sleep, 24,* 591–599.

Espie, C. A. (2002). Insomnia: Conceptual issues in the development, persistence, and treatment of sleep disorder in adults. *Annual Review of Psychology, 53,* 215–243.

Espie, C. A., & Lindsay, W. R. (1985). Paradoxical intention in the treatment of chronic insomnia: Six case studies illustrating variability in therapeutic response. *Behaviour Research and Therapy, 23,* 703–709.

Goodwin, F. K., & Jamison, K. R. (1990). *Manic-depressive illness*. New York: Oxford University Press.

Harvey, A. G. (2000). Pre-sleep cognitive activity: A comparison of sleep-onset insomniacs and good sleepers. *British Journal of Clinical Psychology, 39*, 275–286.

Harvey, A. G. (2001). Insomnia: Symptom or diagnosis? *Clinical Psychology Review, 21*, 1037–1059.

Harvey, A. G. (2002). A cognitive model of insomnia. *Behaviour Research and Therapy, 40*, 869–894.

Harvey, A. G. (2003a). The attempted suppression of presleep cognitive activity in insomnia. *Cognitive Therapy and Research, 27*, 593–602.

Harvey, A. G. (2003b). Beliefs about the utility of presleep worry: An investigation of individuals with insomnia and good sleepers. *Cognitive Therapy and Research, 27*, 403–414.

Harvey, A. G. (2005a). A cognitive theory of and therapy for chronic insomnia. *Journal of Cognitive Psychotherapy, 19*, 41–60.

Harvey, A. G. (2005b). Unwanted intrusive thoughts in insomnia. In D. A. Clark (Ed.), *Intrusive thoughts in clinical disorders: Theory, research, and treatment* (pp. 86–118). New York: Guilford Press.

Harvey, A. G. (in press). Sleep and emotion. In D. Sander & K. Scherer (Eds.), *Oxford companion of affective sciences*. Oxford, England: Oxford University Press.

Harvey, A. G., Hairston, I. S., Gruber, J., & Gershon, A. (in press). Anxiety and sleep. In M. M. Antony & M. B. Stein (Eds.), *Handbook of anxiety and the anxiety disorders*. New York: Oxford University Press.

Harvey, A. G., Mullin, B. C., & Hinshaw, S. P. (2006). Sleep and circadian rhythms in children and adolescents with bipolar disorder. *Development and Psychopathology, 18*, 1147–1168.

Harvey, A. G., & Payne, S. (2002). The management of unwanted pre-sleep thoughts in insomnia: Distraction with imagery versus general distraction. *Behaviour Research and Therapy, 40*, 267–277.

Harvey, A. G., Schmidt, D. A., Scarna, A., Semler, C. N., & Goodwin, G. M. (2005). Sleep-related functioning in euthymic patients with bipolar disorder, patients with insomnia, and subjects without sleep problems. *The American Journal of Psychiatry, 162*, 50–57.

Harvey, A. G., Sharpley, A., Ree, M. J., Stinson, K., & Clark, D. M. (2007). An open trial of cognitive therapy for chronic insomnia. *Behaviour Research and Therapy, 45*, 2491–2501.

Harvey, A. G., & Tang, N. K. J. (2003). Cognitive behavior therapy for insomnia: Can we rest yet? *Sleep Medicine Reviews, 7*, 237–262.

Heidenreich, T., Tuin, I., Pflug, B., Michal, M., & Michalak, J. (2006). Mindfulness-based cognitive therapy for persistent insomnia: A pilot study. *Psychotherapy and Psychosomatics, 75*, 188–189.

Hoban, T. F. (2004). Sleep and its disorders in children. *Seminars in Neurology, 24*, 327–340.

Hudson, J. I., Lipinski, J. F., Keck, P. E., Jr., Aizley, H. G., Lukas, S. E., Rothschild, A. J., et al. (1992). Polysomnographic characteristics of young manic patients: Comparison with unipolar depressed patients and normal control subjects. *Archives of General Psychiatry, 49*, 378–383.

Hyman, S. E. (2000). Goals for research on bipolar disorder: The view from NIMH. *Biological Psychiatry, 48*, 436–441.

Jackson, A., Cavanagh, J., & Scott, J. (2003). A systematic review of manic and depressive prodromes. *Journal of Affective Disorders, 74*, 209–217.

Kasper, S., & Wehr, T. A. (1992). The role of sleep and wakefulness in the genesis of depression and mania. *Encephale, 18*, 45–50.

Kryger, M. H., Roth, T., & Dement, W. C. (2005). *Principles and practice of sleep medicine* (4th ed.). Philadelphia: WB Saunders.

Leibenluft, E., Albert, P. S., Rosenthal, N. E., & Wehr, T. A. (1996). Relationship between sleep and mood in patients with rapid-cycling bipolar disorder. *Psychiatry Research, 63*, 161–168.

Martin, S. A., Aikens, J. E., & Chervin, R. D. (2004). Toward cost-effectiveness analysis in the diagnosis and treatment of insomnia. *Sleep Medicine Reviews, 8*, 63–72.

McCrae, C. S., & Lichstein, K. L. (2001). Secondary insomnia: Diagnostic challenges and intervention opportunities. *Sleep Medicine Reviews, 5*, 47–61.

Means, M. K., Lichstein, K. L., Epperson, M. T., & Johnson, C. T. (2000). Relaxation therapy for insomnia: Nighttime and daytime effects. *Behaviour Research and Therapy, 38*, 665–678.

Morin, C. M., Blais, F., & Savard, J. (2002). Are changes in beliefs and attitudes about sleep related to sleep improvements in the treatment of insomnia? *Behaviour Research and Therapy, 40*, 741–752.

Morin, C. M., Bootzin, R. R., Buysse, D. J., Edinger, J. D., Espie, C. A., & Lichstein, K. L. (2006). Psychological and behavioral treatment of insomnia: An update of recent evidence (1998–2004). *Sleep, 29*, 1396–1406.

Morin, C. M., Culbert, J. P., & Schwartz, S. M. (1994). Nonpharmacological interventions for insomnia: A meta-analysis of treatment efficacy. *The American Journal of Psychiatry, 151*, 1172–1180.

Morin, C. M., & Espie, C. A. (2003). *Insomnia: A clinical guide to assessment and treatment.* New York: Kluwer Academic/Plenum Press.

Morin, C. M., Stone, J., Trinkle, D., Mercer, J., & Remsberg, S. (1993). Dysfunctional beliefs and attitudes about sleep among older adults with and without insomnia complaints. *Psychology and Aging, 8*, 463–467.

Murtagh, D. R., & Greenwood, K. M. (1995). Identifying effective psychological treatments for insomnia: A meta-analysis. *Journal of Consulting and Clinical Psychology, 63*, 79–89.

National Institutes of Health. (2005, June). National Institutes of Health State of the Science Conference Statement: Manifestations and management of chronic insomnia in adults. *Sleep, 28*, 1049–1057.

Neitzert Semler, C., & Harvey, A. G. (2005). Misperception of sleep can adversely affect daytime functioning in insomnia. *Behaviour Research and Therapy, 43,* 843–856.

Ohayon, M. M., Caulet, M., Philip, P., Guilleminault, C., & Priest, R. G. (1997). How sleep and mental disorders are related to complaints of daytime sleepiness. *Archives of Internal Medicine, 157,* 2645–2652.

Perlis, M. L., & Lichstein, K. (Eds.). (2003). *Treating sleep disorders: Principles and practice of behavioral sleep medicine.* New York: Wiley.

Perlis, M. L., & Nielsen, T. A. (1993). Mood regulation, dreaming and nightmares: Evaluation of a desensitization function for REM sleep. *Dreaming, 3,* 243–257.

Perlis, M. L., Smith, L. J., Lyness, J. M., Matteson, S. R., Pigeon, W. R., Jungquist, C., et al. (2006). Insomnia as a risk factor for onset of depression in the elderly. *Behavioral Sleep Medicine, 4,* 104–113.

Pilcher, J. J., & Huffcutt, A. I. (1996). Effects of sleep deprivation on performance: A meta-analysis. *Sleep, 19,* 318–326.

Ree, M. J., & Harvey, A. G. (2004). Insomnia. In J. Bennett-Levy, G. Butler, M. Fennell, A. Hackman, M. Mueller, & D. Westbrook (Eds.), *Oxford guide to behavioural experiments in cognitive therapy* (pp. 287–305). Oxford, England: Oxford University Press.

Ree, M. J., Harvey, A. G., Blake, R., Tang, N. K. Y., & Shawe-Taylor, M. (2005). Attempts to control unwanted thoughts in the night: Development of the Thought Control Questionnaire-Insomnia Revised (TCQI-R). *Behaviour Research and Therapy, 43,* 985–989.

Riedel, B. W., & Lichstein, K. L. (2000). Insomnia and daytime functioning. *Sleep Medicine Reviews, 4,* 277–298.

Rombaut, N., Maillard, F., Kelly, F., & Hindmarch, I. (1990). The Quality of Life Insomniacs Questionnaire. *Medical Science Research, 18,* 845–847.

Roth, T., & Ancoli-Israel, S. (1999). Daytime consequences and correlates of insomnia in the United States: Results of the 1991 National Sleep Foundation Survey: II. *Sleep, 22*(Suppl. 2), S354–S358.

Rybarczyk, B., Lopez, M., Schelble, K., & Stepanski, E. (2005). Home-based video CBT for comorbid geriatric insomnia: A pilot study using secondary data analyses. *Behavioral Sleep Medicine, 3,* 158–175.

Saper, C. B., Cano, G., & Scammell, T. E. (2005). Homeostatic, circadian, and emotional regulation of sleep. *Journal of Comprehensive Neurology, 493,* 92–98.

Smith, M. T., Huang, M. I., & Manber, R. (2005). Cognitive behavior therapy for chronic insomnia occurring within the context of medical and psychiatric disorders. *Clinical Psychology Review, 25,* 559–592.

Spielman, A. J., Saskin, P., & Thorpy, M. J. (1987). Treatment of chronic insomnia by restriction of time in bed. *Sleep, 10,* 45–56.

Tang, N. K. Y., & Harvey, A. G. (2006). Altering misperception of sleep in insomnia: Behavioural experiments versus verbal explanation. *Journal of Consulting and Clinical Psychology, 74,* 767–776.

Van Dongen, H. P. A., Maislin, G., Mullington, J. M., & Dinges, D. F. (2003). The cumulative cost of additional wakefulness: Dose-response effects on neurobehavioral functions and sleep physiology from chronic sleep restriction and total sleep deprivation. *Sleep, 26*, 117–126.

Walker, M. P., Brakefield, T., Morgan, A., Hobson, J. A., & Stickgold, R. (2002). Practice with sleep makes perfect: Sleep-dependent motor skill learning. *Neuron, 35*, 205–211.

Watkins, E., & Baracaia, S. (2001). Why do people ruminate in dysphoric moods? *Personality and Individual Differences, 30*, 723–734.

Wegner, D. M., & Schneider, D. J. (1989). Mental control: The war of the ghosts in the machine. In J. S. Uleman & J. A. Bargh (Eds.), *Unintended thought* (pp. 287–305). New York: Guilford Press.

Wehr, T. A., Sack, D. A., & Rosenthal, N. E. (1987). Sleep reduction as a final common pathway in the genesis of mania. *The American Journal of Psychiatry, 144*, 201–204.

Wells, A. (1995). Meta-cognition and worry: A cognitive model of generalized anxiety disorder. *Behavioural and Cognitive Psychotherapy, 23*, 301–320.

Wicklow, A., & Espie, C. A. (2000). Intrusive thoughts and their relationship to actigraphic measurement of sleep: Towards a cognitive model of insomnia. *Behaviour Research and Therapy, 38*, 679–693.

Wu, J. C., & Bunney, W. E. (1990). The biological basis of an antidepressant response to sleep deprivation and relapse: Review and hypothesis. *The American Journal of Psychiatry, 147*, 14–21.

Yoo, S. S., Hu, P. T., Gujar, N., Jolesz, F. A., & Walker, M. P. (2007). A deficit in the ability to form new human memories without sleep. *Nature Neuroscience, 10*, 385–392.

14

ANGER

HOWARD KASSINOVE AND RAYMOND CHIP TAFRATE

Anger is a normal and a psychopathological emotional response. In that sense, it is similar to anxiety. Both are hard-wired, previously useful responses, which are part of humans' evolutionary history. They cannot be totally eliminated. Anger responses represent the "fight" side of the fight-or-flight reaction, and from a historical perspective, it was the wise animal that knew when to fight and when to flee. Of course, we now live in civilized societies, and responses in the fight spectrum are needed much less often for survival. Yet, strong anger reactions have persisted and are quite frequent. They become clinical problems when they are too frequent, too intense, or endure too long. In this chapter, we deal with the treatment of anger problems using typical anger reactions as a backdrop against which to judge clinically significant anger. Given that anger is an emergent area of research focus, this chapter covers fundamental aspects and recent research findings regarding this emotional state before discussing factors that lead to poorer treatment response.

To set the stage for understanding and reducing anger reactions from a cognitive–behavioral therapy (CBT) perspective, it is important to begin with a comprehensive definition and to differentiate anger from similar responses. This is critical because lay definitions of anger are often inadequate. For example, one online dictionary simply defines *anger* as "a strong feeling of displeasure or hostility" (Anger, n.d.b). This suggests that anger is strong and represents the same response as hostility. On a medically oriented dictionary Web site, *anger* is defined as "an emotional state that may range in intensity from mild irritation to intense fury and rage. Anger has physical effects including raising the heart rate and blood pressure and the levels of adrenaline and noradrenaline" (Anger, n.d.c). This limited definition suggests that anger is an emotion of variable intensity that causes physical effects. It makes no mention of its cognitive, motivational, or behavioral characteristics. Another definition suggests that *anger* is "a strong emotion; a feeling that is oriented toward some real or supposed grievance" (Anger, n.d.a). In this case, readers are left with the belief that an emotion and a feeling are the same phenomenon.

On the basis of interactions with the lay public, patients, and media reporters, it seems that the most common error related to definitional clarity is to consider anger as the equivalent of aggression. This seems to occur because aggression is often sensational (as in cases of assault and murder) and readily visible to others, whereas anger has private elements known only to the angry person.

In our work with adults (Kassinove & Tafrate, 2006a), we have considered anger to be a multidimensional construct that consists of a private awareness, motor behaviors, and physiological responses. We suggest the following definition:

> *Anger* is a negative feeling state that motivates desires for actions, usually against others, that aim to warn, intimidate, control, attack, or gain retribution. It is variable in terms of frequency, intensity, and duration and is associated with perceived injustices, cognitive distortions and misappraisals, morally based justice-oriented demands, global evaluations of others, and attributions of blame. As a personal experience, anger is subjectively labeled according to the language of the speaker and is often associated with thoughts about revenge and punishment, physiological changes, and patterns of behavior that define how to act when angry.

This definition begins with the private event and clearly places anger as an experience within the person. Whereas psychodynamic formulations assume that patients are often unaware of their repressed feelings, in CBT we believe that adults are typically aware of their anger and its various elements. Thus, anger is often brought up during verbal interactions with patients, and it can be reliably measured with paper-and-pencil tests. We are aware, of course, of the long and disappointing history of introspection as a scientific tool (Skinner, 1974) and the care that has to be taken when patients tell their life stories. Nevertheless, for CBT practitioners, verbal reports of anger often begin the chain of assessment and intervention activities.

Some parts of the anger construct consist of motor behaviors (e.g., waving a fist, throwing a book against a wall, taking a domineering physical posture, driving recklessly) that can easily be seen by others. These actions that intimidate or warn others about an agitated internal state can be reliably observed and measured. This is also true for verbal behaviors. We can count the number of times that patients use verbal threats, curse words, put-downs, and so forth. We can also measure the volume of the profanities and catalog the stimuli that elicit them. These motor behaviors are motivated by other, perhaps cognitive, elements of the internal feeling state.

Anger is also associated with moderate to strong hormonal and physiological changes. Persistent anger triggers are perceived as stressors and, as such, Selye's (1956, 1971, 1974) general adaptation syndrome can be evoked to explain part of the internal anger response. In his model, an alarm is first sounded (e.g., a threat to the marriage precipitated by an affair, repeated unfair evaluations by a supervisor at work) that leads to a mobilization of coping resources. This mobilization leads to autonomic system arousal, hormonal fluctuations, and neurochemical changes. The hypothalamic–pituitary–adrenal gland axis is energized, which results in the release of epinephrine, norepinephrine, and cortisol from the adrenal gland. The pituitary gland secretes adrenocorticotropic hormone ACTH, which in turn leads the adrenal cortex to secrete corticosteroids that result in increased access to energy stores and reductions in body inflammations. At the same time, there are increases in catecholamine in the adrenal medulla, which lead to increases in cardiovascular responding, respiration and perspiration, blood flow to active muscles, and strength and mental activity. During the second stage of resistance, people successfully cope with the stressor for some period of time. However, the cost of this coping is significant because of the depletion of bodily resources. It eventually leads to the final stage, exhaustion, when physical functioning deteriorates.

The specific effects of this process and of prolonged anger seem to be on a number of systems, including the cardiovascular, immune, digestive, and central nervous systems. Thus, prospective studies show that enduring anger is associated with stroke, hypertension, coronary artery disease, and perhaps even Type 2 diabetes (see Golden, Williams, Ford, & Yeh, 2006; Matthews, 2005; Williams et al., 2000; Williams, Nieto, Sanford, Couper, & Tyroler, 2002). However, the relationship of anger to cardiovascular problems may not be linear, as some studies find moderate anger expression to be protective (Eng, Fitzmaurice, & Kubzansky, 2003). No studies, to our knowledge, have found intense and enduring anger to be useful.

In a CBT model, anger experiences are associated with a variety of cognitive distortions about the triggering event or person. These include misappraisals about the importance of the event (e.g., "It's truly awful that my son lied to me," "It's absolutely terrible that he cheated on her") or about the capacity to cope (e.g., "I just can't deal with my son anymore," "I can't take her nonsense any more"). Because anger is a moral emotion, it is typically associated with justice-oriented demands (e.g., "She should treat her students fairly and with more respect," "She ought to watch what she says"). When adults are angry, they don't simply engage in conditional thinking (e.g., "Students will perform better if she treats them with more respect," "If he is careful with his words, then he is less likely to offend others"). Rather, they change their preferential ideas to those that are dogmatic and demand oriented. These demands are linked to evaluations of others (e.g., "Look at the way she acts. She's a real dope!"). In addition, when angry, adults often make overgeneralizations about the meaning of behaviors shown by others (e.g., "Since he didn't call me, it means he doesn't like me"), and they limit their options with dichotomous thinking (e.g., "Either he's my friend or he's not. It's just that simple! Is he with me or against me?"). These kinds of distortions are part of CBT models promoted by Ellis (1973, 1994) and A. T. Beck (1999) and have been supported empirically (Eckhardt, Barbour, & Davison, 1998; Kassinove & Eckhardt, 1993; Tafrate & Kassinove, 1998; Tafrate, Kassinove, & Dundin, 2002; Zwemer & Deffenbacher, 1984).

The cognitions exhibited by angry adults differentiate anger from anxiety and depression. With anger, there are typically attributions of blame that involve behavior that has already occurred (e.g., "He made me angry. It's his fault that I'm acting this way. Why don't you just fix him, Doc? Then, I would be calm"). In contrast, although anxiety attributions may be about other people (e.g., "My son frightens me when he yells at me"), they can also be about inanimate objects (e.g., "Elevators frighten me"), and they are future oriented. People rarely attribute their anger responses to elevators, supermarkets, tall buildings, and the like. Anger attributions are sometimes expanded to include beliefs about preventability and/or intentionality (e.g., "It's my boss who made me angry. If she had really thought about it, she would not have put me down in front of the other workers. I think she did it on purpose, just to show how important she is"). Anger is also associated with fantasies of revenge and punishment (e.g., "I'll teach her a lesson! I can really make her life miserable by working slowly. Then, *her* supervisor will yell at *her*").

Finally, anger can be purposely held in, controlled and reduced, or expressed outwardly. When it is expressed outwardly, it is associated with specific patterns of motor behavior that are either part of our evolutionary history or have been learned and reinforced. Thus, we know how to act in order to show our anger to others. These motor behaviors may include using a loud and intimidating voice, along with sarcastic or demeaning comments and the use of profanity. Angry behaviors include pointing fingers, glaring, crossing arms, smirking, stomping, and banging. Anger behaviors may also include physical aggression. In contrast, anger does not usually include singing, asking for forgiveness, smiling, placing a finger in the ear, and so on. The constellation of behaviors that define anger can be easily catalogued and are quite reliable.

Anger is also defined and differentiated by subjective and verbal labeling of the feeling (e.g., "I feel angry," "I feel annoyed," "I feel really pissed"). Patients may be able to verbally communicate the intensity of their personal anger through the use of different verbal labels, although this may require some clarification on the part of the practitioner.

EMPHASIZING STATES OVER TRAITS IN PRACTICE

Personality researchers often examine the role of traits as causal agents of human behavior. Traits, however, are hypothetical constructs that refer simply to the cross-situational stability of behaviors. They don't exist but, instead, are reference points for behaviors in multiple situations. For the clinician, it is more useful to consider individual behaviors that compose the anger syndrome. With regard to anger, the CBT clinician will typically consider it as a state of being at a moment in time. Patients bring in specific episodes of anger and ask for our help. We analyze the chain of events that led to the anger and develop an intervention plan based on the specific problem. Certainly, traits and hypothetical constructs have their utility and some paper-and-pencil tests (e.g., DiGiuseppe & Tafrate's 2004 Anger Disorders Scale, Novaco's 2003 Novaco Anger Scale and Provocation Inventory, Spielberger's 1999 State-Trait Anger Expression Inventory) assess them rather well. Unfortunately, traits are often used to both categorize and blame people for their anger and may be of little help in the psychotherapy office. Consider, for example, the statements in Table 14.1.

Trait-oriented statements are certainly useful in research, to determine whether there are group changes in relevant anger variables. However, they do not help us understand the unique situations that our patients experience and that they report in the consulting office. Traits simply label the person as having a certain degree of something. In contrast, state-oriented statements describe the specific problem and may lead to specific interventions by helping the CBT clinician understand the context of the anger.

USING PATIENT ANGER EPISODES TO GUIDE INTERVENTIONS

Anger episodes consist of various components that make up the larger chain of events. Interventions can be targeted at each part of the chain. For the CBT clinician, understanding the chain in context provides the best chance of developing a specific intervention.

In Kassinove and Tafrate's (2002) five-stage anger episode model (see Figure 14.1), the anger chain begins with a trigger. Most of the time, the trigger is objectively negative. Common triggers include real or perceived verbal insults (e.g., "You are just plain stupid"), neglect by friends or family

TABLE 14.1
Trait- and State-Oriented Anger Statements

Trait oriented	State oriented
"He's so hostile."	"His behavior this morning seemed to be hostile since he was ready to blame her before she told him what happened."
"She is an annoying person."	"I felt annoyed when she kept asking questions about my past."
"They tell me that I'm an angry person."	"They said I yelled and screamed when I received that poor evaluation at work."
"My brother said I'm a maniac."	"My brother said that yesterday when I was cut off by that other driver, I glared at him, flipped him the bird, and drove on his tail."
"He's like a wild dog that can't control itself."	"When he was fired, he showed intense anger and yelled at his children."
A clinician talking to a parent: "Your daughter Carmen scored quite high on trait anger. That means she likely gets angry really often."	A clinician talking to a parent: "Carmen seems to become angry when you ask her to come home by 10 p.m."
A clinician talking to an adult patient: "You scored at the 93rd percentile on the Anger Reactivity and Expression factor. This indicates anger pathology. When you become angry, you may react with verbal attacks or nasty responses."	A clinician talking to an adult patient: "I heard you say that when your boss loaded you with those new work responsibilities, you felt angry and told him to 'screw off.' I'd like to talk with you about better ways to handle your boss."
Report written about an unhappy factory worker: "Jane scored at the 90th percentile on the Vengeance factor. Thus, she may experience persistent thoughts about revenge and may seek retribution through physical, passive, indirect, or relational aggression. Her aggression often interferes with her functioning. Therefore, I do not recommend a promotion for her at this time."	Report written about an unhappy factory worker: "When I spoke to Jane about her unhappiness, she said she was denied a salary raise she thought she deserved. In response, she said she considered spreading a rumor that her boss was having an affair with his secretary. However, she was willing to discuss this problem further. Anger management counseling is recommended to help her become a better employee."
From a computer-generated report: "You frequently react in an angry way to life's many annoyances. You are substantially more irritable than the average person."	From a clinical interview: "John said he often wakes up feeling irritable and that it gets worse after he eats breakfast. I suggested that he switch to decaffeinated coffee to see if that helps."

members (e.g., as when a person is not invited to a cousin's wedding), rejections by lovers, memories of neglect or abuse, unfair negative feedback from supervisors, inconsiderate behavior by others (e.g., driving slowly in the fast

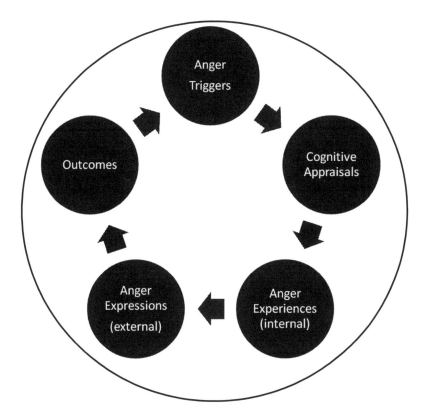

Figure 14.1. Kassinove and Tafrate's (2002) five-stage anger episode model. Adapted from *Anger Management: The Complete Treatment Guidebook for Practitioners* © 2002 by Howard Kassinove and Raymond Chip Tafrate. Reproduced for the American Psychological Association by permission of Impact Publishers, P.O. Box 6016, Atascadero, CA 93423-6016, http://www.impactpublishers.com. Further reproduction prohibited.

lane), failures at work or school, and so on. In some cases, the trigger is objectively neutral, as when a patient reported to us that he became furious when his wife asked him to blow his nose. Sometimes, anger can be triggered by a behavior that would be considered to be objectively positive. Consider, for example, the anger (and anxiety) that might emerge from repeated, unwanted compliments or from receiving unwanted flowers on a daily basis.

When considering an intervention plan, it is sometimes possible to work on changing the ways in which a person relates to an aversive trigger. The CBT practitioner might teach a parent or supervisor to give negative feedback in a more palatable manner, thus not eliciting a negative reaction that would start the anger chain. Or a person might be taught how to avoid aversive interactions with colleagues by writing an e-mail rather than by meeting face-to-face. Another example might be to have a patient avoid traffic jams by leaving earlier for work, thus eliminating the trigger.

In a purely stimulus–response (S-R) behavior therapy model (O'Donohue & Krasner, 1995), the trigger is thought to predict and control the occurrence of the anger response because of the consequences that follow. However, in the CBT model, it is thought that a stimulus is interpreted in some way so that its aversive magnitude is greatly increased. CBT practitioners believe that patients take neutral or moderately aversive events (e.g., "My wife seems uninterested in working more hours at her job") and misinterpret them in ways that lead to anger (e.g., "This is going to be a total disaster. We won't be able to afford buying a home. She lied to me about her intentions. What a bitch she is.").

What is the evidence for the CBT model? The CBT practitioner observes that adults have different responses to the same stimulus. When given poor feedback from a supervisor, for example, one person cries, another pouts and becomes angry, another plans revenge, and another quits the job. This observation is used to support the hypothesis that cognitive appraisals about the event are different (leading to different reactions). Thus, a successful intervention would help angry patients change their appraisals. Indeed, appraisals are the second stage in our anger episode model.

The CBT practitioner, however, may be wrong in this interpretation. Other factors may account for the variable responses to aversive stimuli both between and within patients. Simple conditioning (e.g., reinforcement, extinction, observational learning) may lead some to become angry when cut off on the highway, whereas others just ignore the other driver's behavior. Alternatively, people may be born with differing levels of autonomic system reactivity, and this may account for their native reactions to aversive stimuli and to the degree to which they are conditionable. Or patients may react with an intense anger response to a rejection that occurs when they are fatigued or have used alcohol, whereas they respond with less anger to a rejection that occurs when they are well rested.

These possibilities do not negate the hypothesis that it is cognitive interpretations that lead to anger reactions. The problem, rather, is that the entire field of CBT is built on introspection. Psychologists cannot actually assess cognitions. As a remedy, it has been suggested (Kassinove, 2007a, 2007b) that verbal behavior therapy would more correctly describe what CBT practitioners do. We listen to the patient's verbalizations, believe that they represent his or her thoughts, interpret them according to Ellis's (1973, 1994) or A. T. Beck's (1976) model, and modify the patient's verbalizations about the anger triggers.

Because there are a number of possible explanations that describe what may happen in CBT, the appraisal portion of the anger episode model remains a viable explanation. However, if it is wrong, then so-called difficult or refractory cases may not improve simply because we are spending too much time on cognitive restructuring and not enough time on well-supported, time-tested S-R behavior therapy interventions such as assertiveness training or relaxation training. Nonetheless, the theories of Ellis and A. T. Beck, as well as the developing literature on forgiveness, offer practitioners a range of intervention strategies that specifically target the appraisal stage of the model.

Anger experiences, the third stage of the model, are the personal, private events about which we are told by our patients. Anger-related physiological reactions may be perceived and described by patients as their subjective descriptions of intensity and duration. Relaxation and exposure interventions can both be useful in reducing the intensity of the internal experience.

Anger expression represents the fourth component of anger episodes. Here, we are talking about motor actions that can be seen by others. These include verbal behaviors such as a raised voice, accusatory content, name calling and direct personal insults, gossiping, nagging, expressions of hatred and contempt, sarcastic content, a harsh tone, and profanity. Gross motor behaviors that indicate anger include facial expressions, gestures, breaking objects, throwing objects, and hitting or kicking objects such as walls, automobile tires, or computers. These behavioral actions are responses to triggers that are appraised as frustrating, unfair, unwanted, wrong, and intolerable.

Anger can be expressed openly, controlled and reduced, or consciously held in (see Spielberger, 1999). When it is expressed openly, and others feel threatened, referrals to CBT professionals may come from the criminal justice system, marital partners, teachers, supervisors at a work setting, and so on. When it is held in and suppressed, it may show itself as skepticism and distrust of others, oppositional argumentativeness, resentment and envy, sullenness, cynicism, or even the adoption of a superior attitude. Alternatively, anger may not emerge at the conscious level. It may simply fester silently and lead to passive behaviors such as arriving late, not answering questions, and poor work or school performance. Interventions targeted at this stage of the model include social problem-solving, skills training, and assertiveness training.

The final stage of the model is outcomes, long-term and short-term. Some of these are positive, and along with our genetic fight-or-flight history, they account for the continuation of our anger responses because of their reinforcing properties that led to survival of the human species. Thus, anger may serve to alert us to problems. It may lead to better compliance by others with our wishes (as when a parent yells at a child) or an improved attention to, and understanding of, the position of another person during a discussion. Anger also adds a positive, zestful feeling to life. At the same time, some of the negative short-term outcomes are interpersonal conflicts, negative evaluations by others, verbal and physical assault, erratic driving, property destruction, occupational maladjustment, inappropriate risk taking, substance abuse, accidents, and physical injury to oneself. When anger continues over the years, negative long-term outcomes (e.g., ongoing relationship difficulties; disruption of career paths; the increased probability of hypertension, stroke, or other cardiovascular events) are more likely. Helping patients examine both the short- and long-term outcomes of their anger episodes is often a practical place to begin building awareness of the costs associated with anger.

MEASURING ANGER

As noted previously, the central core of anger is private. It consists of thoughts and appraisals about the triggering event, desires for retribution, and plans to make the outcome fair. In clinical practice, we are also interested in many behaviors that we do not or cannot observe in the consulting office. For example, we are interested in what the patient thinks about his or her coping ability, how often anger has occurred over the lifetime, and what triggers initiate anger episodes in a specific patient.

Although clinicians often rely on simple, narrative self-reports that can be presented by patients in an anger episode record (Kassinove & Tafrate, 2002), paper-and-pencil psychometric tests are also used to improve reliability that may be lacking in narratives. These measures still rely on introspection rather than observation. Yet, they are popular in practice and are linked to specific conceptions of anger. Three are worth noting.

Spielberger's (1999) State-Trait Anger Expression Inventory—2 (STAXI–2) measures anger from the perspective of states and traits. Adults with high trait anger become angry in response to many relatively mild negative stimuli, such as a slight insult, a small frustrating delay, lack of recognition, or any level of negative feedback. Persons high on trait anger are known as quick tempered, explosive, fiery, and hotheaded. Their anger emerges when interacting with a variety of others, such as peers or parents or children, colleagues, sales personnel, students, or strangers in anonymous environments such as buses or supermarkets. In addition to assessing this general propensity to become angry, the STAXI–2 asks for reports about specific angry states. Patients can be asked to recall a specific anger event and rate the intensity of their anger.

The theory underlying the STAXI–2 also notes that adults have a typical manner of dealing with anger. Anger-out expressers are people who argue and yell, are sarcastic, emit nasty put-downs, and throw or break objects. In contrast, some adults have a normative pattern of held-in anger. They are aware of their anger but do not show it to others. They ruminate and have long-term fantasies of revenge, but others do not generally know how angry they are. Finally, some people engage in constructive actions. They may try to breathe deeply or relax, or they may try to engage in private thinking or discussions with friends that increase tolerance and understanding. Support for the STAXI–2 model has been generally good (Deffenbacher, Oetting, & Thwaites, 1996; Forgays, Spielberger, & Ottaway, 1998; Lindqvist, Dåderman, & Hellström, 2003).

The Novaco Anger Scale and Provocation Inventory (NAS-PI; Novaco, 1975, 2003) is a second well-standardized, research-based, self-report instrument. On the basis of theory, it assesses a general tendency to respond with anger across three subscales. The cognitive subscale assesses the likelihood of ruminating about anger triggers, justifying personal anger reactions, and suspicious or hostile attitudes. The arousal subscale measures the intensity and duration of anger, as well as irritability and somatic tension. On the behavior subscale, items address a tendency to respond impulsively, to become verbally nasty, to physically confront others, and to indirectly express anger by smashing objects and so on. Central to Novaco's model, the scale also assesses anger-regulation strategies such as engaging in anger-reducing thoughts, calming down, and behaving constructively when provoked. With regard to provocations, respondents report "how true" it is that various trigger classes are likely to evoke anger. These potential provocations are disrespectful treatment, unfairness, frustration, annoying behaviors of others, and irritations such as being slowed down by another person's mistakes. The specificity of the Novaco scale makes it particularly useful for the clinician who wants to identify triggers, appraisals, experiences, and expressive patterns of anger. Again, research support for the Novaco scale has been positive (Jones, Thomas-Peter, & Trout, 1999; Mills, Kroner, & Forth, 1998).

Finally, DiGiuseppe and Tafrate (2004) developed the Anger Disorders Scale (ADS) to measure clinically relevant dimensions of anger. A total anger score is based on items from five domains that are thought to represent different aspects of human emotion. These are provocations, cognitions, arousal, motives, and behaviors. *Provocations* refers to the scope of triggers and may be helpful for the CBT practitioner who wants to differentiate situationally limited anger (e.g., that might only appear within the family) from anger that is more generalized. The items also assess disrespect and social rejection as specific, narrow-scope anger triggers. In the arousal domain, reported physiological arousal as well as length of the episode and the duration of anger problems are assessed. As noted elsewhere (DiGiuseppe & Tafrate, 2007), duration of clinical problems is important, because a *Diagnostic and Statistical Manual of Mental Disorders* (DSM–IV–TR; 4th ed., text rev.; American Psychiatric Association, 2000) criterion for some emotional disorders is that they have to exist for 6 months or longer. Anger episode length is also important as adults higher on trait anger show longer episode lengths and, thus, are likely to suffer more negative consequences (Deffenbacher, Oetting, Lynch, & Morris, 1996; Tafrate, Kassinove, & Dundin, 2002). In the cognitions domain, suspiciousness, resentment, impulsivity, and rumination are assessed. Impulsivity, or the lack of thoughtful delay in responding, has been conceptualized for a long time to be part of the anger response and is part of various anger control programs, in particular by building in a relaxation component (Deffenbacher & McKay, 2000; Feindler, 2005; Kassinove & Tafrate, 2002; Novaco, 1975). It is interesting that although the cognitions domain of the scale was intended to reflect both attitudinal and appraisal aspects of anger episodes, items that assess stimulus appraisals according to Ellis's (1973, 1994) and A. T. Beck's (1976) theories are absent. Such items did not successfully load on the proposed factors and were not retained on the scale. In the motives domain, characteristics such as a desire for revenge and using anger to reduce tension or for coercion of others are examined. Finally, the behaviors domain includes engaging in aversive verbal behavior and acting with aggression.

Each of these measures has strengths and weaknesses. In particular, each allows for quick, psychometrically sound assessments across a wide age range. On the other hand, the STAXI–2 does not follow an anger episode model, which makes it less useful for the CBT practitioner, the ADS measures traits but not states, and both the NAS-PI and the ADS do not follow A. T. Beck's and Ellis's theories, which are practiced by many CBT clinicians.

Although standardized measures add much to our understanding, it is the anger state within an individual anger episode that is typically brought into the clinician's office. Richer information for the CBT practitioner may be obtained by an individualized, clinical analysis of specific anger episodes. For this reason, the anger episode model can be paired with anger episode analysis self-monitoring forms, which can add much to clinical work (Kassinove & Tafrate 2002). In this model, patients consider specific anger episodes and analyze them with their CBT practitioner to examine triggers, appraisals, experiences, expressive actions, and outcomes. For practitioners, we recommend using both standardized and idiographic approaches to assessment.

ANGER IN THE CURRENT DIAGNOSTIC SYSTEM

Effective treatment is based on reasonable and agreed-upon classification of a patient's problem. Clinicians require criteria to help them distinguish normal and adaptive anger from disruptive anger. Failure of a CBT intervention program may not be a function of a "difficult patient" but of misdiagnosis.

Unfortunately, neither the *DSM–IV–TR* (American Psychiatric Association, 2000) nor the *International Classification of Diseases* (ICD-10; World Health Organization, 1992) contains any diagnoses in which anger is the primary problem. As DiGiuseppe and Tafrate (2004) wrote, the "*DSM–IV–TR* fails to address the presence of anger consistently or systematically. Anger is mentioned only as a symptom that occasionally appears across divergent disorders" (p. 2). Similar conclusions were reached in 1995 by Eckhardt and Deffenbacher when they examined the 1994 version of the *DSM–IV* (American Psychiatric Association, 1994). They wrote, little progress has been evidenced in the assessment of anger in what is the most common form of clinical measurement—*diagnosis*. The most obvious indication that contemporary psychology and psychiatry have neglected anger as a clinically-relevant problem is the absence of a diagnostic category with anger as the central and defining feature. (p. 35)

Eckhardt and Deffenbacher (1995) noted that on Axis I, the *DSM–IV* contained 11 anxiety-related disorders and 9 mood-related disorders. However, none were available for parallel conditions of chronic, moderate, and pervasive anger. For example, categories existed for situational anxiety reactions (i.e., phobias) but not for situational anger reactions. This might refer to the intense anger that occurs in the presence of criticism at home or at work. In the *DSM–IV–TR* (American Psychiatric Association, 2000), anger symptoms appear only as part of other Axis I and Axis II diagnoses such as generalized anxiety disorder, posttraumatic stress disorder (PTSD), borderline personality disorder, antisocial personality disorder, and manic phases of bipolar disorder. Although anger is recognized as important in Axis III problems, such as high blood pressure, stroke, and cardiovascular disease, it is considered as one of the many possible symptoms of these disorders. Of interest is the observation that all of the previously mentioned disorders may be diagnosed without anger. Thus, anger is not a necessary component of any current diagnoses. The same situation exists with regard to the ICD-10.

If clinicians working with angry patients must use the *DSM*, they have to approximate the problem and will most likely use the category of intermittent explosive disorder (IED; Lachmund, DiGiuseppe, & Fuller, 2005). However, the criteria for IED include inability to resist aggressive impulses and engaging in violent assaults or the destruction of property. For the CBT practitioner, impulses represent an unmeasurable, hypothetical construct, an especially problematic issue for applied behavior analysts. In addition, the latter criterion of engaging in assaults or destruction rules out patients who hold their anger in, ruminate for years about perceived mistreatment and injustice, become sullen and noncooperative with others, and eventually develop medical problems such as heart disease or stroke.

Because official attention has not been paid to this problem, some researchers have generated anger diagnoses that they hope will be included in future revisions of diagnostic systems. Eckhardt and Deffenbacher (1995), for example, proposed five anger diagnoses that reflect the general or situational nature of the anger, as well as whether aggression was also present. A criterion used by Eckhardt and Deffenbacher to make an anger diagnosis centers on the adaptive versus the disruptive nature of a patient's anger. For example, it would have to be evident that the anger disrupts social, work, or school activities; impairs interpersonal relationships; and/or causes significant personal distress. The following are their anger diagnoses: (a) adjustment disorder with angry mood, (b) situational anger disorder without aggression, (c) situational anger disorder with aggression, (d) general anger disorder without aggression, and (e) general anger disorder with aggression.

More recently, DiGiuseppe and Tafrate (2007) proposed diagnostic criteria for an anger regulation-expression disorder. Similar to that of Eckhardt and Deffenbacher (1995), the diagnosis could not be made unless the anger experiences had negative and lasting effects on important areas of life functioning. In this model, patients can meet the criteria for an anger disorder through several paths: (a) predominately subjective type, (b) predominately expressive type, or (c) combined type. The subjective subtype emphasizes the internal emotional experience. Patients can meet the criteria by experiencing anger episodes that are intense, frequent, or long lasting but with moderate or low levels of expressive or aggressive behaviors. The second type calls attention to verbally expressive behaviors and aggressive reactions associated with anger experiences. The outward reactions associated with anger are the main focus. Finally, the third subtype is for patients who meet the criteria for both the subjective and expressive subtypes. Intense and frequent internal anger experiences along with expressive patterns that are associated with poor outcomes characterize this proposed diagnosis.

COMORBIDITY

Another issue that may affect treatment relates to comorbidity. Patients treated by CBT practitioners may not be simply difficult or refractory types. Rather, treatment effectiveness may be impaired by other problems. Certainly, anger problems exist as independent phenomena. Nevertheless, addressing problematic anger reactions may be just one step in an overall treatment plan. Disordered anger may overlap with many other disorders. Kassinove and Tafrate (2006b) provided a data set of scores from the Millon Clinical Multiaxial Inventory (MCMI–III) for high-trait anger (HTA) and low-trait anger (LTA) adults from a community sample (n = 87). Their first finding was that greater overall levels of psychopathology were found among the HTA subjects. In terms of specific patterns, HTA subjects reported significantly more drug and alcohol problems and generalized anxiety. Anxiety appeared to be more prevalent than mood related symptoms. A second data set that examined anger and comorbidity patterns was reported by DiGiuseppe and Tafrate (2007) and was obtained from 25 patients who sought therapy for anger-related problems. Therapists and patients completed a computer-based program to determine DSM diagnoses. Again, the largest comorbid group included patients with a history of substance abuse. A second group displayed significant symptoms of attention-deficit/hyperactivity disorder as adults. This sample reported more overlapping mood difficulties compared with anxiety problems.

Returning to Kassinove and Tafrate's (2006b) MCMI–III data, it was also found that HTA adults presented with a wide range of Axis II profiles. The HTA group was not captured by any one personality disorder. Rather, there was overlap with antisocial, borderline, dependent, narcissistic, and paranoid personalities. Patterns not formally part of the current diagnostic systems also emerged as common in HTA adults. For example, the negativistic pattern on the MCMI–III corresponds to the *DSM–IV–TR* passive–aggressive personality disorder (American Psychiatric Association, 2000) and was among the most common experienced by HTA adults. These individuals experience periods of explosive anger or stubbornness intermingled with guilt, disappointment, and passive resistance to demands for adequate performance.

DiGiuseppe and Tafrate (2007) used their data set from an outpatient sample ($n = 230$) to examine correlations between personality patterns using the MCMI–III and scores on ADS. The highest correlations were found between ADS scores and passive–aggressive personality disorder. Borderline, sadistic, paranoid, schizotypal, and antisocial produced the next highest correlations. Because anger is a core symptom of borderline personality, this finding was not surprising. Sadistic and antisocial are among the most aggressive personality patterns, and their association with anger was also not unexpected.

The presence of personality pathology may influence the way therapists interact with patients and the types of interventions used in treatment. Patients with a paranoid personality disorder, for example, might require greater focus on the therapeutic relationship in addition to specific anger reduction techniques. Antisocial patients, given their typical continuing history of problems, may do better with decision-making strategies that emphasize long-term consequences, such as social problem solving. Dependent patients, who typically cling and seem primed to misinterpret the actions of others, may require greater focus on angry thoughts related to friends, family members, and colleagues who do not meet their strongly perceived desires. Finally, borderline patients may benefit from a broader, long-term approach that emphasizes stability in relationships.

We recognize the limitations that exist in the data sets described above. More extensive research examining larger samples across different settings would allow for stronger conclusions. Because angry patients are likely to present with a wide range of both Axis I and Axis II pathology, screening to detect other disorders seems warranted.

EFFECTIVE TREATMENT PROGRAMS

A number of treatment programs that are based on scholarly works currently exist for the CBT practitioner to follow. Modern programs owe much to the pioneering research by Novaco (1975), who, working with 34 adults, showed that cognitive control procedures could be used to regulate anger arousal. His recent works have centered on the treatment of adults with dysregulated anger (Novaco, 2007), anger in adults with developmental disabilities (Taylor & Novaco, 2005), the role of anger in combat-related PTSD (Novaco & Chemtob, 2002), and anger in offender populations (Novaco, Ramm, & Black, 2000).

Some of the available treatment programs are session-by-session and manual focused (e.g., Deffenbacher & McKay, 2000; Reilly & Shopshire, 2002), whereas others are menu based and clinically driven, allowing for flexibility by the practitioner (e.g., Kassinove & Tafrate, 2002; Tafrate & Kassinove, 2006). Some programs have been developed for persons with general anger disorders (e.g., Deffenbacher & McKay, 2000; Kassinove & Tafrate, 2002, 2006a), whereas others are customized for specific populations (e.g., Reilly & Shopshire's 2002 program is tailored to substance abusers; Feindler's 1995, 2005 program is for adolescents). Williams and Williams (1994) have focused on the negative medical outcomes of anger, whereas other programs focus simply on the techniques necessary to reduce anger. Anger is also addressed in many popular books, which are often based on limited evidence (for an evidence-based self-help program, see Tafrate & Kassinove, 2009). What, then, makes for a good intervention program? Although it is beyond the scope of this chapter to review all of the evidence, the majority of programs contain similar elements.

First, it seems to be important to create awareness among those entering, referred, or coerced into treatment that they indeed have an anger problem and would benefit from an anger management program. Many people seem unaware of the extent of their anger. Particularly if they are high on the trait of anger, or have been brought up in a discordant family, they think that everyone is angry much of the time. They may normalize their experiences and reactions. Thus, good intervention programs begin by building awareness of anger. This can occur by giving standardized tests and providing feedback that indicates that the patient's self-reported anger is very high by comparison with that of others. Motivational interviewing strategies are also useful in the engagement process. However it is done, building awareness of the costs associated with anger is the first step in successful interventions.

Second, awareness is followed by the development of personal responsibility for the anger. Most adults blame others for their anger. Common statements heard in the office are, "My kids make me so angry" or "My wife continually pisses me off" or "Those other drivers infuriate me." Following anger awareness, therefore, effective programs develop a sense that we are all (at least partially) in control of our own emotional reactions. Unless there is awareness of anger and acceptance of personal control, treatment failure is likely. Although some models for successful engagement and motivational enhancement for angry patients have been presented elsewhere (DiGiuseppe,

Tafrate, & Eckhardt, 1994; Tafrate & Kassinove, 2003), a scientific literature on this topic has yet to be developed.

Third, once the patient is on board, the literature has provided a number of effective interventions for the CBT practitioner to use. Some involve simple instructions to remove patients from aversive situations and are based on avoidance or escape maneuvers. Many programs have elements related to relaxation or meditation and are geared toward helping patients reduce arousal. Given the current focus on cognitive mechanisms, it is not surprising that most programs have intervention elements based on the premise that anger is caused by inappropriate thinking. The goal of these interventions is to help patients reduce patterns of catastrophic thinking, to improve beliefs about their ability to cope, to view the perceived transgressions of others in a more accurate manner, and to understand the differences between desires and demands. In each case, the goal is to give patients appropriate language skills to think about anger triggers. Some form of assertiveness training is also central to anger management programs because the belief is that anger would diminish and conflict resolution would increase with more appropriate expression of emotion. CBT practitioners have recognized that some problems that have led to anger can be effectively resolved, leading to better functioning, whereas others cannot be resolved because the offending person may be uninterested in working on the problem or may even have died. Abusers, for example, may be in prison and uninterested in admitting their role in harmful actions. Victims are left to manage their ongoing anger without being able to express their feelings to those who caused them harm. In these cases, anger management programs have modules geared toward acceptance and forgiveness interventions. Finally, given the likelihood that patients will reexperience anger, some attention is usually paid to relapse prevention strategies.

Fortunately, on the basis of four meta-analytic reviews (R. Beck & Fernandez, 1998; DiGiuseppe & Tafrate, 2003; Edmondson & Conger, 1996; Tafrate, 1995), there is evidence that anger management programs for adults are reasonably effective. In the majority of studies, treated research subjects showed moderate to large improvement when compared with untreated controls. Approaches that emerged with empirical support include cognitive, relaxation-based, skills training, and multicomponent interventions. A single CBT approach for anger management has not emerged as the treatment of choice. Rather, an assortment of CBT techniques has begun to form the foundation of an evidence-based approach. For example, most studies that used cognitive interventions focused on a self-instructional training model (Meichenbaum, 1985; Novaco, 1975). Several investigations showed support for Ellis's (1973, 1994) rational-emotive behavior therapy model, and the cognitive therapy model as formulated by A. T. Beck (1976). Thus, there is optimism about these approaches (Deffenbacher, Dahlen, Lynch, Morris, & Gowensmith, 2000; Tafrate & Kassinove, 1998).

FACTORS THAT LEAD TO A POOR RESPONSE TO TREATMENT

What, then, accounts for the observation that some patients do not improve? On the basis of our review of the field, we note that there are some clear roadblocks to successful anger treatment. These include a lack of awareness of the dysfunctionality of personal anger reactions and the associated low motivation for change. Even when there is awareness and motivation, establishing a therapeutic relationship can sometimes be difficult if patients see themselves as being coerced into treatment. We also note that cognitive challenges to irrational and dysfunctional beliefs, a common element in anger intervention programs, are easily viewed as invalidating to patients. Patient responses to irrational thinking challenges are often met with statements such as, "You seem to be in my wife's corner" or "You don't understand how difficult it is." Other causes of a poor response to anger management interventions include the presence of co-morbidity problems that are common in practice. Clinical outcome research is often based on pure cases, whereas CBT clinicians see highly complex cases that are likely to present personal and diagnostic issues that distract from, or interfere with, treatment.

In our experience, it also seems true that CBT has become a wastebasket category that many untrained clinicians use. Although the issue of therapist competence in experimental studies is often addressed, it is not typically done in clinic, criminal justice, or private practice settings. In case notes, therapists simply note that they did assertiveness training or systematic desensitization or cognitive restructuring with no check on how well it was done. Most CBT techniques require precise administration, and some, such as barb exposure (Tafrate & Kassinove, 1998) require careful training. The education, training, and skills of practitioners who routinely deliver anger treatment across diverse settings vary considerably. We believe that lack of training and effective administration of the anger management procedures is a clear reason for some treatment failures.

Finally, we note that in this era of managed care, almost everyone's public goal has been to provide short-term efficient treatment. Relatively few clinicians are currently willing to admit that they practice long-term psychotherapy. That leads to the question of how many sessions of anger management are required for effective intervention. Research studies typically use 8 to 12 sessions in their protocols. However, they use selected cases with less severe comorbid problems. Both of the present authors work with court-mandated anger management cases, and they seem to us to be quite different from what is described in the scientific literature. In our cases, common triggers are perceived disrespect by a lover or spouse, or an argument that ensues about property issues. The anger is often expressed by yelling and cursing, accompanied by a violent outburst. Patients often have long histories of anger problems that began in their adolescent years. After a judge requires 8 to 15 sessions of anger management as an alternative to incarceration, patients often come into treatment justifying and minimizing their anger reactions. In one recent case, a probationer told us, "I didn't do nothing wrong. She just exploded and came running at me with a box cutter. She tripped and cut her own ear off." In another case, a probationer told us that during an argument a woman was swinging her cell phone and she hit herself in the head. Then she said, "I got put on probation even though I did nothing to her." These cases often fail because the patient spends much of the time trying to convince the therapist that there is no anger problem.

We have made the case that anger is part of the fight-or-flight reaction and, thus, it can never be totally eliminated. At the same time, its expression is partially learned and can likely be modified by CBT interventions. But how many sessions are required in true clinical work? We often ask students the following question: "Consider that you want to teach a well-adjusted English-speaking adult from New York to speak Portuguese. How far would you get in 8 to 15 sessions?" The reader can also answer this question. When anger-evoking language, attitudes, ideas, and so forth have been ingrained for 25, 35, or 55 years, it is almost impossible to make changes in a short period of time.

When presented with the learning of Portuguese question, students often ask if the learning will occur in a group or individual setting. They think that learning in a group is easier because of the opportunity for interpersonal practice. Unfortunately, group interventions for anger, which are very common, also offer the opportunity for participants to practice and learn bad responses from each other. What they seem to learn best is how to justify their ideas and to normalize their angry and aggressive behaviors. Simply being in group treatment may lead to a poor outcome. In fact, group CBT interventions have been shown to be iatrogenic (Dishion, McCord, & Poulin, 1999; Poulin, Dishion, & Burraston, 2001).

CASE EXAMPLE

Mark, age 44, came into treatment as a self-referral. His goal was to better manage anger in order to have a more peaceful marriage and home life. He readily acknowledged that anger had been a long-term problem, and his standardized test scores confirmed that view. He scored above 75% on the ADS expression/reactivity score. Mark had gone through a difficult divorce 3 years earlier, and he described his previous marriage as full of conflict. Somewhat surprisingly, Mark's ex-wife did not wish to retain custody of their two children (an 11-year-old boy and a 7-year-old girl), and Mark became the custodial parent.

Six months before arriving in treatment Mark had married Kim. Kim had also been through a difficult divorce, and she had a 6-year-old daughter from that marriage. Unfortunately, her custody battle with her ex-husband was still ongoing. Kim reported that the reason she left her first marriage was that her ex-husband was frequently verbally and physically abusive. After their marriage, Mark and Kim moved in together, along with their respective children.

Individual treatment began well, with Mark having some awareness of the negative consequences associated with his anger reactions. However, as he began to discuss his anger episodes in sessions, it soon became clear that he blamed Kim and her behavior for their problems. Good awareness did not translate into a sense of personal responsibility for his anger reactions.

Mark complained bitterly that the children did not get along with each other and that constant bickering was the norm. To make matters worse, his son showed dislike and disrespect for Kim. However, in Mark's view, Kim did not show enough patience with the boy and had too much of an obvious preference for her own daughter. This was another example of Mark blaming Kim for his anger. Kim was also preoccupied with her ongoing legal situation and feared losing custody of her daughter. Mark complained that much of her energy was still focused on the ex-husband and not on their current marriage. The ongoing legal battle was also creating financial stress due to the mounting attorney's fees. From Mark's perspective, he had plenty of reasons to be angry.

Attempts to build anger management skills, such as relaxation, improved problem solving and decision making, and assertive responses, did not succeed. This seemed to be mostly attributable to Mark's belief that his anger was completely justified and morally appropriate. Thus, he would rarely practice the skills rehearsed in treatment. Rather, he would spend much of his time fuming about Kim's behaviors. After seven sessions, Mark insisted that Kim join him in treatment. She was agreeable, and the sessions became refocused on the couple.

Once Kim became involved in the sessions, it became clear that she was also angry. Her standardized assessment indicated high anger, generalized anxiety, and PTSD symptoms. In addition, it was revealed that she drank heavily at home in order to deal with anxiety about losing custody of her daughter. During the couples sessions, she often reacted strongly to minor disagreements. This set the stage for Mark to react angrily. Thus, the cycle of anger, resentment, and verbal arguing continued.

Attempts to build new skills to help them respond to each other in more effective ways failed. The ongoing chaos of the marriage and household ensured that the time in sessions was focused repeatedly on the most urgent "crisis of the week" and damage control. After nine couples sessions it was agreed that treatment was not helping to restore peace in the marriage. With the full agreement of the couple and the therapist, the case was transferred to another practitioner who specialized in troubled marriages.

This case failed for a number of reasons. In the first phase of treatment with Mark, not enough time was spent building his motivation to change.

Mark's awareness about the destructive impact of his anger was enough to make him seek treatment but was not sufficient for him to follow through and practice new CBT skills. This seemed clear in retrospect, but not at the time of treatment. Mark's justification for his anger reactions was also an obstacle. Low motivation meant that new skills were not practiced to the point at which they produced tangible benefits. A second problem had to do with the chaotic nature of the environment and the number of practical problems that emerged each week. It takes a certain amount of stability to learn and practice new CBT skills. These skills are less likely to be mastered in an unstable home environment that is filled with daily conflicts.

Adding Kim to treatment made the situation more chaotic and the sessions nonproductive. In addition to anger, she had comorbid PTSD, anxiety, and substance use problems. It would have been better to have her focus independently, with her own practitioner, on those issues. Couples counseling was certainly important, but it would likely have been more productive after the partners learned to handle their own emotional reactions.

Other reasons for failure included a limited number of sessions (16) for a couple with complex problems (e.g., anxiety, financial problems, legal concerns, physical abuse, PTSD, substance abuse, three children to care for) and Mark's inability to overcome his blaming orientation. Finally, there is the age-old clinical issue of attempting to do couples work after seeing one of the partners in psychotherapy. The partner added to the sessions often wonders whether the therapist's allegiance is to the original partner.

In hindsight, several additional components would have likely improved the treatment for Mark's anger. Instead of attempting to build anger management skills at the start, initial treatment sessions could have focused more on building awareness, motivation, and commitment to change. Establishing a greater awareness of the costs associated with his anger reactions and being able to envision a better way of interacting with Kim might have been better preliminary goals, after which active behavior change strategies would follow.

The motivational interviewing approach developed by Miller and Rollnick (2002) is a useful way to engage adults who, on the one hand, recognize the personal costs connected with their anger and yet, at the same time, feel justified in their excessive reactions. Early sessions might have explored Mark's reasons for continuing with his usual anger patterns as well as developing reasons to bring his anger under better control. The responsibility for articulating a rationale for less anger and improved conflict resolution behaviors would be left to Mark, hopefully changing the decisional balance toward wanting to change. An approach that emphasizes reflective statements (e.g., "Sounds like your kids are really suffering with all of the conflict in the house"; "So, developing a more peaceful home life is an important goal for you") and open-ended questions (e.g., "What is at stake if you don't change your anger?"; "What are the best reasons for you to work on new ways of responding to Kim?") would have allowed Mark to solidify his own arguments for anger reduction and improve his commitment to learning and practicing new skills in the next phase of treatment.

Another additional treatment component might have focused on fostering a forgiving attitude about some of the behaviors that routinely triggered Mark's anger. Mark spent a good deal of time recalling negative interactions and rehearsing his perceptions of unfair treatment. This, in turn, led to continued high emotional arousal and self-defeating behaviors. Forgiveness interventions would have included perspective taking exercises to help him adopt understanding, compassion, and good will toward Kim and her daughter. Our five-stage treatment model of forgiveness consists of uncovering anger, making a direct and thoughtful decision to forgive, defining forgiveness, understanding why others behave poorly, and giving something of value to the wrongdoer to help that client move out of the victim role (Kassinove & Tafrate, 2002; Tafrate & Kassinove, 2009).

In Mark's situation, we would spend time acknowledging his frustration related to Kim's behaviors. We would ask him to consider forgiveness as a path to allow him to let go of the past and move forward, in order to achieve his goal of creating a calmer and happier home life. Forgiveness would then be discussed further and differentiated from related concepts such as forgetting, excusing, condoning, and justifying. Mark would be asked to verbally elaborate about daily home life from Kim's perspective (e.g., her previous abusive marriage, concerns about losing custody of her child) and to help him develop an understanding of why she acted as she did. Finally, Mark would be asked to suggest ways to be giving toward Kim, in order to create good will in their relationship. Readers interested in video demonstrations of motivational interviewing and forgiveness interventions for the reduction of anger are directed to Kassinove and Tafrate (2007).

CONCLUSIONS AND FUTURE DIRECTIONS

Treatment concerns about anger-related disorders are unique because of the lack of official *DSM* or ICD-10 anger disorders. Until we add anger diagnoses to our classification systems, with inclusionary and exclusionary criteria, we will be unsure of the exact phenomenon being considered across research studies and clinical case reports. This is not meant to indicate that a formal diagnosis will ensure appropriate treatment, as this may occur with a proper functional analysis of anger problems. Rather, the goal of adding anger diagnoses is to build awareness of anger as a possible central problem in patients who present in clinics, hospitals, criminal justice settings, and private practices. Acceptance of primary anger diagnoses will also increase research funding so that we can better understand internal and externally expressed anger. This would likely lead to the development of empirically supported intervention programs.

At present, it is probable that practitioners treat clinical problems with techniques with which they feel comfortable. Frontline clinicians continue, in our judgment, to engage in descriptive analyses and trait-oriented interventions. The future for anger-disordered adults, we believe, is likely to be improved with greater use of an anger-episode model. There are usually many anger events in the patient's life, each beginning with a trigger and ending with an outcome. CBT practitioners would be wise to return to their original learning theory roots and to focus on concepts such as trials to criterion. What is the anger trigger? How frequent, intense, and enduring is the anger response? What better response is desirable for patients who often reside in chaotic environments and who may have a variety of comorbid problems? What empirically validated techniques are likely to lead to that better response? How many trials are required to achieve the better response? And, it is certainly wise for clinicians to self-monitor and ask if they are qualified to administer the empirically supported procedures or if continuing professional education is called for.

If there is but one conclusion we would like the reader to take away from this chapter, it is this: Anger is part of the evolutionarily useful, fight-or-flight reaction. In cases of disordered or excessive anger, it generally cannot be treated with short-term 10- or 15-session solutions. Truly successful CBT for anger problems is likely to be based on the systematic application of empirically supported techniques for the modification (not elimination) of maladaptive reactions to aversive triggers. The reader will likely notice the similarity of our recommendation to Wolpe's (1969) original definition of behavior therapy.

REFERENCES

American Psychiatric Association. (1994). *Diagnostic and statistical manual of mental disorders* (4th ed.). Washington, DC: Author.

American Psychiatric Association. (2000). *Diagnostic and statistical manual of mental disorders* (4th ed., text rev.). Washington, DC: Author.

Anger. (n.d.a). In *Die.net online dictionary*. Retrieved March 11, 2009, from http://dict.die.net/anger

Anger. (n.d.b). In *The free dictionary*. Retrieved March 11, 2009, from http://www.thefreedictionary.com/anger

Anger. (n.d.c). In *MedicineNet.com*. Retrieved March 11, 2009, from http://www.medterms.com/script/main/art.asp?articlekey=33843

Beck, A. T. (1976). *Cognitive therapy and the emotional disorders*. New York: International Universities Press.

Beck, A. T. (1999). *Prisoners of hate: The cognitive bases of anger, hostility, and violence.* New York: HarperCollins.

Beck, R., & Fernandez, E. (1998). Cognitive–behavioral therapy in the treatment of anger: A meta-analysis. *Cognitive Therapy and Research, 22,* 63–74.

Deffenbacher, J. L., Dahlen, E. R., Lynch, R. S., Morris, C. D., & Gowensmith, W. N. (2000). Application of Beck's cognitive therapy to general anger reduction. *Cognitive Therapy and Research, 24,* 689–697.

Deffenbacher, J. L., & McKay, M. (2000). *Overcoming situational and general anger.* Oakland, CA: New Harbinger.

Deffenbacher, J. L., Oetting, E. R., Lynch, R. S., & Morris, C. D. (1996). The expression of anger and its consequences. *Behaviour Research and Therapy, 34,* 575–590.

Deffenbacher, J. L., Oetting, E. R., & Thwaites, G. A. (1996). State-trait anger theory and the utility of the Trait Anger Scale. *Journal of Counseling Psychology, 43,* 131–148.

DiGiuseppe, R., & Tafrate, R. (2003). Anger treatment for adults: A meta-analytic review. *Clinical Psychology: Science and Practice, 10,* 70–84.

DiGiuseppe, R., & Tafrate, R. C. (2004). *Anger Disorders Scale.* New York: Multi-Health Systems.

DiGiuseppe, R., & Tafrate, R. (2007). *Understanding anger disorders.* New York: Oxford University Press.

DiGiuseppe, R., Tafrate, R., & Eckhardt, C. (1994). Critical issues in the treatment of anger. *Cognitive and Behavioral Practice, 1,* 111–132.

Dishion, T. J., McCord, J., & Poulin, F. (1999). When interventions harm: Peer groups and problem behavior. *American Psychologist, 54,* 755–764.

Eckhardt, C. I., Barbour, K. A., & Davison, G. C. (1998). Articulated thoughts of maritally violent and nonviolent men during anger arousal. *Journal of Consulting and Clinical Psychology, 66,* 259–269.

Eckhardt, C. I., & Deffenbacher, J. L. (1995). Diagnosis of anger disorders. In H. Kassinove (Ed.), *Anger disorders: Definition, diagnosis, and treatment* (pp. 27–48). Washington, DC: Taylor & Francis.

Edmondson, C. B., & Conger, J. C. (1996). A review of treatment efficacy for individuals with anger problems: Conceptual, assessment, and methodological issues. *Clinical Psychology Review, 16,* 251–275.

Ellis, A. E. (1973). *Humanistic psychotherapy.* New York: McGraw-Hill.

Ellis, A. E. (1994). *Reason and emotion in psychotherapy: Revised and updated.* New York: Carol.

Eng, P. M., Fitzmaurice, G., & Kubzansky, L. D. (2003). Anger expression and risk of stroke and coronary heart disease among male health professionals. *Psychosomatic Medicine, 65,* 100–110.

Feindler, E. L. (1995). "Ideal" treatment package for children and adolescents with anger disorders. In H. Kassinove (Ed.), *Anger disorders: Definition, diagnosis, and treatment* (pp. 173–196). Washington, DC: Taylor & Francis.

Feindler, E. L. (2005). CBT and adolescent anger management. In *Encyclopedia of cognitive behavior therapy* (Vol. 8, pp. 11–14). New York: Kluwer Academic.

Forgays, D. K., Spielberger, C. D., & Ottaway, S. A. (1998). Factor structure of the State-Trait Anger Expression Inventory for middle-aged men and women. *Assessment, 2,* 141–155.

Golden S. H., Williams, J. E., Ford, D. E., & Yeh, H. C. (2006). Anger temperament is modestly associated with the risk of Type 2 diabetes mellitus: The atheroslcerosis risk in communities study. *Psychoneuroendocrinology, 31,* 325–332.

Jones, J. P., Thomas-Peter, B. A., & Trout, A. (1999). Normative date for the Novaco Anger Scale from a non-clinical sample and implications for clinical use. *British Journal of Clinical Psychology, 38,* 417–424.

Kassinove, H. (2007a, May). *Cognitive–behavior therapy: Origins, scope, and relationship to faith, philosophy and science.* Paper presented at the 15th World Congress of the World Association of Dynamic Psychiatry, Bekhterev Psychoneurological Institute, St. Petersburg, Russia.

Kassinove, H. (2007b). Finding a useful model for the treatment of anger and aggression: Comments on Novaco's "Anger dysregulation: Its assessment and treatment" and DiGiuseppe, Cannela, and Keller's "Effective anger treatments require a functional analysis of the anger response." In T. A. Cavell & K. T. Malcolm (Eds.), *Anger, aggression, and interventions for interpersonal violence* (pp. 77–96). New York: Erlbaum.

Kassinove, H., & Eckhardt, C. I. (1993). Irrational ideas and self-reported affect in Russia and the USA. *Personality and Individual Differences, 16,* 133–142.

Kassinove, H., & Tafrate, R. (2002). *Anger management: The complete treatment guidebook for practitioners.* Atascadero, CA: Impact.

Kassinove, H., & Tafrate, R. (2006a). *Anger management video program: An instructional guide for practitioners.* Atascadero, CA: Impact.

Kassinove, H., & Tafrate, R. (2006b). Anger-related disorders: Basic issues, models, and diagnostic considerations. In E. Feindler (Ed.), *Comparative treatments of anger disorders* (pp. 1–27). New York: Springer.

Kassinove, H., & Tafrate, R. (2007). *Treating angry adults: Preparation, change, and forgiveness strategies* (Clinical Grand Rounds, DVD). New York: Association for Behavioral and Cognitive Therapies.

Lachmund, E., DiGiuseppe, R., & Fuller, J. R. (2005). Clinicians' diagnosis of a case with anger problems. *Journal of Psychiatric Research, 39,* 439–447.

Lindqvist, J. K., Dåderman, A., & Hellström, Å. (2003). Swedish adaptations of the Novaco Anger Scale-1998, the Provocation Inventory, and the State-Trait Anger Expression Inventory—2. *Social Behavior and Personality, 31,* 773–788.

Matthews, K. A. (2005). Psychological perspectives on the development of coronary heart disease. *American Psychologist, 60,* 783–796.

Meichenbaum, D. H. (1985). *Stress inoculation training.* New York: Pergamon.

Miller, W. R., & Rollnick, S. (2002). *Motivational interviewing: Preparing people for change* (2nd ed.). New York: Guilford Press.

Mills, J. F., Kroner, D. G., & Forth, A. (1998). Novaco Anger Scale: Reliability and validity within an adult criminal sample. *Assessment, 5,* 237–248.

Novaco, R. W. (1975). *Anger control: The development and evaluation of an experimental treatment.* Lexington, MA: D.C. Heath.

Novaco, R. W. (2003). *The Novaco Anger Scale and Provocation Inventory.* Los Angeles, CA: Western Psychological Services.

Novaco, R. W. (2007). Anger dysregulation. In T. Cavell & K. Malcolm (Eds.), *Anger, aggression, and interventions for interpersonal violence* (pp. 3–54). Mahwah, NJ: Erlbaum.

Novaco, R. W., & Chemtob, C. M. (2002). Anger and combat-related posttraumatic stress disorder. *Journal of Traumatic Stress, 15,* 123–132.

Novaco, R. W., Ramm, M., & Black, L. (2000). Anger treatment with offenders. In C. Hollin (Ed.), *Handbook of offender assessment and treatment* (pp. 281–296). London: Wiley.

O'Donohue, W. T., & Krasner, L. (1995). Theories in behavior therapy: Philosophical and historical contexts. In W. T. O'Donohue & L. Krasner (Eds.), *Theories of behavior therapy: Exploring behavior change* (pp. 1–22). Washington, DC: American Psychological Association.

Poulin, F., Dishion, T. J., & Burraston, B. (2001). 3-year iatrogenic effects associated with aggregating high-risk adolescents in cognitive–behavioral preventive interventions. *Applied Development Science, 5,* 214–224.

Reilly, P. M., & Shopshire, M. S. (2002). *Anger management for substance abuse and mental health clients.* Washington, DC: U.S. Department of Health and Human Services.

Selye, H. (1956). *The stress of life.* New York: McGraw-Hill.

Selye, H. (1971). *Hormones and resistance.* New York: Springer-Verlag.

Selye, H. (1974). *Stress without distress.* Philadelphia: J. B. Lippincott.

Skinner, B. F. (1974). *About behaviorism.* New York: Random House.

Spielberger, C. D. (1999). *Manual for the State Trait Anger Expression Inventory—2.* Odessa, FL: Psychological Assessment Resources.

Tafrate, R. (1995). Evaluation of treatment strategies for adult anger disorders. In H. Kassinove (Ed.), *Anger disorders: Definition, diagnosis, and treatment* (pp. 109–130). Washington, DC: Taylor & Francis.

Tafrate, R., & Kassinove, H. (1998). Anger control in men: Barb exposure with rational, irrational, and irrelevant self-statements. *The Journal of Cognitive Psychotherapy, 12,* 187–211.

Tafrate, R., & Kassinove, H. (2003). Angry patients: Strategies for beginning treatment. In R. Leahy (Ed.), *Overcoming roadblocks in cognitive–behavioral therapy* (pp. 295–317). New York: Guilford Press.

Tafrate, R., & Kassinove, H. (2006). Anger management for adults: A menu-driven cognitive–behavioral approach to the treatment of anger disorders. In E. L. Feindler (Ed.), *Anger related disorders: A practitioner's guide to comparative treatments* (pp. 115–138). New York: Springer.

Tafrate, R., & Kassinove, H. (2009). *Anger management for everyone: 7 proven ways to control anger and live a happier life*. Atascadero, CA: Impact.

Tafrate, R., Kassinove, H., & Dundin, L. (2002). Anger episodes in high and low trait anger community adults. *Journal of Clinical Psychology, 58*, 1573–1590.

Taylor, J. L., & Novaco, R. W. (2005). *Anger treatment for people with developmental disabilities: A theory, evidence, and manual based approach*. London: Wiley.

Williams, R., & Williams, V. (1994). *Anger kills*. New York: HarperCollins.

Williams, J. E., Nieto, F. J., Sanford, C. P., Couper, D. J., & Tyroler, H. A. (2002). The association between trait anger and incident stroke risk: The atherosclerosis risk in communities (ARIC) study. *Stroke, 33*, 13–19.

Williams, J. E., Paton, C. C., Siegler, I. C., Eigenbrodt, M. L., Nieto, F. J., & Tyroler, H. A. (2000). Anger proneness predicts coronary heart disease risk: Prospective analysis from the atherosclerosis risk in communities (ARIC) study. *Circulation, 101*, 2034–2039.

Wolpe, J. (1969). *The practice of behavior therapy*. New York: Pergamon.

World Health Organization. (1992). *International classification of diseases (ICD-10)*. Geneva, Switzerland: Author.

Zwemer, W. A., & Deffenbacher, J. L. (1984). Irrational beliefs, anger, and anxiety. *Journal of Counseling Psychology, 31*, 391–393.

III

TREATING REFRACTORY POPULATIONS AND CLINICAL PROBLEMS

15

HYPOCHONDRIASIS AND SEVERE HEALTH ANXIETY

JONATHAN S. ABRAMOWITZ, STEVEN TAYLOR, AND DEAN McKAY

The essential feature of *hypochondriasis* (HC), according to the *Diagnostic and Statistical Manual of Mental Disorders* (4th ed., text rev.; American Psychiatric Association, 2000), is a preoccupation with the (inaccurate) belief that one has, or is in danger of developing, a serious illness. Whereas most people evince occasional passing health concerns, the disease conviction in HC is intense, frequent, and persistent. Moreover, it endures despite appropriate (even excessive) medical evaluations and reassurance of good health. Furthermore, the health preoccupation results in functional disability. Traditionally considered a somatoform disorder because of the focus on bodily symptoms, recent conceptualizations of HC have emphasized the role of health anxiety (e.g., Taylor & Asmundson, 2004). This approach has transformed what was once considered a treatment-refractory problem into one with a broader conceptualization and a wider range of treatment options and therapy response.

We begin this chapter by introducing the reader to the cognitive–behavioral approach to HC (and other forms of health anxiety). We next describe the treatment based on this approach and evidence supporting the use of this treatment. An important obstacle to successful treatment of health anxiety is that many patients have poor insight into their condition and believe strongly that they require medical, as opposed to psychological, interventions. Using a case example, we illustrate the use of motivational interviewing principles (Miller & Rollnick, 2002) to help health anxious patients embrace and engage in effective psychological treatment.

The cognitive–behavioral model of HC (Salkovskis, Warwick, & Deale, 2003; Taylor & Asmundson, 2004) views this clinical condition as a form of excessive health anxiety. This model is among the best empirically supported accounts of HC (Taylor & Asmundson, 2004). It proposes that excessive health anxiety arises from dysfunctional beliefs about sickness and health, including beliefs that lead people to misinterpret the significance of bodily changes and sensations. Bodily sensations are common occurrences even in people who do not have life-threatening diseases (Pennebaker, 1982). Such sensations may arise for a variety of reasons, including minor diseases or autonomic arousal associated with stress. People with excessive health anxiety believe that these bodily changes and sensations have catastrophic consequences; for example, abdominal pain may be misinterpreted as a ruptured appendix, or exercise-related shortness of breath may be misinterpreted as an indication of lung disease. People with excessive health anxiety also tend to believe that they are healthy only when they do not have any bodily sensations and that worrying about their health will keep them safe (Taylor & Asmundson, 2004). As a result of these various types of dysfunctional beliefs, the person tends to focus on his or her body, which increases the chance of detecting—and misinterpreting—minor bodily changes or sensations.

Maladaptive coping behaviors associated with health-related dysfunctional beliefs can perpetuate excessive health anxiety. Such behaviors include persistent reassurance seeking (from physicians or family members), other forms of repetitive checking (e.g., bodily checking, searching the Internet for disease-related information), and avoidance of behaviors that elicit bodily sensations (e.g., physical exertion). Reassurance seeking can prolong a person's preoccupation with disease, expose him or her to frightening information about health conditions, reduce his or her sense of independence (e.g., by repeatedly turning to others for help), and lead to iatrogenic effects (e.g., potentially hazardous invasive medical tests). Maladaptive coping behaviors persist in HC because they are reinforced by reduced anxiety in the short term. In the long term, however, they are not only ineffective in producing lasting reductions in anxiety, but they actually serve to perpetuate health anxiety.

The following example illustrates the interplay between dysfunctional beliefs, selective attention, health anxiety, and maladaptive coping behaviors. A person who complains of chronic unexplained dizziness might come to believe that he or she is actually suffering from an undiagnosed serious neurological condition. Thoughts about the seriousness of this imagined condition will lead to anxiety and evocation of the fight or flight response, which naturally produces feelings of dizziness and unreality (which the individual will misinterpret as further signs of a serious problem). He or she might also begin paying attention to dizziness sensations—looking for them and noticing even slight (normal) variations in vestibular system functioning that most people simply ignore (e.g., turning the head quickly normally produces a brief sensation of dizziness). These sensations are subsequently taken as evidence for a medical problem. Finally, he or she might frequently consult with physicians, conduct research online for information about symptoms, or ask friends or relatives about the suspected illness. These behaviors might result in brief reductions in anxiety (hence they are negatively reinforced), but they have the long-term effect of producing more anxiety or distress because they result in upsetting interactions with doctors and relatives, unnecessarily focus the person on grave illnesses that are not present (e.g., learned from the Internet), and maintain the self-focused attention that leads to the exaggerated sensitivity to innocuous bodily sensations. Thus, the problem is maintained by vicious cycles resulting from excessive responding to ostensibly harmless body sensations.

EFFECTIVE PSYCHOLOGICAL TREATMENTS FOR HEALTH ANXIETY

Historically, the conditions now collectively called *health anxiety* (primarily HC and somatization disorder) were considered highly treatment-resistant problems. This speaks to the relative ineffectiveness of psychoanalytic and psychodynamic treatments, which were the treatment of choice yet were also based on speculative theories that were unhinged from behavior and physiology. Even among behaviorally oriented psychologists, it was believed that these conditions were based to a large extent on rigid personality features and would not respond as well to goal-oriented interventions. For example, Eysenck (1982) referred to these conditions as *secondary anxiety disorders*, which conferred on this class of disorders a primary personality feature. The development of cognitive–behavioral conceptualizations and treatments of anxiety and symptoms associated with biases toward misinterpreting the risk of harm over the past 20 years has begun to change this notion of health anxiety as an intractable set of problems (Taylor, Asmundson, & Coons, 2005). The sections that follow describes the current psychological treatment of health anxiety and presents a succinct review of the treatment-outcome literature.

Psychoeducational Treatments

Barsky, Gerringer, and Wolf (1988) developed a course comprising six weekly sessions of education about the factors that maintain or exacerbate medically unexplained bodily sensations and symptoms (e.g., faulty symptom attribution, dysphoric mood). The role that faulty psychological and medical information plays in health anxiety was emphasized. Two studies found this program helpful in reducing health anxiety severity and medical consultation frequency (Avia et al., 1996; Stern & Fernandez, 1991). Another psychoeducation program based on the notion that stress exacerbates the presence of, and vigilance to, bodily sensations was found to be effective in reducing health anxiety complaints in a preventative medicine unit when compared with a wait-list control group (Lidbeck, 1997). Bouman (2002) later modified the Barsky et al. program and reported significant reductions in health anxiety, depressive symptoms, trait anxiety, and medical consultations.

Buwalda, Bouman, and van Duijn (2007) compared psychoeducation based on the cognitive–behavioral model of health anxiety with a problem-solving focused therapy. Both treatments were delivered in a 6-week group format and both included didactic lectures, demonstrations, informational videos, focused group discussions, in-class assignments, and optional homework. Results indicated that immediately after treatment and at 6-month follow-up, the treatments were equally effective in reducing health anxiety, depressive symptoms, trait anxiety, and the number of daily stressors. Taken together, the findings for psychoeducation suggest this intervention is a viable treatment for health anxiety.

Exposure and Response Prevention

Exposure and response prevention (ERP) is a behavior therapy technique that involves confrontation with stimuli that provoke phobic anxiety but that objectively pose a low risk of harm (e.g., Foa & Kozak, 1986). For example, a health anxious individual who fears books about cancer would be helped to read such books even if they provoke fears about getting this disease. Because individuals with health anxiety experience excessive fear as provoked by bodily sensations (e.g., stomach bloating), external stimuli (e.g., reminders of a feared illness), and thoughts and images (e.g., thoughts of dying from some dreaded disease), three forms of exposure are used for such patients: (a) repeated actual encounters with the feared situations (i.e., *situational* or *in vivo exposure*), (b) imaginal confrontation with anxiety-provoking thoughts and images (i.e., *imaginal exposure*), and (c) confrontation with feared bodily stimuli (i.e., *interoceptive exposure*).

Guided by the therapist, the patient practices confrontation with each type of feared stimulus and remains exposed instead of engaging in escape or avoidance behaviors. As would be expected, when an exposure task is begun, the patient experiences anxiety. Patients are encouraged to engage in the exposure task fully and allow him- or herself to experience this distress. Over time, the distress (and associated physiological responding) naturally subsides—a process known as *habituation*. With repeated exposure, habituation occurs more rapidly (for a detailed discussion of this process, see Richard & Lauterbach, 2007).

Response prevention is an important component of ERP. This entails refraining from any behaviors (e.g., reassurance seeking or avoidance) that serve as an escape from anxiety and that would terminate exposure de facto. Response prevention therefore is a necessary component of behavior therapy because it is required to bring about the natural extinction of anxiety. These treatment techniques have been described in detail elsewhere (e.g., Abramowitz & Braddock, in press; Taylor & Asmundson, 2004); thus, we provide only a brief description here.

ERP for health anxiety begins with the patient and therapist constructing a fear hierarchy—a list of the patient's feared stimuli (i.e., situations, stimuli, thoughts, and body sensations) rated from least to most anxiety inducing. Gradually, and with the help of the therapist, the patient uses the three exposure media (i.e., situational, imaginal, and interoceptive) to confront these stimuli. In addition to observing the natural decrease in anxiety that occurs with prolonged exposure, the patient and therapist use exposure tasks to test out (and disconfirm) the basis for the patient's health-related dysfunctional beliefs. For example, a patient with excessive fears of contracting blood-borne illnesses through coincidental skin contact would walk through an emergency room or medical inpatient floor, touching objects feared to be "contaminated," such as walls and doorknobs. An explicit hypothesis regarding the fear would be tested (i.e., "By merely being in the hospital, I'm going to get HIV; the only way I can prevent HIV and reduce my anxiety is to avoid hospitals and wash my hands").

During and following the exposure, response prevention strategies are used where the patient is discouraged from engaging in his or her typical maladaptive coping behaviors (e.g., checking body for possible open sores, asking for reassurance). Instead, the patient is helped to experience the anxiety induced by the exposure and allow it to subside naturally. With repeated and prolonged exposures, the basis for the irrational fear is disconfirmed, and the patient learns that the anxiety does subside even without safety-seeking behaviors.

The aim of imaginal exposure for health anxiety is to foster habituation to fear-evoking thoughts or images and to help patients correct how they misinterpret the presence and significance of such thoughts. The technique may be used in different ways depending on the patient's symptom presentation. In *primary* imaginal exposure, the patient directly confronts anxiety-provoking thoughts and images via methods such as looped (repeating) audiotapes or written scripts containing the upsetting material. For example, a man whose anxiety is triggered by intrusive images of his "enlarged prostate" would practice visualizing what the swollen and diseased organ might look like in his body. A woman with upsetting thoughts of her own death by cancer might be exposed to vivid stories of this event taking place. Following the imaginal exposure, the patient would be helped to refrain from engaging in any anxiety-reducing behaviors such as bodily checking or seeking medical reassurance.

Secondary imaginal exposure is a technique for helping patients with health anxiety confront fears of diseases that might not occur until the distant future. Usually, the imaginal exposure is begun during or after situational exposure (hence it is secondary to situational exposure) and involves visualizing the feared outcomes (or uncertainty) associated with the situational exposure task. For example, a patient with fears of losing his hearing from attending a sporting event might attend a game for situational exposure, refrain from wearing ear plugs (response prevention), and then focus on being uncertain about whether hearing loss has (or will) occur. Thus, secondary imaginal exposure involves amplifying the uncertainty about possible negative outcomes of situational exposures.

Finally, confrontation with anxiety-evoking bodily stimuli is accomplished via interoceptive exposure. As we have discussed, health anxious individuals typically associate certain bodily sensations with anxiety. Accordingly, the aim of this exposure medium is to help the patient reduce this association and learn that such sensations are not dangerous. Interoceptive exposure is often used in the treatment of panic disorder in which patients exhibit a fear of their own physiological response to anxiety (Craske & Barlow, 2007; Taylor, 2000). Interoceptive exposure exercises are individualized to mimic the patient's feared body sensations. Table 15.1 describes some common interceptive exercises and the physical symptoms they seek to elicit.

Leonhard (1961) anecdotally reported success using ERP for health anxiety, yet it would be almost 30 years later that the first empirical studies would be conducted (Logsdail, Lovell, Warwick, & Marks, 1991; Visser & Bouman, 1992; Warwick & Marks, 1988). A recent controlled trial demonstrated that ERP was significantly more effective than a wait-list control condition, with gains maintained at 7-month follow-up (Visser & Bouman, 2001). Presently, ERP occupies a central role in the treatment of health anxiety, as is discussed in several volumes on the topic (e.g., Abramowitz & Braddock, in press; Taylor & Asmundson, 2004).

Cognitive–Behavioral Therapy

Cognitive–behavioral therapy (CBT) for health anxiety is based on the cognitive–behavioral model of health anxiety described earlier in this chapter. The primary aims of CBT are to (a) help patients recognize and modify faulty health-related beliefs and perceptions and (b) eliminate safety-seeking behaviors and other barriers to correcting these faulty beliefs. A range of methods are used to achieve these aims, including psychoeducation, cognitive therapy (CT) techniques, and exposure methods such as behavioral experiments.

TABLE 15.1
Examples of Techniques for Provoking Body Sensations During Interoceptive Exposure

Technique (instruction)	Body sensation(s)
Hyperventilation (breathe deeply and rapidly for 90 seconds)	Shortness of breath, sense of unreality, tingling, sweating, dizziness, lightheadedness, dry mouth/throat, light sensitivity, chest tightness, racing heartbeat, exhaustion
Body tensing (tense muscles in arms, legs, abdomen, neck, face, etc., or do push-ups for 60 seconds)	Muscle tension, sweating, racing heart, pain
Head lifting (place head between legs for 30 seconds, then lift head quickly to normal position; repeat)	Lightheadedness, head rush, disorientation
Swallowing (attempt to swallow five times in quick succession)	Throat tightness, lump in throat, breathlessness
Run in place (lift knees up to chest or step up on stairs for 60 seconds)	Shortness of breath, racing heartbeat
Staring intensely (stare intensely at a small spot in the corner for 2 minutes)	Sense of unreality
Spinning (for 60 seconds, spin either in a standing position or while seated in a revolving chair)	Dizziness, disorientation
Straw breathing (breathe rapidly through a very thin straw for 60 seconds)	Shortness of breath, chest tightness, smothering sensations
Hot shower (take a hot shower with the door closed)	Weakness, disorientation, hot flash
Gag (use toothbrush to brush the back of the tongue)	Nausea
Caffeine (drink highly caffeinated beverage, or take caffeine pills, e.g., NoDoz).	Racing heart, sweating, hot flash

Following a careful assessment of the triggers, faulty beliefs, and behavioral aspects of the patient's particular health anxiety symptoms, the therapist creates an individualized case conceptualization to specify the erroneous illness-related beliefs and the relationship among physiological, cognitive, and behavioral factors that maintain these beliefs. Typically, patients feel discounted by their medical doctors; therefore, a thorough and open consideration of their feelings, thoughts, and behaviors fosters an acceptance of the conceptual model and treatment plan (Walker, Vincent, Furer, Cox, & Kjernisted, 1999).

Patients are then provided with psychoeducation about anxiety. This emphasizes how anxiety is a normal and adaptive reaction to perceived threat that involves behavioral, mental and physiological responses aimed at preparing the body for fight or flight. Patients are also taught about the numerous sources of normal "body noise," some common physiological explanations for benign body sensations, and the detrimental effects of various forms of checking and reassurance seeking.

Cognitive restructuring (Beck, 1976; Beck & Emery, 1985) is a set of verbal techniques that help the patient identify objective evidence for and against faulty beliefs about health and illness, and faulty interpretations of specific body sensations and other stimuli. The therapist helps the patient to (a) identify the basis for these beliefs, (b) recognize contradictory events or experiences, and (c) understand the significance of contradictory evidence. The goal is to help the patient adopt rational responses to normal physiological sensations.

Behavioral experiments, some of which approximate ERP exercises, are also used to help patients deepen their convictions in their new rational responses to health relevant stimuli. These experiments might involve confronting feared stimuli and noting the effects on health, dropping safety behaviors to examine whether confrontation with the feared stimulus leads to illness, as well as other techniques for testing out the logic of new beliefs (for examples, see Abramowitz & Braddock, 2008; see also Taylor & Asmundson, 2004).

Strong evidence is emerging in favor of the efficacy of CBT for health anxiety (for a meta-analytic review, see Taylor et al., 2005). Several controlled studies indicate clinically significant and lasting improvements after less than 20 sessions (e.g., Clark et al., 1998; Visser & Bouman, 2001). In a wait-list controlled study, Warwick, Clark, Cobb, and Salkovskis (1996) found that CBT produced significant reductions in reassurance seeking, overall health anxiety, and checking frequency. General anxiety was reduced by approximately 70%, and depressive symptoms were reduced by 53%. Moreover, CBT was acceptable to patients; only 6% of those recruited into the study refused to begin therapy, and another 6% dropped out of treatment prematurely.

A controlled study of 16 weekly cognitive–behavioral sessions demonstrated short- and long-term (1 year) efficacy in reducing fears of illness, as well as unnecessary medical visits (Clark et al., 1998). Additionally, CBT tended to be more effective than stress management techniques, which also had beneficial effects. Thus, the specific procedures of CBT for health anxiety, as opposed to nonspecific factors (i.e., attention from the therapist), are important for treatment. Refusal and dropout rates were low in this study (4%), suggesting acceptability and tolerability.

In a study by Barsky and Ahern (2004), a six-session CBT program that focused on psychoeducation and correcting dysfunctional health-related beliefs was more effective than medical care as usual in reducing health anxiety and had beneficial effects on various behavioral, cognitive, affective, and functional domains. Treatment gains were maintained at both 6-month and 1-year follow-ups. A limitation of this study, however, was that many otherwise eligible patients declined to participate. Thus, it cannot be ruled out that the effects of CBT have something to do with the patient's willingness to engage in this treatment. We believe that motivation for change is a critical component of treatment for health anxiety, as we discuss in the sections that follow.

FACTORS ASSOCIATED WITH POOR TREATMENT RESPONSE

Research has yet to closely examine which factors predict success and failure in the psychological treatment of health anxiety. As alluded to previously, however, our observations suggest a positive correlation between the strength of disease conviction (i.e., how strongly the person believes he or she has a medical disease) and willingness to consider and engage in psychological treatment. Those with moderate or low conviction might view therapy in a more favorable light than those with very strong disease conviction. Individuals who strongly believe they have a serious undiagnosed medical condition are often quite adamant about seeking further medical assessment to confirm the origin and authenticity of their physical complaints. Consistent with our clinical observations, research has suggested that poor treatment outcome is associated with severe, chronic HC, especially when there are complicating factors that strengthen or maintain dysfunctional health-related beliefs, such as comorbid general medical conditions and environmental contingencies (i.e., secondary gains) that reinforce health anxiety and sick-role behavior (Taylor & Asmundson, 2004).

Given that CBTs rely on learning and practicing new (and often challenging) skills, willingness to embrace and participate in treatment is an important predictor of outcome. In the next section, we describe a case illustrating health anxiety with strong disease conviction, and the management of this problem in therapy by drawing on the principles of motivational interviewing (MI; Miller & Rollnick, 2002). Although the efficacy of MI for HC is currently limited to only a handful of encouraging case studies (e.g., McKay & Bouman, 2008), our clinical experience is that this is a very promising intervention that clinicians may want to consider using to improve the odds that a patient with HC will remain in, and benefit from, CBT.

CASE EXAMPLE

Yolanda was 29 years old and had suffered with HC for 10 years. She believed her body was "falling apart" and had consulted more than 10 doctors in her hometown. Yet numerous head computed tomography scans, cardiac work-ups, and gastrointestinal studies revealed no serious medical conditions. On more than one occasion, psychotherapy had been suggested, and Yolanda had accumulated a file of referral information and other handouts on psychological treatments for medically unexplained symptoms. Occasionally, when worrying about her physical symptoms, she would open the folder and start to read this material. However, instead of feeling hopeful that she might get relief with psychological treatment, reading the material evoked feelings of agitation and the sense that she was misunderstood by her doctors. She created mental pictures of a therapist trying to convince her that her problems were "all in her head." A part of her understood that doing psychotherapy would probably not be harmful and could, perhaps, be beneficial in light of the results of her medical tests. But there was another part of her that believed her symptoms were "real" and should only be managed from a medical standpoint.

Yolanda's story illustrates how health-anxious patients with poor insight into the psychological basis of their difficulties typically harbor at least some degree of ambivalence. That is, Yolanda at once recognized the possible benefits of psychological treatment, yet also viewed this approach as admitting that her problems were mental and not medical. One aspect of Yolanda's ambivalence concerned the general idea of seeing a psychologist for a "medical" problem. She also had ambivalence about the specifics of psychological treatment—she was concerned that by focusing on psychological issues, her dire medical concerns would be overlooked.

A key assumption in MI is that the responsibility for a positive patient–therapist relationship lies with the therapist, not with the patient. This departs from a traditional-thinking approach in which it is common for a therapist to say, "This patient is just not motivated." Accordingly, when Yolanda finally decided to see what psychological treatment would be like, the therapist, Dr. Smith, worked to help Yolanda keep an open mind about treatment using the perspective, "What must I do to help Yolanda decide to engage in therapy?" Dr. Smith utilized a number of communication strategies during the initial sessions. These are outlined in the sections that follow.

Demonstrating Empathy

Dr. Smith expressed interest in understanding Yolanda's dilemma without being critical or judgmental. He used reflective listening strategies, as described by Carl Rogers (1951), to gain a thorough understanding of the problem while also deepening Yolanda's experience of ambivalence. The hope was that this would lead Yolanda to question her status quo and move toward accepting treatment. In addition, this communicated to Yolanda that Dr. Smith respected her point of view, which is particularly crucial with health anxious individuals who often feel they (and their complaints) are not taken seriously. Specific strategies of reflective listening Dr. Smith used were as follows:

- Asking genuine open-ended questions about the problem: "What do you like and dislike about going for all of these medical tests?"
- Making reasonable guesses as to how the patient is thinking or feeling: "It must be frustrating when your family harps on you to see a psychologist."
- Eliciting self-motivational statements by selectively reinforcing certain aspects of what the patient says: "Why do you think your partner is upset with how you've handled your health concerns?"
- Giving affirmation with compliments, appreciation, and statements of understanding: "I know it's not easy to talk about this with a psychologist, and I wanted you to know I appreciate your willingness to share this information with me."
- Summarizing material that has been discussed, particularly self-motivational statements: "So as you pointed out, going for another medical test would have some advantages and disadvantages. On the one hand, you feel you cannot go on without getting to the bottom of what is causing the physical symptoms. But on the other hand, you think more tests are not going to show anything new."

Avoiding a Lecture

Miller and Rollnick (2002) suggested that ambivalent patients are most likely to engage in treatment when they hear themselves arguing for change. Rather than lecture or persuade Yolanda to begin treatment (e.g., "Let me tell you all the reasons why you should do therapy . . ."), Dr. Smith elicited and reinforced self-motivational statements from Yolanda. Miller and Rollnick listed four categories of self-motivational statements: *problem recognition* (e.g., a statement that one has a problem), *expression of concern* (e.g., a statement that the problem is serious and that help is needed), *intention to change* (e.g., a statement that one has decided to do something about the problem), and *optimism* (e.g., a statement that the problem can be changed).

Medicalizing (Instead of Psychologizing)

Dr. Smith referred to Yolanda's complaints using medical terms—the same terms Yolanda used. He told Yolanda he understood that her complaints were genuine and avoided telling her there was "nothing wrong" or that the symptoms were simply caused by "stress." Instead of referring to "anxiety," he referred to the fight-or-flight response (i.e., the physiological correlate of anxiety), thoughts about symptoms (i.e., the cognitive correlate of anxiety), and taking precautions (i.e., the behavioral correlates). Yolanda responded agreeably to this language and was able to engage with Dr. Smith without feeling defensive.

Avoiding Arguments and Rolling With Resistance

Health-anxious patients sometimes become argumentative and contest the therapist's accuracy and integrity. To offset this, Dr. Smith avoided dynamic and vigorous attempts to push Yolanda into treatment. If patients such as Yolanda perceive their therapists as trying too forcefully to present or argue one side of an issue (e.g., "I've looked over your medical records; there is no sign of any serious disease"), they tend to dig in and generate arguments to the contrary, often indicated by "yes, but . . ." statements (e.g., "Yes, but my doctors haven't conducted the right tests").

Dr. Smith also avoided the following conversational styles:

- ordering, directing, or commanding;
- warning or threatening;
- giving unsolicited advice and suggestions;
- trying to persuade with logic or lecturing;
- moralizing, preaching, or telling Yolanda what she "should" do;
- criticizing, blaming, or labeling;
- interpreting or analyzing;
- asking rapid-fire questions that elicit defensiveness; and
- insisting on talking about the problem behavior when Yolanda raised other concerns.

Again, Dr. Smith kept in mind that instead of directly presenting Yolanda with arguments for changing her position, he would have greater success by helping her to generate her own arguments for change.

When Yolanda did show resistance to the idea of psychological treatment—for example by interrupting Dr. Smith, ignoring his remarks, or minimizing the seriousness of her problem—Dr. Smith responded by raising Yolanda's concerns and desires both for and against change. For instance, he slightly overstated her resistance in a genuine way (a strategy called *amplified reflection*). The dialogue below illustrates how this strategy was used to help Yolanda make her own argument for engaging in therapy.

> Dr. Smith: One of the goals of treatment is to help you learn that you do not need to keep going to doctors to get more opinions about your symptoms. You're going to learn a new approach to—
>
> Yolanda: [*interrupting*] But that doesn't make any sense. I need to get to the bottom of this medically, not psychologically.

Dr. Smith:	Well, I understand how you feel. You're saying you think you should continue going for more tests and exams since this has been so helpful for you in the past. I mean, if it has been helpful to get tests in the past, why should you stop now?
Yolanda:	Well, actually, they haven't been helpful. All that happens is that the tests are negative, and the doctor tells me I'm healthy.
Dr. Smith:	So, then maybe you feel the next test you have will finally be the one to give you all the answers. It sounds like you are pretty confident another test will put you on the right track.
Yolanda:	Well, no. Having more tests will probably be just as frustrating.

Dr. Smith also used a strategy known as *agreement with a twist* (Miller & Rollnick, 2002), in which he let Yolanda know he agreed with her but then also incorporated a slight change of direction. For example,

Yolanda:	[*interrupting*] I need to get to the bottom of this medically, not psychologically.
Dr. Smith:	You're absolutely right that you've got real medical symptoms. And I am not a physician, so I can't give you an explanation for them. But you told me how frustrated you've become with your physicians. If you reduce this frustration, think of how it could help you develop better relationships with your doctors. Perhaps they will be able to help you more effectively that way.

A third technique was to reflect the resistance and pair it with a self-motivational statement. This forced Yolanda to examine the discrepancy in her beliefs.

Yolanda:	[*interrupting*] No, no, that doesn't make any sense. I need to get to the bottom of this medically, not psychologically.
Dr. Smith:	Right, so you have been trying very hard to get a medical diagnosis for your symptoms. After all, they're real. And, as you said before, this approach hasn't been helpful. In fact, it's made you feel very frustrated.
Yolanda:	Yeah, that's exactly my problem.
Dr. Smith:	What are some things you might do about this problem?

Dr. Smith also managed Yolanda's resistance by emphasizing her control and personal choice. This reduced her defensiveness.

Yolanda:	[*interrupting*] No, no, that doesn't make any sense. I need to get to the bottom of this medically, not psychologically.
Dr. Smith:	Well, ultimately, the decision about how to deal with your symptoms is completely yours. I cannot tell you what you should or should not do. What I will point out is that you seem to be

saying that your way of handling this has not been very helpful. Perhaps it's time to try something new.

Yolanda: Well, I guess it can't hurt to hear a little about your therapy, even though I may decide not to come back.

Socialization

Socialization is the process of introducing the patient to the psychological model of treatment. This requires no small amount of tact because there is a risk that the patient will feel labeled as a "hypochondriac," which will almost certainly evoke strong resistance. On the other hand, the patient needs to understand the conceptual model so he or she can benefit maximally from therapy. Dr. Smith used a number of helpful rhetorical maneuvers to socialize Yolanda to the psychological model of health anxiety that guides treatment. These strategies were infused with the MI approach previously described.

Getting a Foot in the Door

To begin with, Dr. Smith endeavored to raise Yolanda's ambivalence about the status quo and help her make an argument for addressing her problem from a new and different perspective. He began by asking her open-ended questions about why she had been referred to a psychologist in the first place and what it was like not to have medical answers. Dr. Smith had an idea of the answer to this question but still inquired in a genuine way about the nature of the referral. This allowed Yolanda to hear herself clarify how her physicians had not found medical problems despite comprehensive testing and how going for medical exams was frustrating for her. Dr. Smith also showed acceptance of Yolanda's physical complaints as authentic.

Next, Dr. Smith began helping Yolanda identify how psychological treatment could be useful. The maneuver illustrated next gives the therapist permission to talk about a psychological perspective without pressuring the patient to change his or her attitude about the medical basis of symptoms. Instead, it helps the patient move from an all-or-none perspective (e.g., "Symptoms are either medical disorders or all 'in my head'") to a more useful continuum approach (e.g., "My symptoms might have both a medical and a psychological basis").

Dr. Smith: I'd like to know your guess as to what percentage of your health issues—out of 100—might be due to medical causes versus what percentage might be due to some sort of psychological factor. So, give me an estimate, like 50/50 or 60/40.

Yolanda: My problems are much more due to medical causes. So, it's probably 90% medical and 10% psychological.

Dr. Smith:	So psychological factors only account for 10%. Why even give them 10%? I mean, why not even less than that? Why not 5% or 0%?
Yolanda:	Well, I've been through so many tests and checkups, and the doctors never find anything. It sometimes makes me wonder about whether there is a psychological cause.
Dr. Smith:	I see. And how do you think psychological factors might play a role here?
Yolanda:	I don't know. Maybe I don't realize how much stress I have.
Dr. Smith:	Well, as you know, I am not a physician. But since I am a psychologist, we could spend some time trying to better understand this 10% of the equation. Would it be OK if we talk some about the 10% that could be psychological?
Yolanda:	I guess so. I've never thought about it like that before.

Presenting the Psychological Model of Health Anxiety

We find it helpful to introduce the psychological (cognitive–behavioral) model of health anxiety by focusing on the patent's tendency to closely monitor his or her body for symptoms of the feared disease. Once this idea is presented, its "side effects" (e.g., sensitivity to innocuous "body noise") can be discussed. Dr. Smith helped Yolanda to understand how even healthy human bodies produce noticeable sensations and perturbations (body noise) and that such body noise is not necessarily an indication of a serious medical illness. However, body vigilance can lead to increased perception of body noise, and this can strengthen the idea that a serious disease is present.

Yolanda's physicians had suggested that her unexplained body symptoms were probably caused by too much stress, or perhaps some traumatic event or history of abuse. Yolanda denied stress and any history of abuse or trauma. Although Dr. Smith was inclined to try to convince Yolanda that she was overlooking how much stress she was under, he recognized this approach would be perceived as advocating a psychological explanation too strongly. Instead, he held out the attention to body noise explanation as a possible alternative way of viewing Yolanda's physical complaints. Yolanda agreed with this explanation more than she agreed with the stress and trauma explanation, which had no historical basis.

Next, Dr. Smith and Yolanda discussed how thinking and acting can influence physical symptoms in the body (i.e., the *mind–body connection*). First, Dr. Smith focused on the relationship between the perception of threat and physiologic arousal. Yolanda's interpretations of body sensations led her to feel as if she was in danger. This leads to activation of the fight-or-flight mechanism, which produces more body noise, increasing the level of "body symptoms." Dr. Smith and Yolanda also discussed how behaviors such as getting frequent medical tests, discussing health issues, looking up information on the Internet, and doctor shopping make health concerns worse, rather than being a solution. Using the MI techniques described earlier, he engaged Yolanda in a discussion of the advantages and disadvantages of these behaviors and the pros and cons of working on ending them. The aim of this discussion was to provide Yolanda with a new way to think about her behaviors and to amplify her ambivalence with regard to using these strategies for managing bodily sensations.

Providing a Rationale for Psychological Treatment

Once Yolanda was introduced to the cognitive–behavioral approach to unexplained medical symptoms, Dr. Smith summarized the conversation and moved the discussion to the possibility of starting psychological treatment. He presented the rationale for treatment in the following way:

> We've covered a lot of ground today, so let's see if we can pull it all together to see where we are and where we're going. It is clear that you're experiencing real physical symptoms that bother you, but it also seems that, at least to some extent, there are things you could do to manage these symptoms in more helpful and healthy ways than you have been. We talked about certain thoughts that trigger your body to produce more physical symptoms. We also talked about strategies such as seeking medical tests and looking up information on the Internet and so on that seem to temporarily work but that backfire in the long run instead of making you feel better. It seems like in the past you've only considered a medical approach to getting help. You've seen lots of doctors and had many, many tests and examinations, but these have left you feeling frustrated and without good, clear answers. How do you feel about us working together to see if we can figure out how to address some of these problems from a new perspective?

Eliciting Change Talk

Yolanda agreed to begin treatment; however, throughout the first several sessions she continued to express arguments against the psychological approach and treatment. Dr. Smith addressed this resistance by helping Yolanda generate her own arguments for treatment (i.e., change talk) without pushing her too strongly in this direction. Change talk includes statements by the patient that reflect commitment, desire, perceived ability, need, readiness, or reasons to change (Amrhein, Miller, Yahne, Palmer, & Fulcher, 2003). Miller and Rollnick (2002) suggested eliciting change talk by asking evocative questions such as the following:

- How have your unexplained symptoms interfered with your life?

- What bothers you the most when your physicians cannot find a medical explanation for your symptoms?
- How would life be different if you didn't need an explanation for every symptom your body produces?
- What are some of the advantages of being medically healthy?
- How important is it for you to get some help for your unexplained medical symptoms?
- What would the rest of your life be like if your doctors never gave you an adequate explanation for these symptoms?
- How much more time and money are you going to spend on doctor appointments that only seem to make you more frustrated?
- How will the other people in your life react when you can manage these symptoms in more helpful ways?

Finally, Dr. Smith, as suggested by Wells (1997), presented psychological treatment as a no-lose opportunity. He brought up the length of time Yolanda had been pursuing a medical explanation for her complaints and asked Yolanda about the effectiveness of this pursuit in solving her problems. He also pointed out that Yolanda had little to lose by engaging in an alternative (or augmentative) psychological treatment approach. If this approach turned out not to be helpful, Yolanda could return to the previous strategy. Yolanda continued in treatment and, following about 20 sessions of CBT involving exposure and response prevention and CT, reported reduced health concerns and less frequent urges to consult medical personnel about her complaints. She continued to experience occasional uncomfortable body sensations, yet was able to manage her responses to these in more useful ways.

CONCLUSIONS AND FUTURE DIRECTIONS

HC and other forms of severe health anxiety can be severe and debilitating. Research has suggested that dysfunctional beliefs play an important role, which can contribute to self-defeating behaviors such as excessive reassurance seeking. Previously, individuals with HC and other forms of health anxiety were considered treatment refractory. A tremendous step forward came with the conceptualization of this problem as akin to an anxiety disorder focused on one's personal health. This framework led to the use of treatment strategies commonly applied (with empirical support) in the treatment of anxiety disorders such as panic disorder and obsessive–compulsive disorder. Evidence now abounds for the efficacy of this cognitive–behavioral approach. A remaining problem, however, is that despite effective treatments, many patients with HC and other forms of health anxiety are resistant to psychological treatment because of their strongly held belief that they have a medical, and not a psychological, problem. Thus, a major roadblock to effective treatment is acceptance of a psychological approach. In this chapter, we have illustrated one approach to this problem and exemplified an MI approach to engaging patients in psychological treatment. Educating primary care physicians in some basic aspects of MI may be helpful in moving health anxious clients from the medical doctor's office to the cognitive–behavioral therapist's office.

The MI strategies described here all involve conveying acceptance and empathy. This helps expand the patient's understanding of the pros and cons of treatment and helps him or her to clarify both the hesitancy and appeal of beginning therapy. It is often a profound experience for patients to air their grievances about physicians and to share their reservations about psychotherapy for health anxiety and still find the therapist listening and responding thoughtfully and compassionately without dismissing these concerns or trying harder to sell CBT. The patient often feels understood and may be more likely to opt to engage in therapy. The alternative is for the therapist to respond with further attempts to persuade the patient to change; yet, as we have mentioned repeatedly, this typically evokes even stronger resistance on the part of the patient.

Despite the early promise of MI, empirical support is currently limited to a handful of case studies. Further research, such as randomized controlled trials comparing MI plus CBT with CBT alone, are needed to evaluate whether MI increases patient engagement in and adherence to CBT. Given that MI methods for HC have now been developed and pilot tested, the time is ripe for more rigorous evaluations.

REFERENCES

Abramowitz, J., & Braddock, A. (2008). *Psychological treatment of hypochondriasis and health anxiety.* Cambridge, MA: Hogrefe and Huber.

American Psychiatric Association. (2000). *Diagnostic and statistical manual of mental disorders* (4th ed., text rev.). Washington, DC: Author.

Amrhein, P. C., Miller, W. R., Yahne, C. E., Palmer, M., & Fulcher, L. (2003). Client commitment language during motivational interviewing predicts drug use outcomes. *Journal of Consulting and Clinical Psychology, 71,* 862–878.

Avia, M. D., Ruiz, M. A., Olivares, M. E., Crespo, M., Guisado, A. B., Sanchez, A., et al. (1996). The meaning of psychological symptoms: Effectiveness of a group intervention with hypochondriacal patients. *Behaviour Research and Therapy, 34,* 23–31.

Barsky, A. J., & Ahern, D. K. (2004). Cognitive behaviour therapy for hypochondriasis: A randomized controlled trial. *JAMA, 291,* 1464–1470.

Barsky, A. J., Gerringer, E., & Wolf, C. A. (1988). A cognitive–educational treatment for hypochondriasis. *General Hospital Psychiatry, 10,* 322–327.

Beck, A. T. (1976). *Cognitive therapy and the emotional disorders*. New York: International University Press.

Beck, A. T., & Emery, G. (1985). *Anxiety disorders and phobias: A cognitive perspective*. New York: Basic Books.

Bouman, T. K. (2002). A community-based psychoeducational group approach to hypochondriasis. *Psychotherapy and Psychosomatics, 71*, 326–332.

Buwalda, F., Bouman, T. K., & van Duijn, M. A. J. (2007). Psychoeducation for hypochondriasis: A comparison of a cognitive–behavioural approach and a problem-solving approach. *Behaviour Research and Therapy, 45*, 887–899.

Clark, D. M., Salkovskis, P. M., Hackmann, A., Wells, A., Fennell, M., Ludgate, J., et al. (1998). Two psychological treatments for hypochondriasis: A randomized controlled trial. *The British Journal of Psychiatry, 173*, 218–225.

Craske, M. G., & Barlow, D. H. (2007). *Mastery of your anxiety and panic*. Oxford, England: Oxford University Press.

Eysenck, H. J. (1982). Neobehavioristic (S-R) theory. In G. T. Wilson & C. M. Franks (Eds.), *Contemporary behavior therapy: Conceptual and theoretical foundations* (pp. 205–276). New York: Guilford Press.

Foa, E. B., & Kozak, M. J. (1986). Emotional processing of fear: Exposure to corrective information. *Psychological Bulletin, 99*, 20–35.

Leonhard, K. (1961). On the treatment of ideohypochondriac and sensohypochondriac neuroses. *International Journal of Social Psychiatry, 7*, 123–133.

Lidbeck, J. (1997). Group therapy for somatization disorders in general practice: Effectiveness of a short cognitive–behavioural treatment model. *Acta Psychiatrica Scandinavica, 96*, 14–24.

Logsdail, S., Lovell, K., Warwick, H., & Marks, I. (1991). Behavioral treatment of AIDS-focused illness phobia. *The British Journal of Psychiatry, 159*, 422–425.

McKay, D., & Bouman, T. K. (2008). Enhancing cognitive behavior therapy for monosymptomatic hypochondriasis with motivational interviewing: Three case illustrations. *Journal of Cognitive Psychotherapy, 22*, 154–166.

Miller, W. R., & Rollnick, S. (2002). *Motivational interviewing: Preparing people for change* (2nd ed.). New York: Guilford Press.

Pennebaker, J. W. (1982). *The psychology of physical symptoms*. New York: Springer.

Richard, D. C. S., & Lauterbach, D. L. (2007). *Handbook of exposure therapies*. Amsterdam: Academic Press.

Rogers, C. R. (1951). *Client-centered therapy*. Boston: Houghton Mifflin.

Salkovskis, P. M., Warwick, H. M., & Deale, A. C. (2003). Cognitive–behavioral treatment for severe and persistent health anxiety (hypochondriasis). *Brief Treatment and Crisis Intervention, 3*, 353–367.

Stern, R., & Fernandez, M. (1991, November 16). Group cognitive and behavioural treatment for hypochondriasis. *BMJ, 303*, 1229–1231.

Taylor, S. (2000). *Understanding and treating panic disorder*. New York: Wiley.

Taylor, S., & Asmundson, G. (2004). *Treating health anxiety: A cognitive–behavioral approach*. New York: Guilford Press.

Taylor, S., Asmundson, G., & Coons, M. (2005). Current directions in the treatment of hypochondriasis. *Journal of Cognitive Psychotherapy, 19,* 285–304.

Visser, S., & Bouman, T. K. (1992). Cognitive–behavioral approaches in the treatment of hypochondriasis: Six single case cross-over studies. *Behaviour Research and Therapy, 30,* 301–306.

Visser, S., & Bouman, T. K. (2001). The treatment of hypochondriasis: Exposure plus response prevention vs. cognitive therapy. *Behaviour Research and Therapy, 39,* 423–442.

Walker, J., Vincent, N., Furer, P., Cox, B., & Kjernisted, K. (1999). Treatment preference in hypochondriasis. *Journal of Behavior Therapy and Experimental Psychiatry, 30,* 251–258.

Warwick, H. M., Clark, D. M., Cobb, A. M., & Salkovskis, P. M. (1996). A controlled trial of cognitive–behavioral treatment of hypochondriasis. *The British Journal of Psychiatry, 169,* 189–195.

Warwick, H. M., & Marks, I. M. (1988). Behavioural treatment of illness phobia and hypochondriasis: A pilot study of 17 cases. *The British Journal of Psychiatry, 152,* 239–241.

Wells, A. (1997). *Cognitive therapy of anxiety disorders.* New York: Wiley.

16

BORDERLINE PERSONALITY DISORDER

ALEXANDER L. CHAPMAN

At first blush, it would seem that, if ever there was a disorder that could be considered *refractory*, it would be borderline personality disorder (BPD). As noted in previous chapters of this book, refractory patients are those that do not respond to usual treatment protocols. Persons with BPD demonstrate many characteristics that would appear to place them into the category of refractory patients. For example, persons with BPD demonstrate instability and dysregulation in a variety of life domains, including interpersonal, emotional, cognitive, identity, and behavior (American Psychiatric Association, 2000). Despite a general prevalence of approximately 1% to 2%, persons with BPD constitute up to 20% of psychiatric inpatients in the United States and they are heavy users of outpatient services (Skodol et al., 2002). In fact, over their lifetimes, 97% of patients with BPD receive outpatient treatment from an average of 6.1 therapists (Perry, Herman, van der Kolk, & Hoke, 1990; Skodol, Buckley, & Charles, 1983). Individuals with BPD demonstrate exceedingly high prevalence rates of severe, self-destructive behaviors, such as suicide attempts (75%) and self-harm (69%–80%; Skodol et al., 2002).

The author expresses appreciation to Kristy N. Walters and Katherine Dixon-Gordon for comments on versions of this chapter.

Perhaps not surprisingly, the term *borderline* strikes fear into the hearts of many clinicians.

Common clinical lore still holds that BPD is difficult, if not impossible, to treat successfully. The term *personality disorder* itself seems to suggest a relatively chronic, debilitating condition not unlike a deep scar that never quite fades, or terminal cancer. Yet despite the obvious severity of the disorder, evidence is accumulating that BPD is treatable, and the course of BPD is characterized by a high rate of diagnostic remission.

There is no doubt, however, that BPD can be a difficult disorder to treat. Indeed, several aspects of BPD create unique clinical challenges. Persons with BPD experience rapidly shifting moods and intense, overwhelming emotional states. They sometimes develop behaviors that are very hard to stop, such as self-harm or drug use. Persons with BPD also, by definition, experience interpersonal problems, characterized by chaotic relationships and vacillation between the idealization and devaluation of other people—even, at times, the therapist. Although work with BPD patients can be very rewarding, it is certainly not for therapists who want a serene professional life.

In this chapter, I discuss the factors that seem to create challenges in the treatment of BPD. I provide information that is accumulating on the course, prognosis, and treatment response of individuals with BPD. Subsequently, I discuss therapist and patient factors related to treatment challenges and present a transactional model. I also discuss how to treat difficult-to-treat problems among persons with BPD, primarily from a dialectical behavior therapy (DBT; Linehan, 1993a) perspective.

IS BORDERLINE PERSONALITY DISORDER REFRACTORY?

The short answer to this question is, no, but it can be difficult to treat. Evidence from research on the course of BPD as well as treatment research on BPD has suggested that individuals with BPD do improve over time and that BPD can be successfully treated. These findings challenge long-standing clinical lore that BPD is a refractory disorder.

Borderline Personality Disorder Is Not a Stable, Intractable Disorder

Emerging evidence from longitudinal studies of BPD has suggested that the course and prognosis of BPD are much more hopeful than previously thought. Zanarini, Frankenburg, Hennen, and Silk (2003) conducted the largest study in this area—a longitudinal follow-up study of patients with BPD who had been hospitalized for psychiatric reasons. After 2 years, 35% of participants with BPD had experienced a full remission from the BPD diagnosis. The numbers at the 4-year (49%) and 6-year (69%) points reflect a disorder that is not as intractable as previously thought. In fact, throughout the 6-year study period, 74% of patients experienced a full remission at some point, and of these individuals, 94% never met criteria again during the rest of the study.

Another study is currently examining the course of BPD in comparison with three other personality disorders and major depression (Gunderson et al., 2000; Skodol et al., 2005). This study has been underway for over 7 years and has found a pattern similar to that found in the Zanarini et al. (2003) study. Specifically, over half of the patients with BPD in their study stopped meeting criteria for BPD at some point within the first 2 years of the study (Grilo et al., 2004). In addition, over 25% of the patients with BPD reported almost no symptoms for more than a year (Grilo et al., 2004). Also, this study found that 10% of patients with BPD stopped meeting criteria for BPD within the first 6 months of the study (Skodol et al., 2005). Across studies in this area, the following findings are consistent (Chapman & Gratz, 2008, p. 3):

1. Most people with BPD experience major reductions in their symptoms far sooner than previously thought.
2. Once people with BPD experience a reduction in their symptoms, these symptoms are very unlikely to return.
3. Once people with BPD stop meeting criteria for BPD, they are very unlikely to meet criteria for BPD again in the future.

Persons With Borderline Personality Disorder Improve With Psychological Treatment

Treatment outcome research has also demonstrated that BPD is treatable. A substantial number of patients with BPD make clinically meaningful improvements with treatment. Moreover, a few different treatments have shown promising outcomes for BPD.

Dialectical Behavior Therapy

Since the early 1990s, several studies have been published on DBT (Linehan, 1993a) for BPD. DBT is based on the theory that BPD results from a transaction of emotion vulnerability with an invalidating rearing environment. Emotion vulnerability consists of a temperament-based propensity toward low-threshold emotional responses (it does not take a strong emotional event to trigger a response) combined with intense emotional responses and a slow return to baseline emotional arousal. An invalidating environment rejects the child's emotional communications as invalid, punishes emotional display and intermittently reinforces emotional escalation, and oversimplifies the ease of problem solving or coping. As a result, individuals with BPD are highly emotional but have great difficulty managing their emotions. DBT largely aims to help patients with BPD learn to effectively regulate emotions.

Standard DBT consists of weekly individual therapy and group skills training sessions, in addition to a therapist consultation team and availability of the individual therapist for telephone contact (or other types of contact, such as e-mail or pager) in between sessions.

To date, numerous studies have been conducted on DBT, with 10 of these consisting of randomized clinical trials focused on BPD. Across studies, findings indicate that DBT reduces some of the most severe behavioral problems in BPD more effectively than do treatments for BPD as they are usually conducted in the community as well as other types of control treatments (for a comprehensive review of the research on DBT, see Robins & Chapman, 2004; see also Lieb et al., 2004). On the basis of the evidence so far, DBT has attained the status of a well-established treatment for BPD (Chambless & Ollendick, 2001). In addition, the findings on DBT do not appear to be accounted for by allegiance effects, as several studies have evaluated DBT outside of the treatment developer's laboratory.

Findings from a recent study have suggested that DBT also appears to have specific effects beyond those of expert treatment in general (Linehan et al., 2006). For instance, the most recent, largest, study of DBT compared the treatment with a condition called *community treatment by experts* (CTBE). CTBE therapists were nominated by mental health directors in the community as experts in treating difficult patients. Compared with CTBE patients, the DBT group had a lower frequency of suicide attempts at all assessment time points (over the 2-year study, including 1-year of follow-up); a lower proportion of suicide attempters, hospitalizations, emergency department visits, and dropouts; and a lower medical risk of parasuicide (i.e., any intentional self-injury). In previous studies comparing DBT with treatment as usual, however, DBT patients did not evidence a lower frequency of nonsuicidal self-injury. On the basis of these and other findings, DBT currently is considered part of the standard of care for BPD patients in many areas.

Other Psychological Treatments

Another encouraging set of findings is emerging from research on alternative psychological treatment approaches. As recently as the late 1990s, the only psychological treatment for BPD that had been tested in rigorous clinical trials was DBT. Although DBT still has the strongest research base, other approaches have also demonstrated promising findings. Recent findings have suggested that a cognitively oriented therapy and two psychodynamically oriented treatments have promise in the treatment of BPD.

Schema-focused therapy (SFT; Young, 1994), a cognitive therapy treatment for BPD, is based on the theory that BPD results from the development of early maladaptive cognitive schemas. These schemas are caused by early interactions with caregivers in which the individual did not receive the necessary support, attention, love, validation, or caring and may have been abused or traumatized. Treatment, therefore, involves cognitive strategies to challenge or modify underlying schemas as well as the development of an intense therapy relationship characterized by *reparenting* of the individual. This latter strategy is thought to "undo" the environmental events that led to maladaptive schemas, thereby causing enduring personality change.

In the first clinical trial of SFT for BPD, the treatment involved two 50-minute individual therapy sessions per week for 3 years (Giessen-Bloo et al., 2006). In this study, the investigators compared SFT with transference-focused psychotherapy (TFP, discussed in this section). Findings indicated that fewer patients in SFT (compared with TFP) dropped out, and that after 3 years, SFT patients showed better improvements in severity of BPD symptoms, general psychopathology, and quality of life (Giesen-Bloo et al., 2006).

Developed by Anthony Bateman and John Fonagy, *mentalization-based treatment* (MBT; Bateman & Fonagy, 1999) is a psychodynamic approach based on the theory that the treatment of BPD must involve increasing the patient's ability to engage in mentalization. Mentalization is the ability to understand that behaviors (both of the patient and of other people) are related to emotions, thoughts, feelings, and desires. As investigated in the original clinical trial (Bateman & Fonagy, 1999), MBT involved 6 hours per week of structured treatment, including individual therapy, group therapy, expressive therapy, and a community meeting. Compared with treatment as usual in the community, MBT had superior outcomes in terms of reducing suicide attempts, self-harm, depression, and anxiety and increasing social functioning. Findings also demonstrated that treatment effects persisted through an 18-month follow-up period.

TFP (Clarkin, Levy, Lenzenweger, & Kernberg, 2007) also has demonstrated some promising effects for patients with BPD. Unlike MBT, which focuses largely on the patient's current experiences, TFP emphasizes transference reactions in the therapeutic relationship. TFP is based on the theory that a primary defense mechanism underlying BPD is that of splitting internal representations of self and other into "good" and "bad." As a result, TFP is an insight-oriented approach that involves the therapist helping the patient to understand and observe the origins and effects of his or her transference reactions.

A recent randomized clinical trial compared TFP with supportive psychotherapy (involving emotional support and advice regarding daily problems) and DBT for 90 patients with BPD (Clarkin et al., 2007). Findings indicated that patients in TFP, DBT, and expressive psychotherapy each showed significant improvements on important clinical outcomes, such as depression, global functioning, anger, suicidality, and depression. Findings also revealed no significant differences among these three conditions on major clinical outcomes for BPD. These latter findings suggest that the specificity of DBT warrants further examination, as DBT may not outperform other manualized treatments for BPD.

A couple of important caveats regarding these findings, however, must be considered. One caveat is that the investigators used a measure of adherence to the DBT treatment manual that was neither approved of nor developed by the developer of DBT. There is a psychometrically sound measure of DBT adherence developed at the University of Washington, and it has been used in other randomized trials of DBT (e.g., Linehan et al., 2006). As a result, it is difficult to know whether the therapists were actually practicing DBT with comparable adherence to that in other studies. Another caveat is that the sample size was relatively small for a head-to-head comparison of bona fide treatments. In this type of study, differences between treatments are likely to reflect small effect sizes, requiring large sample sizes to detect them. Nevertheless, the findings from recent research on psychological treatments are very encouraging, suggesting that a variety of treatment approaches might help people with BPD.

Medication Treatments

In terms of medication treatments, the findings are somewhat less encouraging but still suggest that aspects of BPD are treatable through medications. There have been a few recent, thorough reviews of medication-based treatments for BPD (Lieb, Zanarini, Schmahl, Linehan, & Bohus, 2004; Paris, 2005). These reviews have been remarkably consistent and have suggested the following conclusions about medication treatment of BPD:

1. The strongest evidence exists for selective serotonin reuptake inhibitors (SSRIs) in the treatment of depression, anxiety, and mood shifts. Of the medications that have been examined for BPD, SSRIs are likely to have the fewest serious side effects.
2. There is some evidence that mood-stabilizing medications (particularly divalproate sodium) and certain antipsychotic medications (clozapine and olanzapine) may be helpful in reducing irritability, anger, and general psychiatric symptoms. These medications, however, often have serious side effects, and studies are plagued by high dropout rates (80% and higher in some studies).
3. There is no "anti-BPD" medication. Different classes of medications (e.g., antidepressants, antipsychotics, mood stabilizers) seem to have similar effects. Most experts agree that a solely medication-based treatment for BPD is not advisable.

CHALLENGES IN THE TREATMENT OF BORDERLINE PERSONALITY DISORDER

Despite positive findings about course and treatment response, BPD can be a difficult disorder to treat. The disorder itself does not appear to be refractory, but some individuals with the disorder may not respond to treatment. Moreover, clinical work with patients who have BPD can be stressful and challenging. A variety of patient features and therapist factors can interfere with treatment and limit the effectiveness of therapy.

As mentioned, DBT has garnered considerable evidence for its efficacy in the treatment of BPD through several rigorously controlled randomized clinical trials. In the clinical trials conducted at Linehan's research center, inclusion criteria specify that the individual must meet criteria for BPD and must have engaged in recent suicidal behavior (e.g., over the past 8 weeks). As a result, the persons in these trials are among the more serious cases of suicidal individuals with BPD. Because many patients do improve considerably in treatment, certain aspects of DBT may be particularly effective at treating difficult-to-treat problems. In the following section, I discuss patient and therapist factors that create therapy challenges and some of the treatment strategies used in DBT to address them.

Patient Factors That Create Therapy Challenges

Patient factors include a variety of features and behaviors related to BPD that might put stress on therapy or make it difficult for patients to improve. As shown in recent studies on the course of BPD, the symptoms or features that are least likely to remit over time include the following: (a) emotional instability; (b) fears of abandonment; and (c) emotion-linked impulsive actions, such as binge eating, shoplifting, gambling, and other such difficulties (Zanarini et al., 2003). Additionally, findings have suggested that the presence of eating disorders and substance use disorders predict poorer outcomes for BPD, at least in a naturalistic study of the course of BPD (Zanarini et al., 2003). In contrast, crisis-related behaviors, such as suicide attempts and self-harm, often seem to remit, both in treatment and in naturalistic follow-up studies of BPD (Zanarini et al., 2003). The focus here is on patient factors related to poorer prognosis in BPD: emotional instability; interpersonal difficulties/fears of abandonment; and impulsive, mood-driven behavioral problems (e.g., substance abuse, eating disorders).

Emotional Instability and Dysregulation

Emotional instability, a hallmark feature of BPD, can make therapy feel like a roller coaster ride and can make it difficult to maintain a consistent focus or to teach the patient new skills. Therapy with patients who experience frequent emotional volatility requires therapists who are skillful, knowledgeable about interventions for emotional dysregulation, and able to weather emotional storms and crises while helping the patient make meaningful changes. Chronic life stress and chaos can exacerbate emotional instability and interfere with therapy. As noted by Linehan (1993a), persons with BPD seem to encounter an extraordinarily large number of stressful life events on a regular basis (called *unrelenting crisis*; Linehan, 1993a). The therapist may sometimes feel as if he or she is constantly helping the patient "put out fires" and is not making progress in a consistent, focused manner.

As an emotion-focused cognitive–behavioral therapy (CBT), DBT addresses emotional instability in a variety of ways. The therapist conceptualizes patient problems as related to emotions and difficulty regulating emotions. Within sessions, if a patient appears to be experiencing strong emotional reactions that interfere with the progress of the session, the therapist highlights these emotional reactions and helps the patient to observe, notice, and regulate them. DBT teaches a variety of emotion regulation skills designed to help patients understand their emotions, reduce their vulnerability to overwhelming emotions, and regulate or reduce emotional responses once they have begun. There is also a focus in DBT on the acceptance of emotional responses and on skills that involve the patient mindfully observing the experience of emotions (Linehan, 1993b).

Interpersonal Difficulties

Difficulties with interpersonal relationships and fears of abandonment are among the defining features of BPD, and relationship discord often occurs both outside and within the therapeutic relationship. Frequent crises, interpersonal discord, and dysfunctional social networks (i.e., those that reinforce dysfunctional behaviors and punish adaptive behaviors) can present many challenges for therapy. In addition, frequent stressful events can make therapy like a tug of war between the therapist and the patient's natural environment.

DBT therapists use a variety of strategies to address interpersonal difficulties both inside and outside of the therapeutic relationship. In terms of difficulties inside the therapy relationship, the therapist is open to developing an intense therapeutic relationship in which some of the problems the patient experiences in other relationships may occur. When these problems do occur, the therapist highlights them; discusses them in a direct, matter of fact manner; and discusses any possible association of what is happening inside therapy with what happens in relationships outside of therapy. When relationship problems arise, the primary treatment strategy is straightforward problem solving. If it appears that relationship problems or fears within the therapy relationship are relevant to what happens outside therapy, the therapist's main focus is on helping the patient learn new, effective behaviors. As such, the therapist does not normally "remove the cue" for the patient's distress.

Case Example. John was seeing his patient, Michelle, who had an intense fear of abandonment. After they had worked together for a year and a half and Michelle was showing good progress, John asked her how she would know when she was ready to finish therapy. Michelle panicked. Her face went red, her muscles tensed, and she started shaking and told John that she was very angry with him for bringing up termination. She felt terribly afraid that he would drop her and that she would have no say regarding when therapy was to end. Instead of reassuring Michelle, which would remove the fear cue, John highlighted Michelle's fear, asked her whether this comes up with other people as well, and then asked whether she would like to work on reducing her fear of abandonment.

After she agreed that she would like to work on this fear, treatment involved the therapist presenting the cue repeatedly until Michelle learned alternative responses. For example, John and Michelle completed several role-plays in which John brought up termination, and they gradually increased the intensity of this exposure intervention until the role-play involved John telling her that he thought it was time for therapy to end. After several trials, Michelle's fear of termination reduced significantly, and she and John planned for termination in a productive manner. Because of research suggesting that the learning of new associations to feared stimuli are relatively context de-pendent (i.e., might be restricted to therapy termination discussions; Bou-ton, 2004), the therapist encouraged Michelle to practice her new learning when she felt abandoned by her husband and her daughter. Over time, she reported considerably lower fear in these alternative situations as well.

Impulsive and Mood-Driven Behaviors

Impulsive, mood-driven actions, such as substance use problems or eat-ing disordered behaviors, can interfere with therapy in a variety of ways. The effects of illicit substances can decrease the patient's ability to learn new skills, and the difficulties in living that often accompany substance problems can reduce compliance with, interest in, or attendance at therapy. Indeed, Linehan and colleagues found that a variety of modifications to standard DBT were necessary to address the housing, financial, attendance, and social issues of persons with substance dependence (Dimeff, Rizvi, Brown, & Linehan, 2000; Robins & Chapman, 2004).

Some of these modifications involved what are called *attachment strate-gies*. Attachment strategies are interventions by the therapist to encourage the patient to engage in therapy. As an example, if a patient does not show up for therapy, the therapist might call the patient or actually travel to the patient's home or to other places where the patient might be. Other strate-gies might involve the therapist sending warm notes or cards encouraging the patient to return to therapy (see Dimeff et al., 2000).

Two important principles guide the DBT approach to substance use and eating disordered behaviors (and other such actions that do not involve the intentional infliction of injury or the intent to die). First, such behaviors are only targeted in treatment if the patient's goal is to reduce these behav-iors. The DBT therapist does not work on substance use or eating disordered behaviors by default. Rather, treatment generally focuses on these behaviors only if one of the patient's goals is to reduce them.

Second, unlike psychodynamic approaches, which do not directly address behaviors in favor of addressing the psychological conflicts that presumably underlie these behaviors, DBT therapists directly target behavior change. As a result, substance use and eating disordered behaviors are targeted directly in the same manner as are other behaviors, such as suicidal or self-harm behaviors. The patient monitors the behaviors on a daily basis, and if they have occurred, the patient and therapist conduct a behavioral analysis, generate solutions, commit to implementing these solutions, and troubleshoot potential obstacles that might get in the way. Therapy might also involve the therapist teaching specific behavioral skills that help the patient reduce substance use, eating disordered, or other behaviors. These skills normally are taught in group-based skills training sessions but might also be taught informally in individual therapy sessions. Findings on DBT for substance-using individuals have been promising (Robins & Chapman, 2004), suggesting that a direct-targeting approach might be fruitful.

Therapist Factors That Create Therapy Challenges

Therapy difficulties certainly are not solely related to the features and problems related to BPD. Few studies, however, have examined the association of therapist factors with treatment response in BPD. Nevertheless, anecdotal evidence and theory regarding BPD have suggested that several therapist factors can inhibit therapeutic progress, lead to premature termination, or have iatrogenic effects.

One such factor is emotional distress on the part of the therapist. Because BPD is a particularly stigmatized disorder, irritation, anger, judgmental thinking, pejorative labels, and negative attitudes toward patients with BPD can interfere with therapy. Even therapists who diligently practice a nonjudging attitude might find themselves thinking judgmentally about their patients with BPD and, hence, feeling angry, irritated, overwhelmed, or incapable of providing effective treatment. With patients who frequently attempt suicide, confront the therapist, or experience overwhelming emotional storms, therapists sometimes feel overwhelmed and act ineffectively.

Lack of therapist skill or knowledge can also interfere with treatment. Some therapists may not be aware of the existing interventions that work for people with BPD and instead rely on clinical intuition, "comfortable" treatment approaches that fit their interests (e.g., a purely humanistic approach with a multiproblem suicidal patient), or practices with no empirical support. The treatment with the most empirical support for BPD is DBT, a cognitive–behaviorally oriented approach. Studies of how people practice in community settings, however, have revealed that relatively few clinicians use CBTs. Moreover, actual training in evidence-based CBT is not as common as would be expected given the dominance of CBT approaches in the current armamentarium of evidence-based treatments. A lack of training or skill in the treatment of complex, multiproblem patients can lead to therapeutic errors with potentially disastrous effects.

Finally, another therapist factor is motivation. As noted by Linehan (1993a), effective treatment of patients with BPD requires effective, motivated therapists. It can be difficult, however, for therapists to maintain their motivation in the presence of a seemingly unending onslaught of major life problems, stressors, suicidal ideation, self-harm, drug use, binge eating, relationship discord, and so on. Therapists can end up feeling overwhelmed, stuck, demoralized, and unmotivated to put forth the effort needed to help their patients.

Targeting Therapist Factors in Dialectical Behavior Therapy

The primary therapy mode that targets therapist factors in DBT is the therapist consultation team. Typically, the consultation team occurs once per week for approximately 1 to 2 hours and involves a group of individuals who all utilize DBT. The team may consist of only one type of mental health professional (e.g., all psychologists) or, in some cases, may be interdisciplinary. The consultation team essentially is "therapy for the therapists" and involves the team applying the principles of DBT to each team member. The meeting time is prioritized according to the standard DBT hierarchy of treatment targets (Linehan, 1993a), with life-threatening behaviors given top priority, followed by behaviors that interfere with therapy, and behaviors that interfere with the patient's quality of life. The therapy-interfering category, elaborated further later in the chapter, includes behaviors on the part of the patient or the therapist that might interfere with therapeutic progress. The team also might involve a didactic component on DBT as well as active practicing of therapy skills.

Unlike most supervision groups, the consultation team focuses on therapist behaviors rather than on patient pathology. Therapists provide each other with support, encouragement, validation, motivational enhancement, and training and practice where needed. Work with multiproblem patients can be challenging; thus, the consultation team can help prevent therapists from going astray in their clinical work.

The therapist consultation team often actively targets the therapist factors noted previously that can limit the efficacy of treatment.

Case Example. Betty was struggling in her work with her patient, Ed. Ed was recently diagnosed with Parkinson's disease, had BPD and major depression, and spent most of his time sitting on the couch staring at the television set. His son had drowned 4 years earlier during a boating trip, his wife was depressed and uninterested in spending time with him, and he had no friends. Additionally, Ed chronically experienced serious suicidal ideation and hopeless thoughts about his life.

As Betty's attempts to help Ed met with limited success, her motivation began to wane, and she was consumed with hopeless thoughts about the likelihood of Ed developing a life worth living. She did not even recognize this problem, however, until the therapist consultation team noticed it one day. She had failed to address frequent therapy absences by Ed, and the team asked her about this. Through further discussion, her hopeless thinking and lack of motivation became apparent, and the team rallied to help her figure out how to renew her hope and enthusiasm. Although Ed never made earth-shattering treatment gains, he had started volunteer work, was significantly less depressed, and was spending more pleasant time with his wife by the time therapy was over.

Therapy-Interfering Behaviors

Behaviors that interfere with therapy, called *therapy-interfering behaviors* in DBT, are by definition those behaviors on the part of the patient or therapist that make it difficult for therapy to progress. In DBT, therapy-interfering behaviors are given high priority in each session, second only to life-threatening behaviors (such as suicide attempts, self-injury, severe suicidal ideation, suicide crises). Therapy-interfering behaviors fall within two main categories in DBT: (a) behaviors that have negative effects on the therapeutic relationship and (b) behaviors that prevent the patient from benefiting from therapy. Each of these types of therapy-interfering behaviors is defined by its effect on therapy, not by the motivation that the individual had for engaging in these behaviors.

One type of behavior that prevents the patient from benefiting from therapy is the failure to show up for therapy sessions. Therapy absences prevent therapy from happening and thereby interfere with therapy. It does not matter whether the patient is absent because of a life-enhancing vacation or volunteer work or is absent because of life chaos, a car breakdown, or a suicide attempt. Absence from therapy, for whatever reason, interferes with therapy. Other behaviors that limit the patient's ability to benefit from therapy include failure to complete homework or fill out self-monitoring forms, showing up late, showing up to therapy intoxicated, or talking too much or too little. Therapist behaviors that fall within this category include inattentiveness, failure to execute the treatment with adherence, frequent absences (e.g., because of out-of-town trips), failure to return calls, and poor management of session time.

Both therapists and patients might also engage in behaviors that have negative effects on the therapeutic relationship. Patients, for example, might display verbal aggression toward the therapist, call the therapist too frequently, make frequent complaints about therapy, or insult the therapist. Therapists might say judgmental things to the patient, fail to comment when their own personal limits are being pushed (e.g., by allowing the patient to continue to call too frequently), blame the patient for his or her problems, engage in invalidating behaviors, and so on.

Targeting Therapy-Interfering Behaviors in Dialectical Behavior Therapy

In DBT, the therapist and patient address therapy-interfering behaviors when they occur. As mentioned, therapy-interfering behaviors are given high priority each session. Therapists are alert to the occurrence of such behaviors, particularly those that burn out the therapist or make it difficult to work with the patient. When a patient is late, absent, or otherwise engaging in therapy-interfering behavior, the therapist highlights this behavior, explains why the behavior interferes with therapy by clarifying the consequences associated with the behavior (e.g., a decrease in the therapist's motivation to work with the client) and often conducts a chain analysis. The chain analysis is a detailed discussion of the events that led up to the behavior (e.g., antecedents), as well as the events that followed the behavior (e.g., consequences). During this discussion, the therapist helps the patient generate solutions, gets a commitment from the patient to implement these solutions, and troubleshoots potential problems that could get in the way. Therapy-interfering behaviors are discussed in a matter-of-fact, open manner, with the therapist expressing willingness to address his or her own therapy-interfering behaviors. As is the practice throughout DBT, the therapist also balances acceptance and validation of the patient with change-oriented interventions geared toward reducing therapy-interfering behaviors.

As this work is challenging, detailed, and time consuming and sometimes elicits negative reactions on the part of the patient, therapist motivation is critical. This is where the consultation team comes in. The therapist consultation team offers support to the therapist and challenges the therapist when he or she is not targeting behavior that needs to be targeted. The team might also help to enhance the therapist's motivation by using the same types of motivational strategies that DBT therapists use with patients: entertaining the pros and cons of doing something different, using the devil's advocate strategy, and asking the therapist for a commitment to do something different (see Linehan, 1993a). In addition, the consultation team regularly inquires as to whether a therapist is experiencing burnout and helps and supports the therapist in her or his efforts to prevent or reduce burnout.

Case Example. Joan called her new therapist every day of the week and multiple times on the weekend. During each call, Joan appeared to be experiencing intense emotional distress and, frequently, urges to engage in self-harm. She had few alternative social supports, and nobody in her social network knew about her self-cutting or her therapy. As a result, she often felt alone in her struggles and was quickly reassured by the presence of the therapist on the phone. It also appeared that the easily accessible, immediate reinforcement associated with talking with the therapist was winning out over the potentially delayed reinforcement (and possible barriers) associated with establishing other social supports. The therapist felt increasingly stressed out as he frequently interrupted his personal activities to take crisis calls from the patient. He noticed himself feeling irritated whenever Joan called and realized that it was time to talk with her about it.

Therapist: Joan, I'm noticing that you have been calling me several times a week over the past couple of weeks. I know that you're going through a very hard time and feel quite alone. I want to be there to help you, but I can't keep up this number of calls. I'm noticing that I'm starting to feel stressed about the calls and having trouble maintaining my personal life in the evenings and on weekends. What do you think we can do about this?

Patient: Oh no, it's happening again. I just know I burned out my other therapist by calling too much; she just never said anything about it, so I kept doing it. I hate talking about this, and I'm actually feeling a little angry that you're bringing it up.

Therapist: I can see that. I'm wondering whether you're also afraid that I'm going to give up on you—like I'm fed up with you, or something?

Patient: Yeah, well, it's happened to me before.

Therapist: That's exactly why I bring it up. I'm not willing to let myself get to that point. I want us to work well together, and the best way to do that is for us both to bring up things that might make it hard to work with each other. I know how much you need help, but are you willing to cut down on the calls?

Patient: Yeah, I can do that. How many calls could you handle?

Therapist: Maybe three per week?

Patient: That sounds really hard. I don't know how I can do that.

Therapist: It might be hard at first. Let's figure out how to make it easier
. . .

A TRANSACTIONAL MODEL: IMPLICATIONS FOR TREATMENT

Although DBT addresses many of the factors that interfere with therapeutic progress, DBT is not perfect, nor is any other treatment. After treatment, a significant proportion of individuals with BPD are still suffering and still engaging in serious behaviors, such as self-injury and suicide attempts. Treatment needs to improve, and for that to occur perhaps we need a fresh perspective on what might keep patients with BPD stuck in the same patterns that bring them to therapy.

One way to think about the processes that keep patients stuck is to conceptualize them as Person × Environment transactions. In personality psychology, researchers have identified several different Person × Environment transactions that might explain the continuity of personality traits over the life span: evocative, proactive, and reactive transactions. As applied to BPD, this means that the patient's behavior influences the therapist's behavior, and the therapist's behavior influences the patient's behavior. Instead of assuming that refractory cases are solely due to therapist or patient factors operating independently, a transactional model can capture the complexities of when and how therapy with BPD patients seems to go awry.

Evocative Person × Environment Transactions

An Evocative Person × Environment transaction is one in which the individual's existing personality traits or features elicit responses from the environment that reinforce or maintain the individual's traits. In this case, the related features and behaviors of a patient with BPD might elicit responses from the therapist that function to maintain the patient's existing problems.

Linehan proposed that this type of evocative transaction influences the development of BPD. Within Linehan's (1993a) biosocial theory, a transaction between emotion vulnerability and an invalidating rearing environment spawns the development of BPD. The invalidating rearing environment punishes, ignores, dismisses, or becomes dysregulated (e.g., the parents become upset and out of control) when the individual expresses strong emotions. Strong emotions on the part of the child elicit negative, invalidating reactions from the caregivers, and in turn, these invalidating responses magnify the child's emotional reactions. For example, the dismissal, punishment, or negation (e.g., "You don't really feel that way. There's no need for that.") of an individual's emotional pain might actually amplify it. Over time, the invalidating environment maintains emotion vulnerability, and emotion vulnerability continues to elicit invalidating responses. As persons with BPD have difficulty regulating their emotions as well, they are left with intense, overwhelming emotional responses and few adaptive means to modulate these responses. A patient with BPD is much like a very powerful car without a functional braking system (Chapman & Gratz, 2008).

Intense emotionality can elicit maladaptive responses from the therapist that amplify or reinforce the patient's emotionality, particularly if the therapist (a) lacks skill or (b) experiences aversive emotional reactions to the patient.

Case Example

Sally was a very "intense" person. When she was upset, she spoke rapidly and loudly and used dramatic gestures and body language. Her therapist often did not know what to do when Sally was distressed about events in her life. He felt uncomfortable, at a loss for words, and distracted by the dramatic, severe, intense things that Sally was saying (e.g., "I just can't stand this anymore. I have to die now!"). As a result, he responded in an invalidating manner, minimizing Sally's pain (e.g., "It's probably not as bad as you think. You're engaging in catastrophizing right now"), ignoring it and focusing on something else, or appearing uncomfortable or distressed. In response, Sally increased her intensity in order to communicate her feelings and be understood, thereby eliciting further distress and further ineffective therapist behaviors.

Evocative Transactions in Therapy

This scenario also characterizes many therapy transactions, treatment settings (e.g., inpatient hospitalization units), and transactions between the individual with BPD and the community at large (which often involves stigmatizing, invalidating reactions to persons with BPD). Persons with BPD may actually act in such a manner that other people in treatment settings and in the community treat them like "mental patients." Dysregulated behavior and verbalization of suicidal thoughts can elicit fear and concern, which in turn can lead people to be very careful about what they say or do around the individual with BPD. Often afraid of "rocking the boat," family members may become very conciliatory, warm, supportive, and attentive when an individual expresses suicidal thoughts. In turn, the patient ends up stuck in a vicious cycle, as this type of concern and support may only be available contingent upon suicidality or severely dysregulated behaviors. Indeed, people with BPD sometimes report that they engage in self-harm in order to communicate with or influence other people (Brown, Comtois, & Linehan, 2002), and there is some evidence that self-harm may be socially reinforced (Nock & Prinstein, 2005).

The often dramatic or frightening behaviors (e.g., suicidal behavior) exhibited by people with BPD can also shape the environment to respond in ways that do not promote adaptive change. Therapists might adopt an approach that is imbalanced, focusing too much on acceptance of the patient or on changing the patient, or reinforcing the very behaviors that need to change.

Clinical Implications

One clinical implication of evocative transactions is that another pathway for change involves focusing on other individuals' reactions to the patient. Currently, in treatments for BPD, the focus is largely on the patient's behaviors, thoughts, emotions, personality, and skills. Changing these factors presumably would result in changes in the environment's response to the patient; however, more of a focus on changing the individual's environment may be needed. Environmental interventions might involve (a) teaching caregivers, family members, and friends different, effective ways to respond to the individual; (b) actively combating stigma regarding BPD through psychoeducation; the use of television, books, or other media; or social psychological methods that have been shown to reduce in-group/out-group biases; or (c) consultation with treatment providers on how best to respond to the patient. Regarding the latter point, in DBT there is a focus on balancing direct environmental interventions by the therapist with consultation with the patient on how to change his or her environments (Linehan, 1993a).

Proactive Person × Environment Transactions

A Proactive Person × Environment transaction is one in which the individual seeks out environments that reinforce or maintain his or her features or problems. In this case, the individual with BPD may actually self-select into environments or choose therapists who are likely to reinforce dysfunctional behaviors and maintain the patient's existing problems or characteristics.

Case Example

Fred always felt like a misfit. He never fit in with his classmates in elementary and high school. In young adulthood, he ended up in relationships characterized by severe conflict, drug and alcohol abuse, and infidelity. He frequently told his therapist how dissatisfied he was with his current partner, George, but expressed fear that he would never "fit in" in a relationship with someone "more normal." He actively sought out people who had had past childhood abuse, alcoholic parents, severe trauma, or drug/alcohol problems (people he described as "screwed up"). Fred felt most comfortable around these people and believed that they, unlike "normal" people, would understand him. Unfortunately, he ended up in relationships that reinforced and exacerbated his existing problems.

Proactive Transactions in Therapy

This type of transaction occurs in therapy as well. Patients with BPD often come to therapy dissatisfied with their previous therapy experiences. In many cases, they report that their previous therapist simply "listened" and did not help them learn anything new. It is quite possible that patients with BPD actually seek out (with or without awareness) therapists who are not likely to help them. This was the case with Fred, who reported three previous therapists who were warm and attentive but who simply listened and offered emotional support without teaching him new skills or ways to think about his difficulties. For a period, Fred felt comfortable with these therapists because they allowed him to be exactly as he was and did not push him to change. In fact, when he saw therapists who suggested behavioral change, he often felt invalidated and quit or became angry and asked the therapist to stop pushing him to change. As a result, Fred's self-selected social environment and therapy environments reinforced his existing difficulties.

Clinical Implications

An important clinical implication stemming from proactive transactions is that treatment might focus more on the individual's selection of particular environments. This is a focus in adaptations of DBT for substance use disorders, whereby the therapist encourages the patient to cut ties with drug-using friends or dealers. There may, however, be a need for a greater focus on the individual's choice of social environments. Perhaps interventions might be developed to help individuals make effective choices regarding social circles, partners, friends, or activities, with an emphasis on those types of environments that would reinforce adaptive behaviors. Theoretically, this type of work might facilitate the generalization of treatment gains beyond therapy, particularly if the individual gravitates toward environments in which treatment gains are reinforced. Additionally, efforts by the mental health professional community might also focus on the education of patients regarding effective treatments and on helping patients figure out how to find treatment providers who will provide treatment that will not reinforce existing problems.

Reactive Person × Environment Transactions

A Reactive Person × Environment transaction is one in which the individual interprets events in the environment in ways that maintain his or her characteristics or problems. In this case, the individual with BPD may actually enter into different environments but respond as if these environments are functionally the same as previously experienced events. This, in some ways, is the phenomenon of transference emphasized in psychodynamic approaches to BPD. The patient might, for example, have had previous experiences of abandonment and rejection and interpret the therapist's behavior (sometimes correctly!) as indicative of abandonment and rejection. In turn, the patient might experience the same types of emotional reactions and thoughts that he or she would experience in an actual abandonment situation. As a result, the patient's problems are maintained.

Case Example

Jane was deathly afraid of abandonment. She was, in fact, hypervigilant to any sign of abandonment on the part of the therapist, her partner, or anyone else who was close to her. Jane's therapist asked her to reschedule their weekly therapy appointment from Sunday to Tuesday to accomplish her goal of stopping weekend work. Jane thought that the therapist was rejecting her, and she was afraid that she would be moved off the schedule altogether, particularly if she could not attend Tuesday appointments. She felt angry and told the therapist that she was being unreasonable. At that point, an evocative transaction occurred, whereby the therapist felt irritated and burned out with Jane and spoke with an irritated tone of voice. Perceiving this as yet another sign of abandonment, Jane felt hurt, thought this was a signal of impending termination, and ended up hurting herself.

Clinical Implications

For reactive transactions, the key problem is that the individual experiences and responds to different environments in similar ways. For this type of problem, refinement of clinical interventions might involve helping the individual become aware of and responsive to differences in current environments. The example above regarding Jane shows one way to do this. For a patient with a history of abandonment and rejection, exposure-oriented approaches might help the individual learn that his or her fears regarding abandonment in the current context are not justified. Other interventions might involve helping the patient remain open to and check out the facts of the current situation in order to determine whether it is, indeed, as he or she perceives it to be. In Jane's case, the patient might be encouraged to ask the therapist whether she is planning to terminate or to ask about what might happen if she were not able to make Tuesday appointments. DBT already includes these types of interventions, but arguably, more work is needed in this area. Perhaps future research might focus on how to help an individual go into a new environment and respond to it as such, breaking long-standing patterns that have become rooted in different contexts.

SUMMARY AND CONCLUSIONS

In sum, BPD presents many clinical challenges and can be difficult to treat. Findings on the course of BPD, however, suggest that this is a disorder with high rates of diagnostic remission. Treatment outcome studies similarly demonstrate hopeful findings, with a strong foundation of evidence for DBT and emerging evidence suggesting that other treatments have promise. The research, however, has not advanced far enough for us to know who does not benefit from DBT or other treatments. As outlined in this chapter, several factors related to patients and therapists might inhibit therapeutic progress. DBT includes several built-in interventions to address factors such as emotional instability, interpersonal problems, impulsive behaviors, therapist distress, and low motivation or skill on the part of the therapist. In addition, DBT targets therapy-interfering behaviors. Nevertheless, further treatment refinement is needed, as not every patient with BPD benefits from DBT or from other psychological treatments. The use of a transactional model might point researchers and treatment developers in directions that will help refine treatments for patients who may be considered refractory.

REFERENCES

American Psychiatric Association. (2000). *Diagnostic and statistical manual of mental disorders* (4th ed., text rev.). Washington, DC: Author.

Bateman, A. W., & Fonagy, P. (1999). Effectiveness of partial hospitalization in the treatment of borderline personality disorder: A randomized controlled trial. *The American Journal of Psychiatry, 156*, 1563–1569.

Bouton, M. E. (2004). Context and behavioral processes in extinction. *Learning & Memory, 11*, 485–494.

Brown, M. Z., Comtois, K. A., & Linehan, M. M. (2002). Reasons for suicide attempts and nonsuicidal self-injury in women with borderline personality disorder. *Journal of Abnormal Psychology, 111*, 198–202.

Chambless, D. L., & Ollendick, T. H. (2001). Empirically supported psychological interventions: Controversies and evidence. *Annual Review of Psychology, 52*, 685–716.

Chapman, A. L., & Gratz, K. L. (2008). *The borderline personality disorder survival guide: Everything you need to know about living with BPD.* Oakland, CA: New Harbinger.

Clarkin, J. F., Levy, K. N., Lenzenweger, M. F., & Kernberg, O. F. (2007). Evaluating three treatments for borderline personality disorder: A multiwave study. *The American Journal of Psychiatry, 164*, 922–928.

Dimeff, L. A., Rizvi, S. L., Brown, M. Z., & Linehan, M. M. (2000). Dialectical behavior therapy for substance abuse: A pilot application to methamphetamine-dependent women with borderline personality disorder. *Cognitive and Behavioral Practice, 7*, 457–468.

Giesen-Bloo, J., van Dyck, R., Spinhoven, P., van Tilburg, W., Dirksen, C., van Asselt, T., et al. (2006). Outpatient psychotherapy for borderline personality disorder. *Archives of General Psychiatry, 63*, 649–658.

Grilo, C. M., Sanislow, C. A., Gunderson, J. G., Pagano, G. E., Yen, S., Zanarini, M. C., et al. (2004). Two-year stability and change of schizotypal, borderline, avoidant, and obsessive–compulsive personality disorders. *Journal of Consulting and Clinical Psychology, 72*, 767–775.

Gunderson, J. G., Shea, M. T., Skodol, A. E., McGlashan, T. H., Morey, L. C., Stout, R. L., et al. (2000). The collaborative longitudinal personality disorders study: Development, aims, design, and sample characteristics. *Journal of Personality Disorders, 14*, 300–315.

Lieb, K., Zanarini, M. C., Schmahl, C., Linehan, M. M., & Bohus, M. (2004, July 31). Borderline personality disorder. *The Lancet, 364*, 453–461.

Linehan, M. M. (1993a). *Cognitive behavior treatment of borderline personality disorder.* New York: Guilford Press.

Linehan, M. M. (1993b). *Skills training manual for treating borderline personality disorder.* New York: Guilford Press.

Linehan, M. M., Comtois, K. A., Murray, A. M., Brown, M. Z., Gallop, R. J., Heard, H. L., et al. (2006). Two-year randomized controlled trial and follow-up of dialectical behavior therapy vs. therapy by experts for suicidal behaviors and borderline personality disorder. *Archives of General Psychiatry, 63*, 757–766.

Nock, M., & Prinstein, M. (2005). Contextual features and behavioral functions of self-mutilation among adolescents. *Journal of Abnormal Psychology, 114*, 140–146.

Paris, J. (2005). Recent advances in the treatment of borderline personality disorder. *Canadian Journal of Psychiatry, 50,* 435–441.

Perry, J. C., Herman, J. L., van der Kolk, B. A., & Hoke, L. A. (1990). Psychotherapy and psychological trauma in borderline personality disorder. *Psychiatric Annals, 20,* 33–43.

Robins, C. J., & Chapman, A. L. (2004). Dialectical behavior therapy: Current status, recent developments, and future directions. *Journal of Personality Disorders, 18,* 73–79.

Skodol, A. E., Buckley, P., & Charles, E. (1983). Is there a characteristic pattern to the treatment history of clinic outpatients with borderline personality? *The Journal of Nervous and Mental Disease, 171,* 405–410.

Skodol, A. E., Gunderson, J. G., Pfohl, B., Widiger, T. A., Livesley, W. J., & Siever, L. J. (2002). The borderline diagnosis: I. Psychopathology, comorbidity, and personality structure. *Biological Psychiatry, 51,* 936–950.

Skodol, A. E., Gunderson, J. G., Shea, M. T., McGlashan, T. H., Morey, L. C., Sanislow, C. A., et al. (2005). The collaborative longitudinal personality disorders study (CLPS): Overview and implications. *Journal of Personality Disorders, 19,* 487–504.

Young, J. E. (1994). *Cognitive therapy for personality disorders: A schema-focused approach.* Sarasota, FL: Professional Resource Press.

Zanarini, M. C., Frankenburg, F. R., Hennen, J., & Silk, K. R. (2003). The longitudinal course of borderline psychopathology: 6-year prospective follow-up of the phenomenology of borderline personality disorder. *The American Journal of Psychiatry, 160,* 274–283.

17

PARAPHILIAS

J. PAUL FEDOROFF AND W. L. MARSHALL

Paraphilic sexual disorders are psychological conditions characterized by persistent, problematic, sexually motivated fantasies or acts (American Psychiatric Association, 2000). More than 100 unique paraphilias have been described, although those most frequently observed in clinical practice are *pedophilia* (i.e., sexual interest in children), *voyeurism* (i.e., sexual arousal from observing unsuspecting victims), *exhibitionism* (i.e., sexual arousal from exposing to nonconsenting victims), and *frotteurism* (i.e, sexual arousal from rubbing against nonconsenting victims). Less frequently, clinicians may see individuals with *transvestic fetishism* (i.e., sexual arousal from wearing clothes typical of the opposite sex), *sexual sadism* (i.e., sexual arousal from nonconsensual domination), and *sexual masochism* (i.e., sexual arousal from nonconsensual submission). By definition, all paraphilias involve repeated conscious, volitional thoughts associated with acts that result in harm. Because cognitive–behavioral therapy (CBT) is based on the premise that thoughts can be intentionally altered to control or modify emotions and behaviors, CBT would appear to be ideally suited to the treatment of paraphilic disorders.

This chapter reviews the most influential published studies concerning CBT and its variant, relapse prevention (RP) therapy, in the treatment of sex offenders. Typical RP treatment methods are briefly described. Concerns about the generalizability of the published studies are reviewed. Finally, recommendations for therapists are discussed together with a discussion about the future of CBT and RP therapy in the treatment of sex offenders and individuals with paraphilic disorders.

TREATMENT OUTCOME FOR PARAPHILIAS: A REVIEW

In a review of treatments for the paraphilias involving 7,156 men (Maletzky, 1998), *success rate* was defined as the participant having met the following criteria: (a) completed treatment, (b) reported no deviant sexual behavior at the end of treatment, (c) demonstrated no deviant sexual arousal on penile plethysmography at the end of treatment and in follow-up sessions, and (d) had no legal charges up to 60 months after treatment. In this review, reported success rates following CBT varied from a low of 75.5% for rapists to 95.6% for situational heterosexual pedophiles. The same review asserted that "a consensus has arisen that cognitive–behavioral therapies are the standard against which other approaches must be judged" (Maletzky, 1998, p. 483).

Such was the hope when researchers selected a version of CBT to test the effectiveness of psychological treatment of incarcerated sex offenders in a prospective random controlled trial (RCT; Marques, Day, Nelson, & West, 1994; Marques, Wiederanders, Day, Nelson, & van Ommeren, 2005). This study, frequently referred to as the Sex Offender Treatment Evaluation Project (SOTEP), involved nonincestuous "child molesters" and nongang "rapists" with a maximum of three felony convictions who were between 18 and 30 months away from being released, with IQs above 80. Only about one third of eligible offenders volunteered to enter the study, and the majority was first-time offenders. These volunteers were assigned to three groups: 259 were assigned to the RP treatment group, 225 were randomly assigned to the volunteer control group (VC), and 220 were selected for inclusion in a "nonvolunteer" control group (NVC).

Participants in the RP group were the only individuals during the study who received a "comprehensive cognitive–behavioral treatment program" that consisted of three 90-minute manualized, videotaped group therapy sessions per week. After release into the community, study participants were followed for between 5 and 14 years. Reoffense was determined by data collected from the United States Federal Bureau of Investigation (FBI) and the California Department of Justice, and from California Department of Corrections records or parole violations, including return to prison. *Reoffense* was defined as information indicating the commission of a new crime was "at least possible."

Follow-up data indicated no significant differences in rates of sexual offense for the RP group (22%), the VC group (20%), or the NVC group (19.1%). In addition, there were no significant differences in survival distributions (i.e., rates of reoffense over time). Nor were significant differences found between subgroups of treated and untreated participants on the basis of offender or victim type, age, race, prior offender status, previous sex offense, intoxication at the time of offense, physical injury to the victim, or whether the victim was a stranger. Although RP participants who were intoxicated at the time of the index offense had a lower rate of sexual reoffense than did those who were not (12.1% vs. 28.6%, respectively), the statistical significance of this finding was eliminated when the effect of multiple comparisons was controlled for mathematically.

The authors of this study considered several explanations for the failure to demonstrate a significant treatment effect. These included the fact that (a) only the RP participants lived in a state hospital rather than in prison; (b) although assignment was random, the RP group were higher risk than the VC or NVC groups; (c) the overall base rate of sexual reoffense (20%) was low; (d) there was a possibility that the treatment intervention was "too intense" (Hanson, 2000; Marshall & Anderson, 2000; Nicholaichuk, 1966); and (e) the authors went to great lengths to avoid excluding anyone who had started the treatment program, even if they showed little evidence of motivation or performance (Mann, 2000; Mann & Thornton, 2000).

The SOTEP authors also speculated on possibly helpful changes to the treatment program itself. These included addition of innovations from addictions research such as motivational interviewing (Miller & Rollnick, 1991), individualization of treatment (Hollin, 2002), homogenization of offender type and offender motivation for treatment (Ward & Hudson, 1998), and establishment on an individualized case management approach with increased levels of surveillance and checks on compliance (English, 1998; Prentky, 2003). The following changes were recommended: (a) Tailor treatment intensity to the offenders' risk levels, treatment needs, and responsivity factors, (b) monitor treatment progress closely, and (c) include an individualized interdisciplinary aftercare model (Marques et al., 2005).

The hypothesis that CBT group therapy does not reduce sex offender recidivism was also reported in the conclusions of an Australian study of sex offenders (Schweitzer & Dwyer, 2003). This prospective study reported sexual reoffense rates for treatment completers (n = 196), treatment dropouts (n = 85), and a matched control group (n = 164; 2.9%, 1.6%, and 2.7%, respectively). Although the reoffense rates were low and the time to reoffense was longer in the treatment completer group compared with the dropout group and control group (3.8 years vs. 2.7 years vs. 1.6 years, respectively), there was no overall statistical difference among groups.

In contrast to the "no differences" outcomes of the SOTEP studies reviewed previously, a comprehensive meta-analysis of psychological treatment studies reported generally positive results (Hanson et al., 2002). This quantitative review, known as the Collaborative Outcome Data Project (CODP), examined the efficacy of 43 treatment programs, 29 of which were described as "cognitive–behavioral." Inclusion in the meta-analysis required that the study compare a group of sex offenders who received predominantly psychological therapy with a group of sex offenders who had not. Sexual recidivism rates for the 5,078 treated sex offenders and 4,376 untreated sex offenders differed in the hypothesized direction (16.8% vs. 12.3%, respectively). The reoffense rate of the treated group was lower when analyses were restricted to currently used treatment programs (mainly CBT), as opposed to programs considered obsolete. It is not surprising that offenders who dropped out of treatment did less well than those who completed the prescribed treatment, although offenders who refused treatment appeared to do as well as those who completed treatment (Hanson et al., 2002, p. 182). The study authors concluded that "current treatments were associated with a significant reduction in both sexual and general recidivism whereas the older treatments were not" (Hanson et al., 2002, p. 187).

One caveat of the CODP meta-analysis that has led some to challenge its main findings is that not all of the studies in the meta-analysis involved truly random assignment to treatment or control conditions. For example, Rice and Harris (2003) correctly pointed out that it is difficult to interpret studies involving comparison of sex offenders identified on the basis of having completed treatment with offenders who were not offered treatment. Rereviewing the studies in the Hanson and Bussiere (1998) meta-analysis, they concluded that the available data "afford no convincing scientific evidence that psychosocial treatments have been effective for adult sex offenders" (Rice & Harris, 2003, p. 437). Similarly, Seto (2008) concluded that the effectiveness of psychological treatments to reduce sex offender recidivism "has not been convincingly demonstrated" (p. 190).

A second contemporaneous meta-analysis of psychological interventions for sex offenders included nine RCTs that reported on 567 male sex offenders, almost half of whom had been followed for 10 years (Kenworthy, Adams, Bilby, Brooks-Gordon, & Fenton, 2003). This study from the Cochrane Library is widely cited for its "plain language" conclusion:

> Behavioral and/or "talking" therapy is often recommended (and provided) to people who have committed sex offenses. However, the effects of such treatments are unclear. This updated review suggests that, based on a small number of reported trials, CBT and general psychotherapeutic groups have been investigated more often than other treatments. Some evidence suggests that CBT may decrease re-offending at a year; however the general approach may contribute to re-arrest levels up to ten years later. This review shows that evaluative studies are possible in this difficult area, and further ones are urgently needed to resolve persisting uncertainties. (Kenworthy et al., 2003, p. 2)

These conclusions not withstanding, Kenworthy et al. (2003) were careful to point out that in their analyses, patients who prematurely discontinued their treatment were conservatively assumed to have had attenuated outcomes. For example, the assumption was made that participants lost to follow-up subsequently reoffended. In addition, studies were excluded from the Kenworthy et al. meta-analysis if more than 50% of participants in any group were lost to follow-up. Given that most sex offenders do not sexually reoffend after being convicted, regardless of whether they receive treatment (e.g., Hanson, Broom, & Stephenson, 2004; Hanson & Bussiere, 1998; Rice, Quinsey, & Harris, 1991), the decision to assume the opposite (that participants lost to follow-up had reoffended) makes the Kenworthy et al. conclusions less compelling.

A more recent meta-analysis of controlled outcome evaluations of sex offender treatments reported a 37% reduction in sexual recidivism in treated groups (Losel & Schmucker, 2005). Whereas surgical castration and hormonal treatments showed the largest beneficial effects, CBT (which was evaluated in 35 independent treatment comparisons) showed the most robust effect among the psychological treatments. Of note, only treatment programs designed specifically for sex offenders had a significant effect, and treatment programs in which participation was voluntary had a statistically significant odds ratio (1:45), whereas nonvoluntary or mixed group participation did not.

Because this meta-analysis included 69 studies involving a total of 22,181 participants, the authors were able to calculate effect sizes (odds ratios) for potentially moderating variables. Factors that significantly predicted positive outcome included treatment programs that were specific for sex offenders, treatment programs in which the study authors were directly involved, use of group therapy, and use of a cognitive therapy orientation.

COGNITIVE–BEHAVIORAL THERAPY OF PARAPHILIAS: RELAPSE PREVENTION

Several general reviews of possible treatment interventions for a variety of paraphilic disorders are now available (Marshall, Marshall, Serran, & Fernandez, 2006). The first comprehensive description of CBT designed specifically for sex offenders was published about 20 years ago (Laws, 1989). The treatment method of RP uses CBT principles to assist the offender in creating a description of the offense as well as the behavioral and cognitive events that preceded it (Jenkins-Hall, 1989b; Nelson & Jackson, 1989). This process is often highly detailed and involves variable amounts of confrontation by the therapist or by group participants who themselves have committed sex offenses as well as written assignments (Long, Wuesthoff, & Pithers, 1989; MacDonald & Pithers, 1989).

Most sex offender RP treatment programs borrow heavily from concepts developed from CBT treatment of other emotional disorders, including mood disorders and addictions. Sex offenders in RP treatment are introduced to the concepts of "cognitive distortions" (Jenkins-Hall, 1989a), the "problem of immediate gratification" (Marlatt, 1989), and the "abstinence violation effect" (Russell, Sturgeon, Miner, & Nelson, 1989).

Modern reviews of RP sex offender therapy have emphasized the importance of individualized treatment and placed an increased emphasis on health goals as opposed to simply avoiding relapse (Laws & Ward, 2006). In traditional RP programs, sex offenders would be required to fully confess their crimes and describe in detail all their past sex offenses. From this, and collateral information, the therapist would assist the offender in creating a "cognitive–behavioral chain" consisting of a series of antecedent events and emotions that linked in a classical or operant stimulus–response chain leading from a "seemingly unimportant decision" to the offense. Next, the offender would be assisted to develop alternative responses to offense-specific stimuli.

For example, in the case of a man with pedophilia who reported a "lapse" consisting of walking across a school yard, the initial task would be to investigate how he ended up in the school yard in the first place. This patient might say, "I was thirsty and wanted some milk. I noticed I was out of milk, and I knew there was a store that sold milk on the other side of the school yard." RP therapists would question the man about his seemingly unimportant decision to buy milk and help him to understand that his decision to keep walking across the school yard even after he realized this was against his probation orders is an example of the abstinence violation effect and of the cognitive distortion that because he had already broken his probation order and did not intend any harm, he might as well continue walking toward a group of children.

Fundamental to traditional RP for sex offenders are the views that (a) sex offenses are planned and (b) offenders are sufficiently motivated to be able to make prosocial choices if they become aware of their patterns of offense early enough in the chain of events. This view, however, has been challenged (Laws & Ward, 2006), and modifications have been proposed (Marshall, Marshall, Serran, & O'Brien, in press). The primary concerns can be summarized as "one size does not fit all" and "focus on the positive."

COMMON OBSTACLES TO THE EFFECTIVE TREATMENT
OF PARAPHILIAS

In this section, we discuss a number of oft-encountered obstacles and common mistakes in the treatment of paraphilias. We also offer some suggestions for therapists working with this client population. Almost everything known about paraphilic disorders, however, is extrapolated from studies or observations involving sex offenders (not all of whom have paraphilias). This is of no small consequence because most CBT protocols take the form of RP programs in which the target of treatment is sexual reoffense. Assuming CBT is indeed effective in altering paraphilic thoughts, feelings, and therefore acts, it would be expected that any effectiveness would be diluted by any nonparaphilic but nevertheless criminogenic, factors. By analogy, the efficacy of a new medication designed specifically for asthma might be obscured if it were tested on a group of smokers with hay fever, especially when the measure of efficacy is decrease in wheezing.

Treatment can also be expected to work optimally only if it is competently delivered to the appropriate cases at the right time and for the correct duration. Returning to the asthma treatment analogy, even the most efficacious inhaler medication that works within an hour in 100% of asthma sufferers would appear ineffective if it were tested with people who (a) do not have asthma, (b) wheeze because of some problem besides asthma, (c) take the medication at the wrong time, (d) refuse to take the medication, or (e) are compared with people with asthma caused by allergies and who are able to move away from the allergen. The treatment effect would be even more difficult to demonstrate if *outcome* was defined as "likelihood of having had a wheezing spell" or if those known to have stopped using the medication were defined as "failures."

Many versions of CBT applied to sexual offenders, especially those used in treatment studies, are delivered in the form of a manual that is closely followed by therapist and client. An advantage of manualized treatment delivery is that adherence to the therapy regime can be monitored for its integrity. However, manualized therapies have limitations. For example, some therapists (and clients) prefer a more flexible approach, rather than one that specifies what is to be done in treatment from session to session. The requirement to restrict therapy to those procedures described in the treatment manual has even been raised as a possible limitation of investigations such as the SOTEP study (described previously). Another possible problem with manualized therapies is the danger of losing the engagement of the person seeking therapy, either by failing to draw the person into treatment or by discouraging the person (see Case A later in this chapter).

A common mistake is to confuse reluctance to commit to a treatment program with reluctance to get help. Individuals with paraphilic disorders typically traverse many obstacles before they arrive at the therapist's door. They usually have an explanation for their sex problems. They likely also have a preferred way of presenting their problem to the clinician. The first job of the therapist is to accurately learn what the client thinks is the cause of his or her problem (Fedoroff, 2003). For example, if a man thinks his sexual interest in children is the result of having been taken to a nude beach by his parents when he was a child, treatment needs to be tailored to avoid making his misconception and consequent responses worse (see Case B).

Accurate diagnosis includes not only identification of any paraphilic sexual disorders but also identification of comorbid medical problems and other static and dynamic factors that could influence prognosis. Especially important is identification of problems that could interfere with the ability to benefit from therapy. This is especially true in the case of manualized therapies, or group therapies in which accommodation for individual vulnerabilities is less likely. Common problems include mood disorders, alcohol or substance abuse disorders, and attention-deficit/hyperactivity disorder and/ or personality disorders (see Case C).

How the therapist chooses to manage comorbid psychological problems depends on a number of factors, such as the nature and severity of problem, as well as how many resources the treatment team can marshal. In most cases the presenting sexual problem requires immediate and definitive attention. Subsequent interventions, however, need to take account of any and all premorbid and newly emerging problems. It is not uncommon for new cases to require individual, couple, and group therapy, often in conjunction with psychological treatment, counseling, or pharmacotherapy for mood disorders, anger management problems, and substance abuse. The point is to target life-threatening and life-endangering problems quickly and aggressively. Once such issues are under control, problems such as nonsuicidal depression or attention-deficit issues that may interfere with the ability to benefit from CBT can be addressed. As people recover, it is not uncommon for new problems to emerge, and therapists must remain aware of this possibility.

Therapists working with individuals with paraphilias should be aware of three additional common mistakes that can unnecessarily attenuate treatment outcome. The first is to accept the patient's (or referring professional's) point of view that stopping criminal sexual activities will take a long time or require some sort of "tapering." CBT, however, clearly distinguishes between thoughts, feelings, and actions; whereas the modification of paraphilic preferences is often a long-term endeavor, it is within the power of most individuals with paraphilias (in the absence of psychosis) to assume full responsibility for their actions and refrain from inappropriate sexual behavior immediately. It is important for CBT therapists to show that they expect this of the patient.

A second common error is a tendency to "pile on" therapies. As a general rule, there is more to be gained by a single treatment session in which therapeutic work is accomplished and taken home by the patient than there is in a regime in which the patient rushes from session to session and therapist to therapist with no time to reflect or work on establishing a normal life. There is no point in daily therapy sessions if they mean that, as a result, the patient loses his or her job or has no time to practice the skills learned in therapy.

Third, it is important to avoid confusing the map for the territory. This error is particularly common in cases involving paraphilias in which the presenting problem can easily mask the true issues and their resolution (see Case D). Regardless of the true cause of the problem, people invariably have their own explanation or suspicion about what is wrong. Some patients attribute their sexual problems to religious transgressions, others to medical or psychiatric disease, and others to early life experiences. Therapists using CBT techniques should be careful to account for formulations of the problem that go beyond cognitive or behavioral dysfunctions, not only because the source of the problem may indeed be caused by something else but also because if the patient's viewpoint is not respected, the patient is more likely to become discontented with therapy and, perhaps, discontinue.

There are a number of limitations of the cognitive–behavioral conceptualization of paraphilias, and these have been reviewed in depth elsewhere (e.g., Laws & Ward, 2006). Moreover, whereas the field of CBT for these conditions has not arrived at the stage of conducting dismantling studies to identify the potent and less potent aspects of treatment, some limitations of CBT seem obvious. The first is that the form of CBT most often used in the treatment of sex offenders derives from an RP model, an approach originally designed for maintenance treatment of detoxified substance abusers (Marlatt & Gordon, 1985). Traditional relapse prevention treatments assume that (a) a goal of complete abstinence is reasonable and (b) minor transgressions or lapses are inevitable.

In contrast, more modern treatment programs for paraphilic sexual disorders aim primarily to increase the use of normal and healthy social and sexual behaviors and to use these to replace pathologic behaviors (Marshall et al., 2005). The expectation is that both lapses and relapses are under the patient's control. Concepts of "addiction," "tapering," and "irresistible urges" are dismissed. The overall approach is to present noncriminal sexual behaviors as not only healthier but also inherently more enjoyable than criminal or paraphilic ones.

Case Examples

In the sections that follow, we present four typical treatment cases involving sex offenses and/or paraphilic sexual disorders.

Case A

Arthur was a self-employed owner of a moving company referred by his parole officer after a penitentiary sentence due to a first-time conviction for sexual assault of an unrelated child. He was described as "difficult," having declined to participate in the CBT program for sex offenders in the prison, even though this meant he spent longer in custody. In fact, Arthur refused to participate in any evaluation within the prison. During his intake interview, he was asked about his refusal to accept treatment. Again, he adamantly insisted that he did not want CBT in spite of appearing to show remorse for his crime and a wish to rehabilitate. As part of the clinic routine, and as a final part of the assessment, he was administered the Mini-Mental State Exam

(Folstein, Folstein, & McHugh, 1975). He scored 28 out of 30, failing only two items: reading a sentence and writing one. The interview quickly confirmed that Arthur was illiterate. He had managed to run his company by delegating paperwork and using his intimate knowledge of the city. When he went on moving consultations he always took along a helper who could read if needed. On the day of his offense he had enlisted the help of a 13-year-old friend of his son.

CBT has a reputation among prisoners as inevitably involving "homework" consisting of reading exercises and writing out "life histories" or RP plans. As a result, CBT is a treatment modality favored by those who are uncomfortable with spontaneous face-to-face interactions, because they can stay focused on their written materials. Conversely, it is rejected by those with dyslexia, intellectual disability, or other causes of illiteracy. Skilled therapists should consider illiteracy as a potential contributing factor to the reluctance to participate in treatment programs, even if written materials do not play a large part. Some offenders would rather admit their sex crime than admit they cannot read.

Case B

Barry was a successful businessman with a secret "compulsion" to expose his genitals to women. He often engaged in this behavior while seated in his expensive sports car. Although he realized what he was doing was illegal, he believed that some (but not all) women "liked it." When asked to explain his problem, Barry reported that it started when he was a teenager:

> Doc, I was by myself in a park sitting on a bench. This beautiful woman saw me, came over to me, and we ended up getting high and having sex right there in the park. It was the best thing that ever happened to me. Doc, I guess since then I have been trying to have the same experience; that is why I have this problem.

Asked what he had been doing in the park, he said he had been masturbating and using illegal drugs.

Clearly, even allowing for exaggeration concerning how successful the encounter had been, there is no question that the exhibitionistic interests preceded the incident (otherwise Barry would not have been masturbating on a park bench). Confronted with this fact, Barry quickly realized that his explanation of his problems must be incomplete. He also admitted that most of his exhibitionism occurred on park roadways.

Barry's behavioral explanation for his exhibitionism was well rehearsed before he presented for treatment. It served not only as an explanation for his paraphilia but was normative because he was able to convince himself that others would be the same as he was if they had been as "lucky" as he had been. Therapy in this case required education about exhibitionism that included nonbehavioral explanations. The point is that effective CBT requires development of alternative cognitive–behavioral schemas, often in conjunction with pharmacologic and lifestyle interventions.

Case C

Craig was referred from a major teaching hospital with a diagnosis of paraphilia and a recommendation to begin anti-androgen medication "without delay." He was accompanied by his mother, who explained that he had a rare genetic condition for which he was being followed by an expert. The reason he came to the teaching hospital's attention was his unusual method of masturbating. She explained that he would climb onto industrial air conditioners and become exited by the vibrations on his genital area. Neighbors had seen him and threatened to call the police. On examination, Craig was found to have low intellectual functioning. Of greater note was his dysmorphic appearance consisting of an elongated torso with very short arms. When asked, Craig explained that he found it difficult to reach his penis with his hands and had eventually discovered that vibrating objects facilitated masturbation. He had never heard of commercial vibrators but was given a recommendation to purchase one. The importance of privacy during masturbation was also explained.

Craig was seen for a follow-up appointment 6 weeks later. On that occasion both he and his mother appeared substantially happier. Craig reported that he had bought the recommended vibrator. When asked whether it had helped, he said, "Doctor, I am cured!" His mother confirmed that there had been no further incidents involving air conditioners or other public sexual activities.

Case D

Sam and Margaret presented at the request of Margaret's therapist with the chief complaint of "sexual incompatibility." The note from the referring therapist indicated that she had learned Sam would habitually "tie Margaret up" before and during sexual activities. The referral was precipitated when Margaret confessed to her therapist that both she and her husband were unhappy with their sex life. Both were seen together at the initial consultation, and both agreed they were unhappy: Sam because he was uncomfortable with "sadomasochistic activities" and Margaret because she was unable to reach orgasm unless there was a sadomasochistic element to the interaction.

The therapist invited the couple to discuss their sexual activities in terms of their interaction and happiness with each other. Sam was very concerned that his wife's behavior was highly pathological and bordered on criminal. Once he understood, however, that his wife's proclivities were fully consensual and highly unlikely to morph into criminal activities, his concerns abated. Margaret, although understanding that treatment is available for inhibited orgasm, elected to forgo treatment for a problem for which she had already found a satisfactory solution.

Additional Explanations for Poor Outcome

False acceptance of the efficacy of CBT (Type 1 error) is as problematic as false rejection of CBT (Type 2 error). It is important to consider factors that may contribute to both false positive and false negative conclusions.

Outcomes Obscured by Comorbid Problems

As we mentioned previously, most studies on the efficacy of CBT for paraphilia have involved samples of individuals who had been arrested for their sexual misconduct. Although CBT is designed to reduce paraphilic behaviors, outcome has often been measured by the rate of re-arrest, including re-arrest for non-sex-related crimes. This artificially deflates the effects of CBT.

Treatment Dropouts

Whereas arguments can be made about the appropriate way to statistically deal with study participants who are lost to follow-up, this is different than the issue of how to deal with study participants who do not complete CBT treatment. If the study question concerns treatment efficacy, it seems unfair to include treatment dropouts in the "failure" category. Not all people with paraphilic disorders wish to be cured, and not all sex offenders wish to stop offending. The palatability of a treatment is different from its efficacy.

Treatment Provided to the Wrong Group

As a general rule, effective treatments are also specific. Demonstration that CBT or some variant of CBT is effective is part of the question. The more important issue is this: For which paraphilic disorders is CBT most effective? Conversely, what factors make CBT contraindicated? An obvious example is a version of CBT dependant on written materials that would be contraindicated for illiterate patients.

Wrong Treatment Provided

CBT therapy for sex offenders is designed to assist in identifying cognitive distortions, apparently irrelevant decisions, risk factors, the cognitive–behavioral chain, and a variety of coping/diverting mechanisms (Laws, 1989). These clearly are important factors in rehabilitation. The most common variation of CBT used in the treatment of sex offenders, however, is RP, which unfortunately often does not emphasize the importance of replacing unhealthy sexual behavior with more healthy and noncriminal ones (Marshall et al., 2006).

Correct Treatment Provided Poorly

The successful administration of CBT requires a number of clinical skills, including having a solid understanding of the cognitive and behavioral basis of behavior and emotion, the ability to apply cognitive and behavioral conceptual models to understanding deviant sexual behavior, and the ability to use this conceptual foundation to plan and execute appropriate treatment strategies. Unfortunately, the fact that CBT often comes "packaged" in the form of treatment manuals increases the chances of it being delivered by those who do not have the appropriate theoretical grounding, leading to decreased effectiveness.

Treatment Not Needed

Evidence-based therapies have encouraged increasingly sophisticated analyses of therapeutic efficacy. It is remarkable that in the case of studies involving treatment of sex offenders and paraphilic disorders, one of the major recurring problems for researchers is the low base rate for reoffense. Future studies could profitably evaluate the newer variants of CBT, which seem to have more promise than the earlier RP programs (see Marshall et al., 2006). However, evidence has also suggested that researchers and clinicians should be examining the reasons why most sex offenders never reoffend sexually after being returned to the community and what it is about the minority who do reoffend that makes them so unique.

CONCLUSIONS

The development of CBT-based RP treatment for paraphilias and sex offenders has occurred within the past 20 years. Over this time, RP has become the standard clinical treatment for sex offenders, likely due to its face validity and conceptually clear treatment approach. However, these same features have allowed RP to be tested in prospective studies that have failed to demonstrate that it significantly decreases reoffense rates to below those of sex offenders who have received alternative interventions.

This chapter has briefly reviewed the evidence for and against the efficacy of CBT interventions for paraphilias and sex offenders. Several recommendations for therapists wishing to use CBT in the treatment of sex offenders also were reviewed. It is important to remember that one of the strongest features of CBT for this population is that it is fully complementary with other treatment paradigms, including other forms of individual, couple and group psychotherapy, occupational therapy, recreational therapy, social work interventions, and pharmacotherapy. Clinicians and researchers can champion CBT for sex offenders and paraphilias as an example of a treatment paradigm based on solid scientific research that has succeeded in providing a common ground on which experts from widely disparate disciplines can collaborate and from which we can develop even more effective interventions for future use.

REFERENCES

American Psychiatric Association. (2000). *Diagnostic and statistical manual of mental disorders* (4th ed., text rev.). Washington, DC: Author.

English, K. (1998). The containment approach: An aggressive strategy for the community management of adult sex offenders. *Psychology, Public Policy and Law, 4,* 218–235.

Fedoroff, J. P. (2003). Paraphilic worlds. In S. B. Levine (Ed.), *Handbook of clinical sexuality for mental health professionals* (pp. 333–356). New York: Brunner/ Routeledge.

Folstein, M. F., Folstein, S. E., & McHugh, P. R. (1975). Mini-Mental State: A practical method for grading the cognitive state of patients for the clinician. *Journal of Psychiatric Research, 12,* 189–198.

Hanson, R. K. (2000). Treatment outcome and evaluation problems (and solutions). In D. R. Laws, S. M. Hudson, & T. Ward (Eds.), *Remaking relapse prevention with sex offenders: A sourcebook* (pp. 485–499). Thousand Oaks, CA: Sage.

Hanson, R. K., Broom, I., & Stephenson, M. (2004). Evaluating community sex offender treatment programs: A 12-year follow-up of 724 offenders. *Canadian Journal of Behavioral Science, 36,* 87–96.

Hanson, R. K., & Bussiere, M. T. (1998). Predicting relapse: A meta-analysis of sexual offender recidivism studies. *Journal of Consulting and Clinical Psychology, 66,* 348–362.

Hanson, R. K., Gordon, A., Harris, A. J. R., Marques, J. K., Murphy, W., Quinsey, V. L., et al. (2002). First report of the collective outcome data project on the effectiveness of psychological treatment for sex offenders. *Sexual Abuse: A Journal of Research and Treatment, 14,* 169–194.

Hollin, C. R. (2002). An overview of offender rehabilitation: Something old, something borrowed, something new. *Australian Psychologist, 37,* 159–164.

Jenkins-Hall, K. D. (1989a). Cognitive restructuring. In D. R. Laws (Ed.), *Relapse Prevention with sex offenders* (pp. 207–215). New York: Guilford Press.

Jenkins-Hall, K. D. (1989b). The decision matrix. In D. R. Laws (Ed.), *Relapse prevention with sex offenders* (pp. 159–166). New York: Guilford Press.

Kenworthy, T., Adams, C. E., Bilby, C., Brooks-Gordon, B., & Fenton, M. (2003). Psychological interventions for those who have sexually offended or are at risk of offending [Review]. *Cochrane Database of Systemic Reviews, 4.*

Laws, D. R. (Ed.). (1989). *Relapse prevention with sex offenders.* New York: Guilford Press.

Laws, D. R., & Ward, T. (2006). When one size doesn't fit all: The reformulation of relapse prevention. In W. L. Marshall, Y. M. Fernandez, L. E. Marshall, & G. A.

Serran (Eds.), *Sexual offender treatment: Controversial issues* (pp. 241–254). Chichester, England: Wiley.

Long, J. D., Wuesthoff, A., & Pithers, W. D. (1989). Use of autobiographies in the assessment and treatment of sex offenders. In D. R. Laws (Ed.), *Relapse prevention with sex offenders* (pp. 88–95). New York: Guilford Press.

Losel, F., & Schmucker, M. (2005). The effectiveness of treatment for sexual offenders: A comprehensive meta-analysis. *Journal of Experimental Criminology, 1,* 117–146.

MacDonald, R. K., & Pithers, W. D. (1989). Self-monitoring to identify high-risk situation. In D. R. Laws (Ed.), *Relapse prevention with sex offenders* (pp. 96–104). New York: Guilford Press.

Maletzky, B. M. (1998). The paraphilias: Research and treatment. In P. E. Nathan & J. M. Gorman (Eds.), *A guide to treatments that work* (pp. 472–500). New York: Oxford University Press.

Mann, R. E. (2000). Managing resistance and rebellion in relapse prevention intervention. In D. R. Laws, S. M. Hudson, & T. Ward (Eds.), *Remaking relapse prevention with sex offenders: A sourcebook* (pp. 187–200). Thousand Oaks, CA: Sage.

Mann, R. E., & Thornton, D. (2000). An evidence-based relapse prevention program. In D. R. Laws, S. M. Hudson, & T. Ward (Eds.), *Remaking relapse prevention with sex offenders: A sourcebook* (pp. 341–350). Thousand Oaks, CA: Sage.

Marlatt, G. A. (1989). Feeding the PIG: The problem of immediate gratification. In D. R. Laws (Ed.), *Relapse prevention with sex offenders* (pp. 56–62). New York: Guilford Press.

Marlatt, G. A., & Gordon, J. R. (1985). *Relapse prevention.* New York: Guilford Press.

Marques, J. K., Day, D. M., Nelson, C., & West, M. A. (1994). Effects of cognitive–behavioral treatment on sex offender recidivism: Preliminary results of a longitudinal study. *Criminal Justice and Behavior, 21,* 28–54.

Marques, J. K., Wiederanders, M., Day, D. M., Nelson, C., & van Ommeren, A. (2005). Effects of a relapse prevention program on sexual recidivism: Final results from California's sex offender treatment and evaluation project (SOTEP). *Sexual Abuse: A Journal of Research and Treatment, 17,* 79–107.

Marshall, W. L., & Anderson, D. (2000). Do relapse prevention components enhance treatment effectiveness? In D. R. Laws, S. M. Hudson, & T. Ward (Eds.), *Remaking relapse prevention with sex offenders: A sourcebook* (pp. 39–55). Thousand Oaks, CA: Sage.

Marshall, W. L., Marshall, L. E., Serran, G. A., & Fernandez, Y. M. (2006). *Treating sexual offenders: An integrated approach.* New York: Routledge.

Marshall, W. L., Marshall, L. E., Serran, G. A., & O'Brien, M. D. (in press). Sexual offender treatment: A positive approach. *Psychiatric Clinics of North America.*

Marshall, W. L., Ward, T., Mann, R. E., Moulden, H., Fernandez, Y. M., Serran, G. A., et al. (2005). Working positively with sexual offenders: Maximizing the effectiveness of treatment. *Journal of Interpersonal Violence, 20,* 1–19.

Miller, W. R., & Rollnick, S. (Eds.). (1991). *Motivational interviewing: Preparing people to change addictive behavior*. New York: Guilford Press.

Nelson, C., & Jackson, P. (1989). High-risk recognition: The cognitive–behavioral chain. In D. R. Laws (Ed.), *Relapse prevention with sex offenders* (pp. 167–177). New York: Guilford Press.

Nicholaichuk, T. (1966). Sex offender treatment priority: An illustration of the risk/need principle. *Forum on Corrections Research, 8*, 30–32.

Prentky, R. A. (2003). A 15-year retrospective on sexual coercion: Advances and projections. In R. A. Prentky, E. S. Janus, & M. C. Seto (Eds.), *Annals of the New York Academy of Sciences: Vol. 989. Sexually coercive behavior: Understanding and management* (pp. 13–32). New York: New York Academy of Sciences.

Rice, M. E., & Harris, G. T. (2003). The size and signs of treatment effects in sex offender therapy. In R. A. Prentky, E. S. Janus, & M. C. Seto (Eds.), *Annals of the New York Academy of Sciences: Vol. 989. Sexually coercive behavior: Understanding and management* (pp. 428–440). New York: New York Academy of Sciences.

Rice, M. E., Quinsey, V. L., & Harris, G. T. (1991). Sexual recidivism among child molesters released from a maximum security psychiatric institution. *Journal of Consulting and Clinical Psychology, 59*, 381–386.

Russell, K., Sturgeon, V. H., Miner, M. H., & Nelson, C. (1989). Determinants of the abstinence violation effect in sexual fantasies. In D. R. Laws (Ed.), *Relapse prevention with sex offenders* (pp. 63–72). New York: Guilford Press.

Schweitzer, R., & Dwyer, J. (2003). Sex crime recidivism: Evaluation of a sexual offender treatment program. *Journal of Interpersonal Violence, 18*, 1292–1310.

Seto, M. C. (2008). *Pedophilia and sexual offending against children: Theory, assessment, and intervention*. Washington, DC: American Psychological Association.

Ward, T., & Hudson, S. M. (1998). A model of the relapse process in sexual offenders. *Journal of Interpersonal Violence, 13*, 700–725.

18

ANTISOCIAL AND PSYCHOPATHIC INDIVIDUALS

MICHELE GALIETTA, VIRGINIA FINERAN, JOANNA FAVA,
AND BARRY ROSENFELD

Few diagnoses generate as much therapeutic pessimism as antisocial personality disorder (APD) or psychopathy. Frequently, clinicians maintain a pervasive belief that individuals with an antisocial or psychopathic personality style cannot be successfully treated. Whether because of these individuals' lack of motivation to change, the absence of psychological distress that typically drives treatment engagement, or an impaired ability to form meaningful relationships, clinicians often assume that treatment will be inherently frustrating and ultimately unsuccessful.

This chapter briefly reviews the nature and distinctions between these related disorders,[1] as well as the research literature pertaining to their treatability. Following this review, an application of dialectical behavior therapy (DBT) is presented as a promising framework for the treatment of individuals with APD or serious antisocial behaviors. The specific adaptation of DBT

---

[1]Although we are aware that psychopathy is not currently classified by the *DSM–IV–TR* (American Psychiatric Association, 2000) as a mental disorder (i.e., it is not one of the 10 personality disorders listed), the language of *disorder* will be used in this chapter both for simplicity and because it accurately captures the nature of this phenomenon.

developed by our research team was intended for treatment of stalking offenders, but the program has gradually expanded to encompass a wide range
of individuals with severe personality disorders who have been referred for
treatment by the court or the department of probation. Thus, although the
case example described in this chapter is a psychopathic individual who was
charged with a stalking offense, the treatment approach and issues described
appear potentially useful for a wide range of offender populations, many of
whom are labeled *psychopathic* or *antisocial personalities*.

ANTISOCIAL PERSONALITY DISORDER AND PSYCHOPATHY

The diagnostic labeling of antisocial behavior has evolved through the
decades using terms such as *psychopath, sociopath, dissocial personality disorder*,
and finally, *antisocial personality disorder* (Cleckley, 1941/1975; Lykken, 1995;
Rogers & Dion, 1991). Although many individuals use the terms *psychopathy*
and *APD* interchangeably, important differences exist. In fact, some writers
argue that although antisocial individuals may be "treatable," psychopaths
are not (Harris & Rice, 2005). We address this important question but cau-
tion that the distinction may reflect one of severity rather than a qualitative
(e.g., biological) difference between the two constructs. Thus, this chapter
addresses a treatment approach that has potential for individuals who engage
in criminal or antisocial behavior regardless of what label is applied, but ad-
mittedly the likelihood of successful outcomes is related to the severity of the
disorder and the associated risk of future antisocial behavior/violence.

Hervey Cleckley (1941/1975) is widely cited as the originator of the
construct of psychopathy, although the term had been widely used, albeit
poorly defined, since the 19th century. Indeed, shortly after the publication
of Cleckley's seminal book, *The Mask of Sanity*, describing the nature of this
personality style, the term *psychopathic personality disorder* was eliminated from
the diagnostic nomenclature and replaced with *sociopathic personality disorder*
(Cleckley, 1941/1975). Following the publication of the third edition of the
Diagnostic and Statistical Manual of Mental Disorders (DSM; 3rd ed.; American
Psychiatric Association, 1980), the name was changed again to *antisocial personality disorder*. These changing labels have not simply been semantic, as
the criteria used to describe this phenomenon have similarly evolved, with
the formal diagnosis becoming increasingly behavioral and more closely linked
to criminality and further away from Cleckley's original description of an
affective and morally stunted, but not necessarily criminal, personality.

The move to the behaviorally defined construct of APD has largely
been premised on the importance of accurate and reliable diagnoses. Early
versions of the *DSM* were plagued by vague descriptions and poor inter-
clinician reliability, leading to increasingly specific and often concrete criteria (Hare, 1996; Wilson, Frick, & Clements, 1999). Some have criticized

this change, citing the expansive nature of the APD diagnosis (which can be applied to the majority of incarcerated felons and chronic drug abusers, for example) and the corresponding loss of the spirit of Cleckley's original conceptualization of psychopathy. Thus, although APD is the diagnosis used by clinicians, treatment providers and researchers often distinguish between individuals who exhibit the pattern of antisocial behaviors that yield an APD diagnosis and those who exhibit both affective components as well as behavioral aspects warranting the label of *psychopath*. Indeed, psychopathy is typically conceptualized as a combination of affective, interpersonal, and behavioral traits rather than just antisocial behaviors alone (Hare, 1996). This construct has largely become synonymous with the rating scale used to assess it: Hare's (1991) Psychopathy Checklist.

Of course, the essential core of both constructs is the predominantly self-centered focus and a disregard for societal norms regarding behavior. The diagnosis of APD is characterized as a "pervasive pattern of disregard for and violation of the rights of others, occurring since age 15 years," with evidence of conduct disorder beginning even earlier (American Psychiatric Association, 2000, p. 706). The overall prevalence of APD is approximately 3% in males and about 1% in females, but is far higher in correctional settings, approaching 90% of incarcerated felons (Hart & Hare, 1997). Psychopathy, on the other hand, is considered much less common, occurring in roughly 30% of prison inmates (Hart & Hare, 1997); the prevalence of psychopathy in the general public is not known.

EFFECTIVENESS OF TREATMENT FOR ANTISOCIAL AND PSYCHOPATHIC PERSONALITIES

The literature on the effectiveness of treatments for antisocial and psychopathic personalities, while substantial, has significant limitations. Because of ethical problems associated with several notable studies involving prisoners, these participants are now afforded enhanced protections in research (see Galietta & Stanley, 2008). Because of this fact, along with practical difficulties associated with conducting research in correctional and forensic settings, the literature is characterized primarily by case studies, retrospective reviews, and quasi-experimental designs. There are few well-controlled, rigorous trials of interventions, and therefore conclusions should be interpreted cautiously. Nevertheless, a review of this literature does reveal important findings that warrant consideration before conducting treatment with antisocial or psychopathic individuals.

One of the most commonly studied approaches is the therapeutic community (TC). TCs emerged as a common form of treatment in the 1950s, typically integrating humanistic, behavioral, psychoanalytic, and often radical treatment approaches to shape the attitudes and behaviors of criminal offenders. In fact, one of the seminal studies cited in support of the perception that psychopaths are untreatable is Harris, Rice, and Cormier's (1994) retrospective analysis of a Canadian TC. These authors analyzed the probability of violent recidivism in four groups: treated and untreated psychopaths and treated and untreated nonpsychopaths. They found that the rate of violent recidivism was actually greater for treated psychopaths than for those left untreated, whereas the reverse was true for nonpsychopaths (i.e., treatment was associated with lower recidivism). However, numerous methodological flaws plagued this frequently cited study, including the questionable nature of the treatment delivered. For example, the authors wrote that "at various times, methedrine, LSD, scopolamine and alcohol were all used alone or in combination to loosen the rigidly implanted patterns of behavior . . ." (Harris et al., 1994, p. 288); little or no traditional mental health treatment was provided by trained clinicians. Despite this and numerous other methodological limitations (e.g., differences in legal status and reasons for detention between treatment and nontreatment groups), the authors concluded that "psychopaths might have learned to be more self-confident criminals who could maintain high self-esteem whilst committing more antisocial acts" (Harris et al., 1994, p. 293).

Other investigators have reached more optimistic conclusions about the "treatability" of individuals with psychopathic and antisocial personality styles. Salekin (2002) reviewed the literature on treatment of psychopathy, examining studies dating back to the 1940s using a wide range of treatment approaches. Several early studies, many of which utilized psychoanalytic or eclectic interventions, described substantial improvement among psychopathic individuals (Salekin, 2002). Critics have challenged this literature, arguing that these early studies applied overly broad diagnostic criteria, used inadequate follow-up periods, and relied on clinician evaluation or patient self-report rather than recidivism as a primary outcome measure (Harris & Rice, 2005). Moreover, virtually none of these studies applied random assignment to treatment conditions, and treatment groups often differed significantly from comparison groups (as was the case with Harris et al.'s 1994 TC study). Moreover, many of these "studies" consisted of single case examples, further limiting the conclusions that could be drawn.

Nevertheless, Salekin (2002) described a number of variables that appeared to moderate the treatment effects across studies involving antisocial or psychopathic populations. He found that behavioral and cognitive–behavioral interventions resulted in better outcomes compared with either no treatment or other, more traditional criminal justice interventions (e.g., TCs). Additionally, programs that used both group and individual treatment methods were more effective than programs that applied only one of these approaches. Another finding across studies was that more intensive interventions (e.g., treatments that involved multiple modalities or those that were longer in duration) were more effective than less intensive approaches.

This finding is consistent with the growing literature on treatment of juvenile offenders, in which the most successful interventions (e.g., multisystemic family therapy) are far more intensive than traditional mental health approaches (Henggeler, Sheidow, & Lee, 2007), and suggests that treatment success for psychopaths may depend more on the intensity of services provided than on the diagnosis per se.

Similar findings are echoed in the recent study by Skeem, Monahan, and Mulvey (2002), who analyzed treatment response in a large sample of psychiatric patients. Skeem et al. analyzed the likelihood of violent behavior as a function of both psychopathy and treatment intensity, analyzing the number of sessions attended during the 10 weeks between the baseline assessment and follow-up evaluation. Among the individuals identified as definitely or probably psychopathic (on the basis of the Screening Version of the PCL, the PCL-SV; Hart, Cox, & Hare, 1995), those who attended fewer than seven sessions were three times more likely to engage in violent behavior than psychopaths who attended at least seven sessions. Although the magnitude of this treatment effect decreased as the follow-up period increased, and they found no effect of treatment for psychopaths who completed six or fewer sessions (e.g., those attending a few sessions were no less violent than those attending none or one), the authors nevertheless concluded that "patients with psychopathic traits appeared as likely to benefit from adequate doses of treatment by becoming less violent as those without such traits" (p. 594). These findings are all the more striking given the ecological validity of the "treatment" under investigation, as psychopathic patients received a wide range of services with no attempt to standardize or control the treatment received. Thus, although this study's findings do not offer support for any particular treatment approach, they do suggest that the conclusion that psychopaths are untreatable may well be premature.

In our treatment program for individuals charged with harassment or stalking-related offenses, we investigated the impact of psychopathy (based on the PCL-SV) on number of sessions attended, program completion versus dropout, and recidivism. We found no relationship between psychopathy and any of these outcome variables, although the small sample limits the conclusiveness of these findings (Galietta, Garcia-Mansilla, & Rosenfeld, 2006).

CHALLENGES TO SUCCESSFUL TREATMENT

Despite the encouraging findings reported by Skeem and others, many obstacles exist to providing successful treatment for antisocial and psychopathic individuals. Although an exhaustive review of each of these obstacles could fill an entire volume, the following section provides a brief overview of several of the major challenges that arise in providing mental health treatment for individuals with an antisocial or psychopathic personality style.

Motivational Deficits

One of the biggest challenges in working with this population has to do with a lack of motivation to engage in treatment. These motivational deficits can be understood in relation to several other characteristics of this population. Psychological distress is often a factor that motivates people to seek treatment and remain in treatment, particularly during difficult periods. Yet many individuals with APD are not distressed by the difficulties they face. Even arrest and incarceration, with all the attendant restrictions, frequently fail to motivate individuals to change their behaviors. Thus, identifying factors that can increase motivation to change problem behaviors is both challenging and frustrating for mental health clinicians but is critical to successful treatment.

Affective and Cognitive Deficits

Another salient finding from the extant literature on the treatment of psychopathy and APD pertains to the affective deficits that characterize these individuals. Several theorists posit that these affective deficits are the result of poor conditioning and modeling during childhood (Eron, 1997; Ullman & Krasner, 1969), leading to a restricted range of emotion in adulthood. This results in cognitive distortions (e.g., the development of automatic antisocial and aggressive approaches to interactions, rather than prosocial ones), blunted affect, and limited cognitive processing about events in their life. This blunted affective and cognitive style hinders treatment engagement and further limits motivation, frequently resulting in an experience of frustration for clinicians and confusion about the treatment focus.

Mandated Treatment

Finally, the issue of mandated treatment, which is a common route to treatment for antisocial and psychopathic individuals, warrants comment. Ironically, mandated treatment often presents a significant impediment to motivation and treatment engagement. Individuals who are mandated to attend treatment often come with extreme anger and resentment about their lack of control, despite frequently presenting with a veneer of cooperation. Thus, not only does mandated treatment often exacerbate treatment resistance, but it also adds a range of complications regarding issues such as confidentiality (e.g., required disclosure of information) or individuals being mandated to treatments that may not be appropriate for them. All of these issues make treatment with this population extremely difficult. We address strategies for addressing these obstacles later in the chapter, after considering some general issues in the treatment of antisocial or high-risk individuals.

GENERAL CONSIDERATIONS IN TREATING INDIVIDUALS WITH ANTISOCIAL OR PSYCHOPATHIC PERSONALITY

Regardless of the therapeutic approach used, a number of general issues arise in the treatment of criminal offenders, particularly those with elevated risk of violence. One of the first tasks to be accomplished during the initial stages of any treatment is to educate the individual regarding the nature and focus of treatment in order to promote realistic expectations. Clinicians should disclose any relevant information regarding the expectations of the clinician or program and time commitment expected, and carefully explain the limits to confidentiality. In addition, explaining the rules for treatment, including criteria for determining successful completion and, conversely, behaviors that will result in termination, is critical, both at the outset and periodically during the course of treatment. Explaining the process and ensuring understanding at the outset of treatment will help to decrease the possibility of behaviors that will interfere with treatment.

Treatment Readiness

Dahle (1997) observed that a primary factor associated with treatment readiness and commitment was the client's trust in the intentions of the treatment provider. Trust in the clinician is a crucial element of change in a wide range of patient populations, although less often studied in offender samples (Marshall et al., 2003). It is not surprising, however, that individuals mandated to treatment often lack trust in those whom they see as representatives of societal authority. Many individuals with antisocial or psychopathic personalities have been repeatedly assessed by mental health professionals, and often these assessments have led to unfavorable (to them) outcomes. Offenders may therefore regard professionals as untrustworthy, and they may adopt a very careful approach when deciding what information to divulge. It takes time, skill, and patience for clinicians to overcome this inevitable distrust and establish an effective working relationship, particularly with an antisocial client who is mandated to treatment by a judge or probation officer. In our experience, predictability (i.e., doing what one promises) and an unyielding respectful and problem-solving approach (e.g., staying on one focus) lead to the development of a working relationship.

Working Alliance and the Issue of Respect

The notion of respect and "being treated fairly" is extremely important for all clients, especially those who are mandated to treatment. There are many reasons why individuals mandated to treatment are at elevated risk of disrespectful or unfair treatment, including the manner in which they relate to others and the nature of the criminal justice system. Often, there is little recourse for individuals who are treated unfairly by treatment providers, given the power differential between client and clinician that exists in any treatment relationship but is magnified in offender treatment settings. Therefore, clinicians should convey respect, as evidenced by clarity in disclosing expectations and rules in advance of initiating treatment and then by avoiding arbitrary decision making throughout the course of treatment.

Confidentiality Issues

Whether or not the client is referred or mandated to treatment by the criminal justice system, limits of confidentiality must be addressed prior to the first session. Although clinics or hospitals may have long-standing relationships with the criminal justice system that outline the nature of confidentiality and disclosures, many individuals are referred for treatment without such guidance. Thus, the clinician must determine what information is expected to be communicated to the referring party versus disclosures that should be considered confidential, and the client must be informed of these parameters before treatment begins. For example, some settings will provide only attendance information to the court, whereas others provide more detailed information regarding the nature and course of treatment. This important question must be resolved in advance. In most cases, treatment records can be obtained by subpoena, but whether such records will be made available without court order is often less clear. If a situation arises that requires the therapist to disclose information that was considered by the client to be confidential, the therapeutic alliance will suffer, if not end. Most important, clients should be made aware of the therapist's duty to warn and protect any potential victims if a serious threat of violence is identified. On the other hand, a frank discussion of confidentiality issues at the outset of treatment can help promote a therapeutic alliance and can serve to reassure the client that the clinician is vigilant to confidentiality concerns.

Risk Management

Perhaps no greater issue exists in the treatment of antisocial or psychopathic clients than the risk of violence—both to the clinician and/or treatment staff as well as to third parties. Managing risk to treatment staff is, of course, intimately intertwined with the setting in which treatment occurs, but clinicians should never assume that no risk exists simply because treatment occurs in a secure facility. Although risks are certainly greater in community-based treatment settings, in which security personnel are less readily available and access to weapons and potential victims is easier, adequate precautions are critical regardless of the setting. Such precautions include both immediate risk management steps (e.g., availability of security personnel, screening for weapons) as well as planning for possible problems. Risk management protocols should be developed and available, and treatment staff should be familiar with these protocols in case high-risk situations arise during the course of treatment.

The Duty to Protect

If a significant risk of violence is identified, as is to be expected when dealing with antisocial and psychopathic individuals, clinicians are faced with the difficult task of determining an appropriate strategy for intervention. Ever since the California Supreme Court's seminal ruling in *Tarasoff v. Regents of University of California* (1976), clinicians have been acutely aware of the need to protect potential victims when their client presents a serious risk of harm. The actions required of treatment providers vary tremendously across jurisdictions, and clinicians are encouraged to familiarize themselves with the specific statutes within their state. For example, some states and jurisdictions interpret the broad parameters established by *Tarasoff* as a "duty to warn," whereas others enforce a "duty to protect," a distinction that can be critical. Regardless of what actions are required, the potential impact on the therapeutic relationship that can result from a breach of confidentiality makes it imperative for clinicians to be vigilant not only to the degree of risk posed by a particular client but of the clinician's own potential bias, as many clinicians are tempted to ignore or minimize warning signs because of concern about jeopardizing the treatment relationship. Although a thorough review of violence risk assessment is beyond the scope of this chapter (cf., e.g., Rosenfeld, Fava, & Galietta, 2009; Werth, Welfel, & Benjamin, 2009), it is critical for the clinician to maintain an adequate level of knowledge regarding current risk assessment techniques and research. In our own treatment setting, a thorough violence risk assessment is conducted at the time of the initial intake evaluation, in part because a community-based setting may not be suitable for managing very high-risk clients.

A second broad parameter, in addition to careful evaluation of the client's violence risk, pertains to potential victim access. In many treatment settings, the clinician will not have direct contact with or access to a potential victim unless the potential victim is another client in the same treatment setting. Thus, notification might entail informing the police, a probation officer, or even the district attorney's office. Because time is often critical once a client expresses a serious intention to harm someone, it is recommended that treatment staff working with antisocial, psychopathic, and potentially violent individuals elicit as much information as possible in the early stages of treatment in order to make informed judgments. Identifying the most appropriate individuals to contact in case of emergency, and maintaining up-to-date contact information, will be crucial if a serious and imminent threat of violence arises. These procedures represent an integral component of the risk management protocol that all clinicians and program staff should be aware of.

Clinician Bias

Another problem that frequently arises in the context of treating individuals with APD has to do with the feelings, attitudes, and behaviors of treating clinicians. Clinicians may experience anger, resentment, judgments, and fears related to their antisocial clients. These feelings may be useful indicators in the treatment, but if unchecked they may also interfere with treatment. Adequate training and supervision is critical to working with such challenging individuals.

Self-Disclosure

A special consideration when working with antisocial or psychopathic individuals involves establishing limits to self-disclosure. In general, we believe that clinicians should always avoid providing unnecessary information about themselves, their family, or their personal background. Although the Internet-savvy client can often acquire considerable information about the clinician, such precautions can help limit the information that is accessible. However, literature has suggested that the appropriate use of self-disclosure can be beneficial to treatment, both in helping solidify treatment relationships as well as a means of modeling effective behavior. Providing the client with information about how one has handled intense emotions or frustrating experiences may be particularly helpful. That said, the clinician working with psychopathic clients should be particularly intentional about which information is disclosed as the potential for manipulation or retribution (if treatment is not "successful") always exists.

Comorbidity

Treatment of psychopathic or antisocial clients is further complicated by the co-occurrence of various other types of psychological difficulties. Without question, one of the most pervasive and serious comorbid factors involved in treating this population is substance abuse. Although a thorough review of substance abuse treatment is also beyond the scope of this chapter, clinicians must be vigilant to the likelihood of substance abuse and integrate steps to monitor and address this common problem. Of course, a wide range of other psychosocial problems are also common among this population, including housing instability, financial and legal problems, and familial discord (Persons & Bertagnolli, 1994). Monitoring and addressing these comorbid problems, when feasible, can be beneficial both in terms of reducing additional stressors and bolstering the therapeutic alliance.

DEVELOPMENT OF AN APPROACH TO TREAT ANTISOCIAL PERSONALITY DISORDER

In selecting an approach to adapt for use with individuals who engage in stalking and harassment behaviors, and for those with antisocial behaviors in general, we began with an examination of theoretical conceptualizations of the target population and the associated pathology. In our judgment, there was not an adequate empirical basis for excluding those with psychopathy, and thus we developed a treatment approach using a wide range of individuals meeting criteria for APD (including those who also exhibit substantial psychopathic traits). Therefore, our starting point was attempting to target the multitude of problems observed in individuals involved in the criminal justice system. The problems exhibited by this population can be divided into affective, cognitive, and behavioral problems (including interpersonal difficulties; impulsive behaviors such as violence, substance abuse, various other criminal behaviors; and intentional self-injury), as well as the motivational deficits previously described. One approach that seemed particularly promising in terms of addressing clients with multiple problems, including comorbid substance abuse and serious chronic behavioral difficulties, was DBT (Linehan, 1993a). DBT already included explicit strategies for addressing many of the obstacles to treatment and provided a framework to address those obstacles that were not specifically addressed in the model. The DBT approach was originally developed for those who are chronically suicidal, primarily women diagnosed with borderline personality disorder (BPD), but it has been adapted to address a wide range of behavior problems and psychological disorders.

The core maladaptive feature of BPD, according to Linehan's theoretical conceptualization, is dysfunction in the emotion regulation system. Hence, DBT incorporates a biosocial framework that explains the pathogenesis of emotion dysregulation, as well as its maintenance. In this model, a biological vulnerability (conceptualized as a high sensitivity to emotional stimuli) exists along with an environment that functions irrespective of the needs of the individual. Pathology develops as the invalidating environment and biological vulnerability interact with one another, with one side magnifying the other as time moves forward. The result is a pattern of escalating negative emotions, limited skills to manage these negative emotions, and extreme behaviors that flow from the emotions or help the individual self-regulate these emotions. As noted above, individuals with APD have difficulties with emotion regulation but develop a blunted affective style in place of the volatility observed in individuals with BPD. Rather than reacting to stimuli immediately and intensely, many individuals with APD have subnormal thresholds for taking in and reacting to emotional cues in their environments. The result is that such individuals show little motivation, experience chronic boredom, and require excessive stimulation to maintain their interest. Additionally, they cannot use emotional responses of others in a way that provides behavioral feedback (e.g., appreciating the feelings of an individual they have hurt as having done damage, and correcting the behavior).

McCann, Ball, and Ivanoff (2000) conceptualized the invalidating environment in individuals with APD as being similarly unresponsive to the emotional needs of the individual, analogous to the model of BPD proposed by Linehan. However, they added the concept of "disturbed caring." They suggested that individuals with APD are often punished for displaying emotions, particularly attachment or care behaviors, and are reinforced for displaying aggression, resulting in an antisocial belief system and a lack of affective connection to others. Deficits in emotional regulation skills, inaccurate perceptions of the environment, limited distress tolerance, and impaired ability to interact effectively with others are all overlapping problems found in individuals with both BPD and APD.

These similarities between theoretical conceptualizations of BPD and APD highlight the seeming appropriateness of DBT as a treatment modality. Both groups display characteristics that make treatment failures common, such as the tendency toward emotional dysregulation that inhibits learning. Thus, DBT was adapted to address potential treatment impediments such as those described earlier. In addition, DBT incorporates the concept of dialectics, an overarching philosophical approach that includes a process of dialogue that seeks to resolve tensions between competing and apparently disparate principles. The approach requires a willingness to search for synthesis by seeking information or perspectives that have been overlooked. Working with antisocial and psychopathic individuals is replete with such tensions and contradictions. For example, the clinician must convey respect in order to facilitate a working relationship, yet attempt to correct antisocial beliefs and behaviors. In DBT, the competing goals of accepting clients while demanding change are facilitated by balancing acceptance strategies (many of which have their roots in Buddhism) with change strategies rooted in learning theory. The notion of balance is embedded in the treatment in many ways, including the types of skills taught (e.g., both acceptance oriented and change oriented); the strategies used by the clinician (e.g., changing the manner in which one communicates with a client to convey acceptance or to apply a contingency in order to facilitate change); the agreement that therapists adopt and use a dialectical approach; and the emphasis on movement, speed, and flow in the treatment. This emphasis on dialectics also guided the treatment adaptations (described in the next section) we developed to accommodate the unique needs of our sample of stalking and harassment offenders.

First, DBT is a staged treatment. The vast majority of treatment for individuals with APD is Stage 1 treatment; thus, the description provided in this chapter refers to Stage 1 DBT treatment for individuals with APD. The goal of Stage 1 treatment is to move clients from behavioral dyscontrol to behavioral control. Targets for behavioral changes are also prioritized across multiple levels. Level 1 targets, which are the most important, include behaviors that involve harm to self or others and threats and urges to harm others. Level 2 targets, referred to as *treatment-interfering behaviors*, include those that have the potential to damage or destroy the treatment. These include missed sessions, failure to complete homework assignments, intimidating behavior, refusal to participate, and superficially "compliant" behaviors. Clinician behaviors can also be considered to be treatment interfering (and these are addressed in the clinician's consultation team). Clinician treatment-interfering behaviors specific to antisocial clients often include expressions of disgust or other negative judgments about clients, fear of clients, using an authoritarian approach or tone, or lack of unavailability. Level 3 targets are those behaviors that impair quality of life, such as unstable housing, frequent nonviolent criminal behaviors (e.g., turnstile jumping), substance abuse, and lack of education or job skills. Although these three levels of target behaviors are addressed hierarchically, skills to address them are taught in four areas: mindfulness, distress tolerance, emotion regulation, and interpersonal effectiveness.

There are four components in DBT, each organized according to function: individual psychotherapy, group skills training, telephone coaching, and a consultation team for therapists. The first component, individual DBT, is behavioral in nature and focuses primarily on motivating the individual to engage in, and remain in, treatment. Additionally, clinicians work to assist individuals in applying skills to particular problems in their lives. Clinicians utilize tools such as diary cards to monitor treatment targets and skillful behaviors and behavioral analysis of incidents involving problem behaviors. Diary cards for APD individuals may track negative behaviors, such as deceitfulness, as well as caring behaviors (which are modeled and shaped in the treatment).

The second component of DBT is group skills training. Utilizing Linehan's (1993b) treatment manual, this weekly group is designed to increase the individual's capacity for responding effectively to situations by teaching him or her new, more skillful, behaviors. This involves teaching, practicing, and exploring problems that arise in implementing new skills. The groups typically begin with a review of previous homework assignments (typically related to skills taught in the previous session), followed by a presentation of new information regarding the topic under discussion. The four group "modules" address specific skills: mindfulness, distress tolerance, emotion regulation, and interpersonal effectiveness. In our application of DBT to stalking and other types of criminal offenders, we have added additional skill exercises and didactic emphasis on validation, problem solving, dialectical thinking, and dealing with obsessive thoughts and compulsive behaviors. Finally, many of Linehan's original handouts and exercises were modified to incorporate and challenge antisocial beliefs (i.e., those supporting taking advantage of others) rather than the original emphasis on self-destructive behaviors.

The third component of DBT, telephone coaching, presented unique challenges when applied to antisocial and psychopathic individuals. The function of this intervention is to facilitate generalization of the skills learned in group into the lives of clients when they are away from the treatment environment. However, many antisocial individuals have frequent disruptions in housing, live in shelters, or do not own phones. Additional concerns include the client discerning information about the home of our clinicians (through identification of the therapist's telephone number). We have addressed these problems by using a phone-in message system that immediately notifies the clinician's cell phone or e-mail that a message exists, allowing the clinician to call the client back from a blocked telephone number. When necessary, we have even provided phone cards to facilitate telephone consultation, which is available 24 hours per day (i.e., clients who do not have funds can still telephone the project hotline at any time and be routed to their individual clinician).

The final component of the treatment exists to increase the skill level of clinicians, ensure that clinicians stay motivated, and ensure adherence to the treatment principles. Clinicians meet weekly as a group for 90 minutes to consult with one another about clients, provide support, and learn new material together. In treating antisocial and psychopathic individuals, clinicians must work to avoid hopelessness, pessimism, and judgment about their clients and their lack of motivation. Much time is spent discussing challenges related to bolstering treatment engagement among difficult individuals, as well as developing strategies for reducing therapy-interfering behaviors. In our experience, it has been essential to have clinicians with knowledge of DBT as well as experience working with forensic populations. The following case example describes the application of DBT to an individual with APD and significant psychopathic traits.

CASE EXAMPLE

At the time he was referred to treatment, Steve was 25 years old and unemployed. He had been arrested after violating an order of protection for the second time, having gone to the apartment of his ex-girlfriend, Wanda, despite a court order requiring that he stay a minimum of 100 yards away from her at all times. Wanda had initially sought the order of protection shortly after her relationship with Steve ended, accusing him of making threatening and intimidating telephone calls to her home and work and on several occasions waiting for her outside the office where she worked. Although no violence had occurred since the order of protection had been issued, Wanda had previously called the police to intervene several times while she and

Steve were living together, typically after he had verbally threatened her. On the day of his last arrest, Steve had broken a window in Wanda's apartment by throwing a rock from the street. At the time of his referral, he was awaiting sentencing for this incident, with a possible range from probation with no incarceration to 5 years in prison.

During his initial intake interview, Steve acknowledged a number of problem behaviors in addition to his harassment of Wanda (which he quickly minimized, claiming that it was "a misunderstanding"). Steve acknowledged a history of aggression, both in intimate relationships and with strangers (e.g., periodically starting fights while intoxicated). He also described himself as being a frequent target of aggression, having to defend himself from the periodic assaults and random violence in his neighborhood. He had been in several drug rehabilitation programs because of cocaine and marijuana abuse and admitted that he continued to smoke marijuana and use prescription sedatives (for "recreational" purposes) regularly. At the time of the intake, he was living with his mother, whom he described as an alcoholic, and his two younger sisters. One sister was disabled and wheelchair-bound and the other, age 15 years, did not attend school and also smoked marijuana daily. A PCL-SV completed at the time of intake indicated a psychopathic personality style, with both interpersonal/affective symptoms as well as significant and long-standing behavioral problems. Nevertheless, Steve agreed to participate in treatment and appeared, at the time of his initial referral, motivated to complete the 6-month program.

Steve was described as a child with learning difficulties. He experienced chronic invalidation as a result of his mother's alcoholism (she was frequently too drunk to care for his needs) and, during periods of sobriety, her highly emotional criticisms of him (e.g., he was frequently told that his difficulties in school were due to his lack of motivation, when in fact he often missed school because his mother was drunk). Additionally, Steve's mother tended to focus on her disabled daughter and attend to her needs, often forcing Steve to manage his own problems and difficulties.

At the start of the treatment, Steve expressed a commitment to attending treatment to avoid further incarceration, but he did not perceive any need for treatment and had no interest in changing his behaviors. He insisted that he had no intention of renewing any contact with Wanda and readily attributed their "relationship problems" to her erratic and aggressive behavior. The therapist used commitment strategies to highlight his goal of avoiding reincarceration and tied that primary goal to other, secondary goals (e.g., not only would he need to stop all contact with Wanda, but he would need to avoid other violent behaviors in order to prevent new criminal charges). Thus, Steve's overarching treatment goal was to develop a life worth living (for him), which primarily involved being free of oversight from the criminal justice system. His Level 1 target was elimination of violence of any kind, including decreases in threats and urges to harm others. His Level 2 targets, those interfering with treatment, included decreasing late arrivals and missed sessions. His Level 3 targets (i.e., those affecting quality of life) included decreasing substance abuse, finding steady employment, and finding a stable living situation.

Steve's attendance during the initial 2 months of treatment was quite poor. The clinician used behavioral analysis each time he was late in order to assess the problem thoroughly; this process enabled the clinician to dissect the influences that led to his problem behavior in order to identify points at which alternative responses might have occurred. The analyses revealed that, at times, he missed sessions because he was using drugs. Although he was not disturbed by his substance use and was not committed to abstinence, he was able, through this nonjudgmental assessment, to see that his drug use made him late for sessions and would lead to additional problems (e.g., termination from the program). He saw that he often intended to come to treatment but smoked marijuana, overslept, and was therefore late; he often made the decision to skip treatment rather than attend late because of fear of being kicked out of treatment. The clinician clarified that being in skills group and individual therapy was a primary goal (having used drugs or not) and that arriving late was far better than missing treatment altogether. The dialectic presented was that one is asked not to come to sessions under the influence of drugs and yet on the other hand, who needs treatment more than someone caught in a cycle of substance abuse? He agreed to refrain from drinking or using drugs on treatment days. He also agreed that if he did slip, that he would make every effort to show up and do what was needed to be present in treatment (e.g., splash cold water on his face, drink coffee).

A second theme that arose in his behavioral analyses was sessions missed because of his financial situation. Steve often panicked about his financial situation and sought last-minute work as a day laborer, even on treatment days. His primary clinician used "pros and cons" to explore the possibility of tolerating his panic about money and turning down work versus acting in response to his fear and working on treatment days. The clinician validated the reasonableness of needing income. The pros for taking work obviously included money. However, the cons included missing treatment and putting his freedom in jeopardy (as he was mandated to treatment and monitored by probation). He came to the realization that the potential consequences of missing sessions outweighed the potential monetary gain. Additionally, he realized that he could take actions to proactively seek work on other days of the week to reduce his vulnerability to impulsively skip sessions in order to work. These interventions dramatically improved his attendance, which by Month 3 had become quite regular.

Another factor interfering with Steve's treatment was his illiteracy. He had little ability to read materials distributed during or after group and struggled to complete the required homework. Initially, rather than acknowledge this limitation, Steve masked his embarrassment by diminishing the importance of assignments and routinely failing to complete the homework. When confronted with the need to participate more fully, Steve often became hostile and argumentative, calling the treatment program "stupid" and "pointless." His deficits in insight and decision making hindered Steve's ability to identify strategies to change or improve his life, leaving him feeling frustrated and hopeless, emotions that seemed to trigger his aggression and substance abuse. One particularly important behavioral analysis revealed a chain that led directly to his harassment behaviors. Being in a group in which he was asked to read prompted thoughts that he was a failure. He ruminated about the fact that his mother thought he was stupid, and he felt hopeless. This was identified as a vulnerability factor for other negative emotions. Steve first identified that he felt physically numb in group but then realized that these feelings led to his desire to see Wanda, who had helped him read while he was attempting to obtain his GED. He identified an urge to contact Wanda and a physical sensation he described as an ache in his chest. These feelings led to the thought, "that bitch is the reason I'm in this stupid group." He had an urge to call her in order to leave a threatening message but was unable to do so as he was in skills group. Skills group leaders noted that he was irritable and refused to speak in group. During the individual session that followed this group, Steve was noticeably dysregulated, saying, "I don't want to be in this stupid-ass program. . . . Kick me out." The clinician conducted the aforementioned chain analysis to understand Steve's current emotions and to determine an appropriate skill on which to coach him. He provided the details described previously, allowing the clinician to inquire whether his urge to threaten Wanda had increased, decreased, or stayed the same since leaving skills group. He noted that it had decreased; he was no longer feeling irritable or hostile by the conclusion of the chain analysis. The clinician taught him the skill of *urge surfing*, observing one's emotions without acting on them to avoid calling her in the future. The clinician also identified Steve's illiteracy and self-invalidation (calling himself stupid) in response to these feelings, agreed to go over homework readings on the telephone, and coached him to negotiate a solution with his skills leaders about public reading. Steve was also referred to a literacy program in which he could receive educational services that were not connected to his criminal case and mental health treatment. Steve responded well to this flexible approach. He began attending treatment more consistently and participating more fully. His disparaging comments gradually decreased, and he began to actively participate in group and individual sessions.

Although a rigid approach to Steve's poor attendance and nonparticipation might have led to a decision to terminate him from the program, or a decision on his part to drop out (no matter what the consequences), DBT favors a problem assessment and collaborative solution approach (i.e., seeking a dialectical synthesis). Treatment targets are organized hierarchically so that whenever Steve reported violent thoughts or behaviors in the previous week, they were analyzed and attended to first. However, at times, Steve's treatment-interfering behaviors jeopardized his status in the program and thus were also given a high priority. The DBT approach to substance abuse is also unique for a criminal justice setting. Although a commitment to abstinence is desirable, DBT favors shaping commitment to decrease substance use by highlighting the manner in which it interferes with the client's own stated goals.

The process of developing an initial commitment to treatment goals and then revisiting this commitment as treatment targets evolve occurs repeatedly during the course of DBT. Using techniques such as "devil's advocate" (e.g., "Why not drop out of treatment?") and connecting easier goals (e.g., not getting high before session) to larger ones (e.g., staying out of jail and accepting help with his relationships) facilitates this process. Highlighting the freedom to choose with the absence of alternatives is another commitment strategy used by the clinician in this treatment. In Steve's case, the clinician repeatedly acknowledged that Steve could choose whether to use drugs and attend treatment and explored the implications of his choices in a nonjudgmental way. In this process, the clinician avoided a power struggle with Steve over whose goals were most important and helped him avoid the self-destructive choices he had so often made in the past.

Perhaps the most important gains were made in helping Steve manage his violent impulses. When his violence was explored using behavioral analysis, it became apparent that Steve had little insight into his emotions and virtually no skills to manage distressing emotions. He was taught to identify his emotions and used telephone coaching when he had an impulse that he did not know how to manage. He was coached in interpersonal skills as well as distress tolerance skills to assist when situations arose that could not be readily avoided or changed (like dealing with his mother when she was intoxicated).

Steve's attention and participation in skills group improved as he began to see the utility of these skills for improving his life. Once his anxiety about his illiteracy decreased (group leaders were careful not to ask him to read aloud), he was better able to learn and practice these skills. He completed all four of the standard DBT skills modules (mindfulness, distress tolerance, interpersonal effectiveness, and emotion regulation) but also appeared to benefit from the additional exercises designed to enhance decision making skills, as Steve was often hindered by indecision and confusion.

Although Steve's progress in this treatment was slow and sporadic, he became increasingly engaged and motivated, developing a strong relationship with his individual therapist. He began arriving on time for his scheduled sessions, readily discussing both his accomplishments and continued problem behaviors. As the Level 1 and 2 target issues receded, Level 3 problems, and the difficulties within Steve's family in particular, became more salient. He continued to occasionally miss scheduled sessions because of "family crises." He was able to identify protective thoughts and feelings toward his mother and disabled sister despite the negative influences associated with these relationships. Although there were certainly reasons to suggest that Steve find another place to live (e.g., his mother's violence when she was intoxicated, his nondisabled sister's drug use, the high level of aggression in his neighborhood), he was unwilling to make such a move at that time. Nevertheless, Steve became increasingly comfortable discussing these family stressors and identifying strategies to minimize their impact on his mood and behavior. At the point of program completion, Steve was still using marijuana with some regularity but had refrained from aggressive behavior and had not initiated contact with Wanda for several months. One year later, he had not been rearrested and was diligently looking for employment.

CONCLUSIONS AND FUTURE DIRECTIONS

Although clinical lore has fueled the belief that clients with psychopathic and antisocial personality characteristics cannot be successfully treated, this conclusion may well reflect the inadequacy of prior treatment efforts rather than the lack of treatment response of this population. With more aggressive treatment efforts, improved treatment outcomes may follow. In particular, creative efforts to enhance motivation, commitment, and treatment engagement, and concrete skill acquisition strategies to improve stress tolerance, decrease impulsiveness, and bolster interpersonal skills may substantially increase the likelihood of change.

The general descriptions and case study described here should not be taken as suggesting that DBT can overcome the multitude of obstacles that exist in treating antisocial and psychopathic personalities. Neither, however, does our clinical experience support the therapeutic pessimism that is so commonly voiced. Clearly, further research is needed to ascertain when, if, and how often such interventions are successful, and what elements of treatment are most critical in accomplishing these goals. In addition, the many caveats detailed in the first half of this chapter require considerable attention, including dealing with issues of confidentiality, violence risk assessment, and therapist fear and resentment. Without adequate attention to these important elements, treatment may well show the damaging effects feared by some clinicians.

REFERENCES

American Psychiatric Association. (1980). *Diagnostic and statistical manual of mental disorders* (3rd ed.). Washington, DC: Author.

American Psychiatric Association. (2000). *Diagnostic and statistical manual of mental disorders* (4th ed., text rev.). Washington, DC: Author.

Cleckley, H. (1941/1975). *The mask of sanity: An attempt to reinterpret the so-called psychopathic personality*. St. Louis, MO: Mosby.

Dahle, K. P. (1997). Therapy motivation in prisons. In S. Redondo, V. Garrido, J. Pérez, & R. Barberet (Eds.), *Advances in psychology and law* (pp. 431–441). Berlin, Germany: Walter de Gruyter.

Eron, L. D. (1997). The development of antisocial behavior from a learning perspective. In D. M. Stoff, J. Breiling, & J. D. Maser (Eds.), *Handbook of antisocial behavior* (pp. 140–147). New York: Wiley.

Galietta, M., Garcia-Mansilla, A., & Rosenfeld, B. (2006). *The relationship between psychopathy and risk, treatment response, and drop-out in a sample of stalking offenders*. Paper presented at the annual meeting of the American Psychology-Law Society, St. Petersburg, FL.

Galietta, M., & Stanley, B. S. (2008). Ethical considerations in conducting randomized controlled trials in psychotherapy research. In A. M. Nezu & C. M. Nezu (Eds.), *Evidence-based outcome research: A practical guide to conducting randomized controlled trials for psychosocial interventions* (pp. 405–424). New York: Oxford University Press.

Hare, R. D. (1991). *The Hare Psychopathy Checklist—Revised*. Toronto, Ontario, Canada: Multi-Health Systems.

Hare, R. D. (1996). Psychopathy: A clinical construct whose time has come. *Criminal Justice and Behavior, 23*(1), 25–54.

Harris, G. T., & Rice, M. E. (2005). Treatment of psychopathy: A review of empirical findings. In C. J. Patrick (Ed.), *Handbook of psychopathy* (pp. 555–572). New York: Guilford Press.

Harris, G. T., Rice, M. E., & Cormier, C. A. (1994). Psychopaths: Is a therapeutic community therapeutic? *Therapeutic Communities, 15*, 283–299.

Hart, S. D., Cox, D. N., & Hare, R. D. (1995). *The Hare Psychopathy Checklist: Screening Version* (PCL:SV). North Tonawanda, NY: Multi-Health Systems.

Hart, S. D., & Hare, R. D. (1997). Psychopathy: Assessment and association with criminal conduct. In D. M. Stoff & J. Breiling (Eds.), *Handbook of antisocial behavior* (pp. 22–35). New York: Wiley.

Henggeler, S. W., Sheidow, A. J., & Lee, T. (2007). Multisystemic treatment of serious clinical problems in youths and their families. In D. W. Springer & A. R. Roberts (Eds.), *Handbook of forensic mental health with victims and offenders: Assessment, treatment and research* (pp. 315–345). New York: Springer.

Linehan, M. M. (1993a). *Cognitive–behavioral treatment of borderline personality disorder*. New York: Guilford Press.

Linehan, M. M. (1993b). *Skills training manual for treating borderline personality disorder*. New York: Guilford Press.

Lykken, D. T. (1995). *The antisocial personalities*. Hillsdale, NJ: Erlbaum.

Marshall, W. L., Serran, G. A., Fernandez, Y. M., Mulloy, R., Mann, R. E., & Thornton, D. (2003). Therapist characteristics in the treatment of sexual offenders: Tentative data on their relationship with indices of behaviour change. *Journal of Sexual Aggression, 9*, 25–30.

McCann, R., Ball, E. M., & Ivanoff, A. (2000). DBT with an inpatient forensic population: The CMHIP forensic model. *Cognitive and Behavioral Practice, 7,* 447–456.

Persons, J. B., & Bertagnolli, A. (1994). Cognitive–behavioural treatment of multiple-problem patients: Application to personality disorders. *Clinical Psychology and Psychotherapy, 1,* 279–285.

Rogers, R., & Dion, K. L. (1991). Rethinking the *DSM–III–R* diagnosis of antisocial personality disorder. *Bulletin of the American Academy of Psychiatry & the Law, 19*(1), 21–31.

Rosenfeld, B., Fava, J., & Galietta, M. (2009). Working with the stalking offender: Considerations for risk assessment and intervention. In J. Werth, A. Benjamin, & D. Blevins (Eds.), *The duty to protect: Ethical, legal, and professional considerations for mental health professionals* (pp. 95–110). Washington, DC: American Psychological Association.

Salekin, R. T. (2002). Psychopathy and therapeutic pessimism: Clinical lore or clinical reality? *Clinical Psychology Review, 22,* 79–112.

Skeem, J. L., Monahan, J., & Mulvey, E. P. (2002). Psychopathy, treatment involvement, and subsequent violence among civil psychiatric patients. *Law and Human Behavior, 26,* 577–603.

Tarasoff v. Regents of University of California, 131 Cal. Rptr. 14, 551 P.2d 334 (1976).

Ullman, L. P., & Krasner, L. (1969). *A psychological approach to abnormal behavior.* New York: Prentice-Hall.

Werth, J. L., Jr., Welfel, E. R., & Benjamin, G. A. H. (2009). *The duty to protect: Ethical, legal, and professional considerations for mental health professionals.* Washington, DC: American Psychological Association.

Wilson, D. L., Frick, P. J., & Clements, C. B. (1999). Gender, somatization and psychopathic traits in a college sample. *Journal of Psychopathology and Behavioral Assessment, 21,* 221–235.

AFTERWORD: FUTURE DIRECTIONS IN TREATING REFRACTORY CASES

The marks of maturity for a school of psychotherapy involve many things, including a sound empirical foundation of tests of the theoretical rationale for the treatment, mechanisms of psychopathology that lead to interventions tailored specifically for presenting symptoms, and successfully executed randomized controlled trials to evaluate the efficacy of treatment. Further indications that a school of psychotherapy has matured includes the willingness of its practitioners to (a) take on the difficult-to-treat cases, (b) learn from these challenges in order to improve treatment outcome, and (c) identify and acknowledge the limits of treatment efficacy and applicability. Some psychotherapies clearly do not meet these standards, particularly those therapies in which the empirical foundations are lacking and the claims of treatment efficacy are extravagant. In comparison, cognitive–behavioral therapy (CBT) would seem to have all the marks of maturity. The various forms of CBT have a firm empirical basis, although there continues to be research to deepen and broaden our understanding of the mechanisms underlying the disorders to which CBT is applied and the mechanisms of treatment response.

On the whole, those who practice CBT also appear willing to think critically about this form of therapy and to concede that it is by no means a panacea. As the chapters in this volume indicated, they are also eager to take on challenging cases. Indeed, there have been several books devoted to CBT for difficult or complex cases (e.g., Foa & Emmelkamp, 1983; Leahy, 2003; Tarrier, 2006; Tarrier, Wells, & Haddock, 2000). Many CBT practitioners and researchers are also willing to examine their treatment failures in an attempt to learn from these cases. Indeed, it seems that cognitive–behavioral scientists and practitioners have an avid interest in treatment failures and ways to improve outcome, as indicated by the many articles on the topic in, for example, the journal *Cognitive and Behavioral Practice*.

As noted in the preface to this volume, the first book on the issue of CBT refractory cases was Foa and Emmelkamp's (1983) landmark volume *Failures in Behavior Therapy*, which was a brave and frank attempt by practitioners to come to grips with the limitations of their interventions and to conceive methods of improving outcome. This present volume revisited, a quarter of a century later, the important issue of treatment failures for patients receiving CBT. What is the current state of knowledge about the causes of treatment failures, and how might we address the problem? The chapters in this volume examined these questions for most of the common psychiatric disorders. The chapter contributors offered both empirical evidence and clinical wisdom about how to manage treatment-refractory cases. Here we summarize the themes that emerged from these chapters and offer our thoughts on other potentially useful means of improving outcome.

EMERGENT THEMES

Many chapters noted the relationship between pretreatment symptom severity and treatment outcome. For numerous psychological disorders (e.g., social anxiety disorder, panic disorder), people with severe symptoms, compared with those with milder symptoms, make comparable treatment gains. In other words, the magnitude of pre–post symptom reduction is similar across severe and milder groups. This means, however, that for a given course of treatment (e.g., 12 sessions), people who initially have severe symptoms are less likely to have reached "recovered" status. Nonetheless, the accumulating data suggest that clients with all ranges of severity can achieve clinical significance and not merely statistical significance (Jacobson & Truax, 1991). People with more severe psychological symptoms are therefore likely to require a longer course of treatment to achieve the same outcomes that can be achieved more easily in cases of less severe symptoms. This conclusion will come as no surprise to most readers, although health insurance companies and managed care providers who often dictate funding for many patients may need to be educated about the empirical relationship between disorder severity and length of treatment.

A common strategy for improving outcome cited in the chapters in this volume is to identify poor prognostic indicators and then to find ways of modifying or adapting CBT to address the particular problem. Several chapters, for example, noted that treatment outcome for a given disorder is sometimes poorer when a comorbid condition is present. Comorbidity, however, is often an inconsistent predictor of poor outcome, and the literature is not yet clear on how to handle specific comorbid problems in any event (Emmelkamp, 2004; Hollon & Beck, 2004). Nevertheless, it is still important to consider comorbidity in order to avoid potential problems that can arise in such instances. For example, the nature of CBT for posttraumatic stress disorder (PTSD) may vary as to whether the person has a comorbid substance use disorder (SUD), especially if the latter is not in remission. A small but growing body of research has suggested that an effective form of intervention is to treat PTSD and SUD simultaneously, using Najavits's (2002) cognitive–behavioral seeking safety protocol.

Another theme that emerged from several chapters was that methods are needed to enhance the patient's motivation for engaging in treatment, particularly for completing homework assignments. Various suggestions were offered in this regard, including the use of methods based on motivational interviewing (W. R. Miller & Rollnick, 2002). A further theme concerned the need to augment CBT by combining it with other inventions. For example, treatment outcome for SUDs (and other disorders) may be augmented by combining CBT with motivational interviewing. The contributors to this volume also suggested other ways of augmenting outcome, such as by combining a CBT protocol for a given disorder with other cognitive–behavioral interventions (e.g., acceptance, mindfulness-based strategies; Hayes, Luoma, Bond, Masuda, & Lillis, 2006; Segal, Williams, & Teasdale, 2002) or by combining CBT with particular medications (e.g., D-cycloserine; Davis, Ressler, Rothbaum, & Richardson, 2006).

One of the significant lessons from this volume lies in the various case vignettes, which emphasized the importance of therapist factors, particularly the ability of the therapist to conduct a thorough assessment, to devise a good case formulation, and to be creative in developing cognitive or behavioral interventions that are best suited to a given patient's problems. This raises the interesting and clinically important question of what makes a stellar CBT practitioner. Clinical researchers who develop and study CBT interventions, who write CBT treatment manuals, and who regularly conduct workshops are, no doubt, highly competent practitioners, but are they the most stellar exemplars? It is quite possible, indeed likely, that some of the most effective CBT practitioners are those knowledgeable and creative individuals in full-time clinical practice settings who work continuously at perfecting their art, without necessarily publishing or disseminating their insights by mean of workshops or professional publications.

It is interesting to consider that the best lessons learned about refractory cases might be obtained by identifying and interviewing clinicians who are not necessarily recognized as experts or who have not conducted the most rigorous or the largest treatment outcome trials. Such individuals, who have no allegiances to particular techniques they have developed or studied but are simply known in their clinical community as having considerable clinical wisdom (and are commonly consulted by colleagues), might hold untapped pearls of clinical wisdom. This is not to say that we should sacrifice empirical rigor; however, a good way of learning from refractory cases is to draw both from the science of CBT (i.e., empirical studies) and from the art of our therapy (i.e., the methods used by unusually effective therapists). Advances in treating refractory cases may benefit, in part, from research efforts to objectively identify stellar CBT practitioners.

FUTURE DIRECTIONS: COGNITIVE–BEHAVIORAL THERAPY IN A BROADER CONTEXT

The themes that emerged from the chapters in this volume tend to focus on the individual, to the neglect of the wider social context. The experts in this volume recommended that treatment outcome could be improved by adapting CBT to particular clinical problems and by combining CBT with other interventions. In our chapter on obsessive–compulsive disorder (see chap. 5), we also discussed the concept of cure therapeutics (Insel & Scolnick, 2006), whereby advances in treatment efficacy may depend on gaining a better understanding of the biological and psychological etiologic factors in a given disorder. But even the concept of cure therapeutics is unlikely to be sufficient because it ignores the broader context in which a given person's psychological problems arise. The media and grant funding agencies commonly call for the development of "magic bullet" treatments of mental disorders. That sort of endeavor would be fine if the disorder was entirely located "in" the individual (i.e., if social factors were irrelevant), but that is unlikely to be the case for the disorders that were discussed in this volume. Indeed, even infectious diseases, which are obviously biological in nature, are strongly influenced by societal factors, such as practices in a given city concerning standards of sanitation and water purity (Morris, 2007).

An important future direction may therefore be to better integrate CBT with community-based programs, such as health education programs and programs designed to reduce stressors that are known to exacerbate various forms of psychology, such as mood and anxiety disorders. With such programs in place, it may be much easier to successfully implement CBT or other treatments for psychopathology. Examples are as follows:

1. *Social programs to reduce poverty, racism, crime, and other community-based stressors.* To illustrate, CBT may not be effective in completely eliminating a person's depressive symptoms if he or she is living in a community in which there are ongoing stressors. In other words, an aversive social environment may continue to trigger symptoms despite the best efforts of the CBT practitioner. Accordingly, treatment outcome may be enhanced if social programs are in place that buffer the person from ongoing stress.

2. *Urban development programs that aim to foster a sense of community among people.* Such plans can serve as alternatives to the isolating and alienating effects of suburbia (for a discussion of the origins and failure of the concept of suburbia, see, e.g., L. J. Miller, 1995). Ideally, urban development programs would foster a sense of belonging and social support, which serves as a buffer against various forms of psychopathology (e.g., Brown & Harris, 1978; Brown & Moran, 1997). The presence of such social supports may make it easier for people to attain a good response to CBT.

3. *Programs that financially reinforce people for staying on welfare.* These programs may reinforce dependency and helplessness (Dalrymple, 2005), thereby making it difficult to treat associated problems (e.g., depression) with CBT. Similarly, if a person's receipt of disability benefits critically depends on whether he or she continues to meet criteria for a given disorder (e.g., PTSD), then this may undermine any efforts to treat the disorder (Taylor, Frueh, & Asmundson, 2007).

4. *Educational programs that inform people about the distinction between mental disorders and ordinary misery.* There has been a growing trend, which some commentators have attributed to the pharmaceutical industry, in which everyday misery is relabeled as a medical condition in need of treatment. Examples include the medicalization of ordinary sadness as depression (Horwitz & Wakefield, 2007) and the pathologizing of mere social reticence as being indicative of social anxiety disorder (Lane, 2007). The CBT practitioner can help to correct these misconceptions in their patients and thereby reduce the chances that the patient will be alarmed by experiencing ordinary misery (for a discussion of the fear of unpleasant emotions, see Salters-Pedneault, Gentes, & Roemer, 2007; Taylor & Rachman, 1991). Unfortunately, the therapist fights an uphill battle as the media continues to portray these mundane miseries as forms of mental illness. Educational programs

may help correct the social trend toward the pathologizing of ordinary misery.

SUMMARY AND CONCLUSION

Over the past quarter century, since the valuable volume by Foa and Emmelkamp (1983), great strides have been made in improving CBT for a range of psychological disorders. The chapters in this volume discussed many different ways in which treatment outcome might be improved. Given the current state of the field, trainees in mental health practice are likely to be frustrated with the current armamentarium of less-than-perfect interventions. But for those of us who are clinical investigators, our treatment limitations are an interesting, indeed exciting, impetus for further investigation. In the coming decades, many of today's refractory cases may well become tomorrow's easy cures, especially when a deeper understanding of the causes of, and mechanisms of treatment for, psychopathology has been attained. Our conviction is that by examining our current treatment failures, we will be better able to facilitate tomorrow's successes.

REFERENCES

Brown, G. W., & Harris, T. O. (1978). *Social origins of depression*. London: Tavistock.

Brown, G. W., & Moran, P. M. (1997). Single mothers, poverty and depression, *Psychological Medicine, 27*, 21–33.

Dalrymple, T. (2005). *Our culture, what's left of it: The mandarins and the masses*. Chicago: Ivan R. Dee.

Davis, M., Ressler, K., Rothbaum, B. O., & Richardson, R. (2006). Effects of D-cycloserine on extinction: Translation from preclinical to clinical work. *Biological Psychiatry, 60*, 369–375.

Emmelkamp, P. M. G. (2004). Behavior therapy with adults. In M. J. Lambert (Ed.), *Bergin & Garfield's handbook of psychotherapy and behavior changes* (5th ed., pp. 393–446). New York: Wiley.

Foa, E. B., & Emmelkamp, P. M. G. (1983). *Failures in behavior therapy*. New York: Wiley.

Hayes, S. C., Luoma, J. B., Bond, F. W., Masuda, A., & Lillis, J. (2006). Acceptance and commitment therapy: Model, processes and outcomes. *Behaviour Research and Therapy, 44*, 1–25.

Hollon, S. D., & Beck, A. T. (2004). Cognitive and cognitive behavioral therapies. In M. J. Lambert (Ed.), *Bergin & Garfield's handbook of psychotherapy and behavior changes* (5th ed., pp. 447–492). New York: Wiley.

Horwitz, A. V., & Wakefield, J. C. (2007). *The loss of sadness: How psychiatry transformed normal sorrow into depressive disorder*. New York: Oxford University Press.

Insel, T. R., & Scolnick, E. M. (2006). Cure therapeutics and strategic prevention: Raising the bar for mental health research. *Molecular Psychiatry, 11*, 11–17.

Jacobson, N. S., & Truax, P. (1991). Clinical significance: A statistical approach to defining meaningful change in psychotherapy research. *Journal of Consulting and Clinical Psychology, 59*, 12–19.

Lane, C. (2007). *Shyness: How normal behavior became a sickness.* Newhaven, CT: Yale University Press.

Leahy, R. L. (2003). *Roadblocks in cognitive–behavioral therapy: Transforming challenges into opportunities for change.* New York: Guilford Press.

Miller, L. J. (1995). Family togetherness and the suburban ideal. *Sociological Forum, 10*, 393–418.

Miller, W. R., & Rollnick, S. (2002). *Motivational interviewing: Preparing people for change* (2nd ed.). New York: Guilford Press.

Morris, R. D. (2007). *The blue death: Disease, disaster, and the water we drink.* New York: HarperCollins.

Najavits, L. M. (2002). *Seeking safety: A treatment manual for PTSD and substance abuse.* New York: Guilford Press.

Salters-Pedneault, K., Gentes, E., & Roemer, L. (2007). The role of fear of emotion in distress, arousal, and cognitive interference following an emotional stimulus. *Cognitive Behaviour Therapy, 36*, 12–22.

Segal, Z. V., Williams, J. M. G., & Teasdale, J. T. (2002). *Mindfulness-based cognitive therapy for depression: A new approach to preventing relapse.* New York: Guilford Press.

Tarrier, N. (2006). *Case formulation in cognitive–behavior therapy: The treatment of challenging and complex cases.* New York: Routledge.

Tarrier, N., Wells, A., & Haddock, G. (2000). *Treating complex cases: The cognitive behavioural approach.* Chichester, England: Wiley.

Taylor, S., Frueh, B. C., & Asmundson, G. J. G. (2007). Detection and management of malingering in people presenting for treatment of posttraumatic stress disorder: Methods, obstacles, and recommendations. *Journal of Anxiety Disorders, 21*, 22–41.

Taylor, S., & Rachman, S. (1991). Fear of sadness. *Journal of Anxiety Disorders, 5*, 375–381.

INDEX

415

Blaszcynski, A., 234
Bleiberg, K. L., 186
BN. *See* Bulimia nervosa
Bodily sensations, 328–329
Body checking, 170
Body dysmorphic disorder, 244
Bootzin, R. R., 279
Borderline personality disorder (BPD), 347–365
    and anger, 311
    challenges in treatment of, 352–360
    and eating disorders, 169
    and refractory disorders, 348–352
    transaction model for, 360–365
Borkovec, T. D., 113, 117, 119
Bouman, T. K., 330
BPD. *See* Borderline personality disorder
Breitholtz, E., 116
Brief interventions, 236
Brofaromine, 71
Brouwers, C., 6, 10
Brown, E. J., 75
Brown, T. A., 45, 46, 50, 89
Browne, G., 186
Buckminster, S., 73
Bulimia nervosa (BN), 155–157
    and cognitive deficits, 171
    and interpersonal relationships, 168
    and motivation to change, 163
Burgard, M., 240
Buspirone, 71–72
Buwalda, F., 330
Buying, compulsive, 239–240
Byrne, D., 56

California Department of Corrections, 370
California Department of Justice, 370
California Supreme Court, 393
Candida albicans, 267
CAPS. *See* Clinician Administered PTSD Scale
Cardiovascular problems (and anger), 299
Caring (disturbed), 396
Carr, A., 56
Castonguay, L. G., 204
Cataplexy, 286
CBASP. *See* Cognitive–behavioral analysis system of psychotherapy for depression
CBGT. *See* Cognitive–behavioral group therapy
CBT. *See* Cognitive–behavioral therapy

CBT-I. *See* Cognitive–behavioral therapy for insomnia
Chain analysis, 359
Chambless, D. L., 48, 51, 73, 75, 117
Change-oriented interventions, 12
Change strategies, 396
Change talk, 342–343
Childhood abuse, 76
Christos, P. J., 186
Chronic depression. *See also* Depression
    CBASP for treatment of, 186–191
    disability with, 184–185
Circadian system, 281
Citalopram, 71
Clark, D. M., 46, 69–70, 334
Clark, M., 56
Classification
    of eating disorders, 155–157
    of sexual dysfunctions, 255–260
Clayborne, J., 235
Cleckley, Hervey, 386
Client-related factors (for poor response to treatment), 4–6, 12–13
Clinical experience, xxi
Clinical Interview Schedule for Personality Disorders (SCID-II), 48
Clinical perfectionism, 169–170
Clinical trials, 44
Clinician Administered PTSD Scale (CAPS), 145–146
Clinician bias, 394
Clomipramine
    for treatment of obsessive–compulsive disorder, 91
    for treatment of trichotillomania, 238
Clonazepam, 71, 72
Clozapine, 352
CMBT. *See* Cognitive motivational behavior therapy
Coaching (telephone), 398
Cobb, A. M., 334
CODP. *See* Collaborative Outcome Data Project
Cognitions (on Anger Disorders Scale), 307
Cognitive and Behavioral Practice (journal), 408
Cognitive appraisals (in anger episode model), 303–304
Cognitive–behavioral analysis system of psychotherapy for depression (CBASP), 186–191
    assumptions and procedures in, 187–189

Faber, R., 240

Failures in Behavior Therapy (E. B. Foa and P. M. G. Emmelkamp), xxii, 408

Failure to engage in treatment, 162–164

Fairburn, C. G., 165

Falloon, I. R. H., 72

FBI (Federal Bureau of Investigation), 370

Fear, 24–25
  of abandonment, 353–355
  of fear, 43
  of gaining weight, 155
  hierarchy of, 51
  of penetration, 265–266
  structures, 141

Federal Bureau of Investigation (FBI), 370

Fedoroff, I. C., 74

Feelings, internal, 52

Fennell, M. J., 168

Feske, U., 73

Fluoxetine, 238
  for treatment of eating disorders, 157
  for treatment of social anxiety disorder, 71
  for treatment of trichotillomania, 238

Fluvoxamine, 71

Foa, E. B., xxii, 6, 8, 92–93, 408

Fonagy, John, 351

Frankenburg, F. R., 348

Franklin, M. E., 76, 95

Freeman, T., 140

Friis, S., 7

Frotteurism, 369

Functional analyses, 8

Furr, J. M., 95

Gabapentin, 71–72

GAD. *See* Generalized anxiety disorder

GAF (Global Assessment of Functioning) scores, 203

Gamblers Anonymous, 235, 246

Gambling, pathological. *See* Pathological gambling

Gauthier, J., 47

Gauthier, J. G., 46

Gender, 66–67

General adaptation syndrome, 299

Generalization phase (of situational analysis), 189

Generalized anxiety disorder (GAD), 111–132
  case example, 120–131
  CBT for, 116–118

defining, 111–112

future directions for treatment of, 131–132

and motivational enhancement, 20

poor response to treatment of, 118–120

treatments for, 112–116

Generalized social anxiety disorder, 66, 77–78

Genetics
  and eating disorders, 161
  and posttraumatic stress disorder, 140–141

Genital pain, 263–267

Gerringer, E., 329–330

Global Assessment of Functioning (GAF) scores, 203

Goals (for therapy), 27

Goldfried, M. R., 204

Goldstein, A., 48

Gordon, J. R., 212

Gould, R. A., 44, 73

Goyer, L. R., 48

Gracely, E. J., 48

Grayson, J. B., 6

Greist, J. H., 95

Group skills training, 397–398

Group therapy
  individual therapy vs., 18
  for treatment of anger, 315
  for treatment of intermittent explosive disorder, 242
  for treatment of panic disorder, 44
  for treatment of pathological gambling, 235

Gruner, P., 97

Habit-reversal therapy, 237–238

Habituation, 68, 331

Hair pulling. *See* Trichotillomania

Hallucinations, hypnogogic, 286

Hamilton Depression scores, 192

Hare's Psychopathy Checklist, 387

Harpin, R. E., 72

Harris, G. T., 372, 388

Hart, H., 140

Harvey, A. G., 286

Hayes, A. M., 204

Health anxiety, 327–344
  case example, 335–343
  CBT model of, 328–329
  future directions for treatment of, 343–344

and treatment of substance use disorders, 220–222
Motivational deficits, 390
Motivational interviewing (MI), 12
    for treatment of health anxiety, 335
    for treatment of paraphilias, 371
    for treatment of pathological gambling, 235, 236
    for treatment of substance use disorders, 221
Motivation enhancement therapy, 75
Motives (in Anger Disorders Scale), 308
Motor behaviors, 298–300, 305
Mountford, V., 169
Multicomponent cognitive–behavioral therapy, 117
Mulvey, E. P., 389
Mutual-maintenance hypothesis, 219–220
Myczcowisk, L. M., 186

Narcolepsy, 286
NAS-PI. *See* Novaco Anger Scale and Provocation Inventory
National Comorbidity Survey Replication (NCS-R), 66
National Health and Social Life Survey, 256
National Institute of Mental Health Collaborative Depression Study, 183
National Institutes of Health State of the Science, 278
National Institutes of Mental Health, 106
NATs (negative automatic thoughts), 282
Natural disasters (and posttraumatic stress disorder), 139
NCS-R (National Comorbidity Survey Replication), 66
Nefazodone, 186–187
Negative automatic thoughts (NATs), 282
Neighbors, C., 163
Nemeroff, C. B., 190
Newman, M., 117
Nonchange, 21
Nongeneralized social anxiety disorder, 66
Nonparaphilic sexual behavior, 244
Noradrenergic reuptake inhibitors (SNRIs), 143
Novaco Anger Scale and Provocation Inventory (NAS-PI), 307–308
Novaco, R. W., 311–312
Numbing, emotional, 142

Oatley, K., 55

Obsessions, 89, 94–96. *See also* Obsessive–compulsive disorder
Obsessive–compulsive disorder (OCD), 89–106
    case example, 99–105
    comorbidity with, 96–97
    defining, 89–90
    and eating disorders, 160–161
    etiology of, 90–92
    exposure with response prevention for, 92–95
    and fear outcomes, 16
    future directions for treatment of, 105–106
    home-based vs. office-based CBT for, 18–19
    and impulse control disorders, 232
    insight of clients with, 13
    intensive interventions for, 18
    poor response to treatment of, 95–99
OCD. *See* Obsessive–compulsive disorder
Oetting, E. R., 242
Olanzapine, 352
Olatunji, B. O., 52
Ooman, J., 6, 10
Orsillo, S. M., 118
Öst, L. G., 116
Otto, M., 73
Otto, M. W., 44, 45
Outcomes (in anger episode model), 305–306
Overvaluation, 156, 158–159, 162
Overvalued ideation
    and obsessive–compulsive disorder, 97
    and social anxiety disorder, 76

Padula, M. A., 51
Pain, genital, 263–267
Panic attacks, 42, 53
Panic disorder, 41–57, 215
    case example, 53–57
    CBT for, 43–45
    comorbidity with, 46–51
    features and *DSM* criteria of, 42–43
    poor response to treatment of, 45–52
    and sexual dysfunctions, 263
    significance of, 41–42
    and social anxiety disorder, 66
Paradoxical intention, 280–281
Paranoid personality disorder, 311
Paraphilias, 369–382
    case examples of, 377–380
    CBT relapse prevention for, 373–374

for treatment of substance use disorders, 215, 220
Psychometric tests, 306–308
Psychopathy, 385–386, 403
   challenges to successful treatment of, 389–390
   general considerations with, 391–394
   as term, 386–387
   treatment for, 387–389
Psychotherapy, 67–71. *See also* Cognitive–behavioral therapy
PsycINFO database, xxii
PTSD. *See* Posttraumatic stress disorder
Puschner, B., 17

Quetiapine, 106

Race, 57, 411
Rachman, S., 91
Rational-emotive behavior therapy model, 313
Raue, P. J., 204
Ravindran, A. V., 185
Reactive Person x Environment transactions, 364–365
Readiness for treatment, 391
Reardon, M. L., 18
Reassurance seeking, 328
Recidivism
   sexual, 372
   violent, 388
Reeves, M. D., 18
Refractory (term), xiii
Regulation. *See* emotion regulation
Relapse prevention, 22
   for treatment of paraphilias, 369–374, 377, 380–381
   for treatment of pathological gambling, 233, 236
Relational frame theory (RFT), 167–168
Relaxation training
   for treatment of generalized anxiety disorder, 113
   for treatment of insomnia, 280–281
   for treatment of intermittent explosive disorder, 242
   for treatment of sexual dysfunction, 264–266
   for treatment of social anxiety disorder, 70–71
Religious beliefs, 97–98
Remediation phase (of situational analysis), 188

Renneberg, B., 48
Reoffense (of sex offenders), 370–371
Reparenting, 351
Rescripting, memory. *See* Memory rescripting
Research Diagnostic Criteria, 278
Respect, 391–392
Responsibility, 312–313
Restless leg syndrome, 285
Reversible MAOIs, 71
RFT. *See* Relational frame theory
Rice, M., 388
Rice, M. E., 372
Risk management, 392–393
Risperidone, 100
Robinson, S., 44
Roemer, L., 118
Rohsenow, D. J., 213
Role plays (in situational analysis), 188
Rollnick, S., 20–21, 317, 337
Roy-Byrne, P., 49
Rule-governed behavior, 171–172
Ruscio, A. M., 8, 117
Russo, J., 49
Rygh, J. L., 124

SA. *See* Situational analysis
Sacks, M., 186
Sadism, sexual, 369
Sadistic personality disorder, 311
Safety behaviors, 66, 68, 69–70, 128, 170
Safety-seeking behaviors
   defining, 52
   in health anxiety, 331, 332
Safety signals, 52–53
Safran, J. D., 15
Safren, S. A., 16
Salekin, R. T., 388
Salkovskis, P. M., 128, 334
Sallaerts, S., 48
Salvatore, N. F., 242
Sanderson, W. C., 124
Sawchuk, C. N., 52
SCD/CT. *See* Self-control desensitization and cognitive therapy
Schema-focused therapy, 350–351
Schemata, 142
Schizotypal personality disorder, 97, 311
Schmidt, N. B., 51
Schneider, D. J., 282
Schwartz, S. A., 95
SCID-II (Clinical Interview Schedule for Personality Disorders), 48

ABOUT THE EDITORS

Dean McKay, PhD, ABPP, is an associate professor in the Department of Psychology at Fordham University. He currently serves on the editorial boards of *Behaviour Research and Therapy*, the *Journal of Clinical Psychology*, and the *Journal of Anxiety Disorders*, and he is associate editor of the *Journal of Cognitive Psychotherapy*. He has published over 120 journal articles and book chapters, is editor or coeditor of 8 published or forthcoming books, and has over 150 conference presentations. Dr. McKay is board certified in behavioral and clinical psychology by the American Board of Professional Psychology (ABPP), is a fellow of the American Board of Behavioral Psychology and the Academy of Clinical Psychology, and is a clinical fellow of the Behavior Research and Therapy Society. His research has focused primarily on obsessive–compulsive disorder (OCD), body dysmorphic disorder and health anxiety and their link to OCD, and the role of disgust in psychopathology. His research has also focused on mechanisms of information processing bias for anxiety states.

Jonathan S. Abramowitz, PhD, ABPP, is a professor and associate chair of the Department of Psychology and a research professor in the Department of Psychiatry at the University of North Carolina (UNC) at Chapel Hill. He is also founder and director of the UNC Anxiety and Stress Disorders Clinic. Dr. Abramowitz is a North Carolina licensed psychologist, and he holds a Diplomate in Behavioral Psychology from the American Board of Professional Psychology. He conducts research on obsessive–compulsive disorder and other anxiety disorders and has authored or edited 5 books and published over 100 peer-reviewed research articles and book chapters on these topics. He currently serves as associate editor of *Behaviour Research and Therapy* and the *Journal of Cognitive Psychotherapy* and on the editorial boards of several other scientific journals. He is a member of the Obsessive Compulsive

Foundation's Scientific Advisory Board and the Anxiety Disorders Association of America's Clinical Advisory Board. He also served on the Anxiety Disorders Work Group for the *Diagnostic and Statistical Manual of Mental Disorders* (2000). Dr. Abramowitz received the Outstanding Contributions to Research Award from the Mayo Clinic Department of Psychiatry and Psychology in 2003 and the David Shakow Early Career Award for Outstanding Contributions to Clinical Psychology from the American Psychological Association's Division 12 (Society of Clinical Psychology) in 2004, and he was elected to the Board of Directors of the Association for Behavioral and Cognitive Therapies (formerly AABT) in 2005. He regularly presents papers and workshops on anxiety disorders and their treatment at regional, national, and international professional conferences.

Steven Taylor, PhD, ABPP, is a professor and clinical psychologist in the Department of Psychiatry at the University of British Columbia, and he is editor-in-chief of the *Journal of Cognitive Psychotherapy*. Dr. Taylor has published over 200 journal articles and book chapters and over 15 books on anxiety disorders and related topics. He is a fellow of several scholarly organizations, including the American and Canadian Psychological Associations and the Association for Psychological Science. His research interests include cognitive–behavioral treatments and mechanisms of anxiety disorders and related conditions, as well as the behavioral genetics of these disorders.